A History of Neuropsychology

Frontiers of Neurology and Neuroscience

Vol. 44

Series Editor

J. Bogousslavsky Montreux

A History of Neuropsychology

Volume Editors

J. Bogousslavsky Montreux
F. Boller Washington, DC
M. Iwata Tokyo

32 figures and 10 tables, 2019

KARGER Basel · Freiburg · Hartford · Oxford · Bangkok · Dubai · Kuala Lumpur · Melbourne · Mexico City · Moscow · New Dehli · Paris · Shanghai · Tokyo

Frontiers of Neurology and Neuroscience
Vols. 1–18 were published as Monographs in Clinical Neuroscience

Julien Bogousslavsky, MD, PhD
Neurocenter
Swiss Medical Network
Clinique Valmont
CH–1823 Glion/Montreux (Switzerland)

Makoto Iwata, MD, PhD
Tokyo Women's Medical University
4-46-19, Hikawadai, Nerima-ku
Tokyo 179-0084 (Japan)

François Boller, MD, PhD
Department of Neurology
George Washington University Medical School
2150 Pennsylvania Avenue NW
Washington, DC 20037 (USA)

Library of Congress Cataloging-in-Publication Data

Names: Bogousslavsky, Julien, editor. | Boller, François, editor. | Iwata, Makoto, 1942- editor.
Title: A history of neuropsychology / volume editors, J. Bogousslavsky, F. Boller, M. Iwata.
Description: Basel ; Hartford : Karger, 2019. | Series: Frontiers of neurology and neuroscience ; vol. 44 | Includes bibliographical references and index.
Identifiers: LCCN 2019005690 (print) | LCCN 2019007438 (ebook) | ISBN 9783318064636 (eBook) | ISBN 9783318064629 (hard cover) | ISBN 9783318064636 (eisbn)
Subjects: | MESH: Neuropsychology--history | Neuropsychology--methods
Classification: LCC RC346 (ebook) | LCC RC346 (print) | NLM WL 11.1 | DDC 616.8--dc23
LC record available at https://lccn.loc.gov/2019005690

Bibliographic Indices. This publication is listed in bibliographic services, including Current Contents® and MEDLINE/Pubmed.

Disclaimer. The statements, opinions and data contained in this publication are solely those of the individual authors and contributors and not of the publisher and the editor(s). The appearance of advertisements in the book is not a warranty, endorsement, or approval of the products or services advertised or of their effectiveness, quality or safety. The publisher and the editor(s) disclaim responsibility for any injury to persons or property resulting from any ideas, methods, instructions or products referred to in the content or advertisements.

Drug Dosage. The authors and the publisher have exerted every effort to ensure that drug selection and dosage set forth in this text are in accord with current recommendations and practice at the time of publication. However, in view of ongoing research, changes in government regulations, and the constant flow of information relating to drug therapy and drug reactions, the reader is urged to check the package insert for each drug for any change in indications and dosage and for added warnings and precautions. This is particularly important when the recommended agent is a new and/or infrequently employed drug.

www.karger.com
Printed on acid-free and non-aging paper (ISO 9706)
ISSN 1660–4431
eISSN 1662–2804
ISBN 978–3–318–06462–9
e-ISBN 978–3–318–06463–6

Contents

Preface

Focused attention and research on higher cortical functions have led to the launch of a new medical "specialty" called either neuropsychology or cognitive/behavioral neurology. These different terms correspond to different interpretations of its contents, emphasizing either testing versus management or processes of cognition versus observable behaviors. Such trends reflected the historical evolution that occurred mainly from the end of the 19th century till the beginning of the 21st century. The history of neuropsychology indeed is based on other historical developments in brain science and clinical neurology, while at the same time it became a separate field of research with its own experts. Nowadays, neuropsychology is largely a specialized field in psychology, rather than a medical discipline, and its use by neurologists has become critically important either in clinical practice or in research.

This book attempts to cover the most important historical development in the field of neuropsychology over a little more than a century, in order to show how the present concepts used in practice originated and were established. There have been strong cultural influences, and for that same reason, the editorship and authorship of the book span across all developmental initiatives in Europe, America, and Asia the countries where most research work has been carried out so far. We are grateful to all contributors who permitted us to present this essay on history of neuropsychology. Although we did not aim at providing exhaustive information on the subject, we are confident that most of the main concepts have been addressed, leading to a better understanding of the development of higher brain function studies in general.

Julien Bogousslavsky, Montreux, Switzerland
François Boller, Washington, DC, USA
Makoto Iwata, Tokyo, Japan

Bogousslavsky J, Boller F, Iwata M (eds): A History of Neuropsychology.
Front Neurol Neurosci. Basel, Karger, 2019, vol 44, pp 1–14 (DOI: 10.1159/000494938)

The Discovery of Cerebral Specialization

Lauren Julius Harris

Department of Psychology, Michigan State University, East Lansing, MI, USA

Abstract

Of the main principles of human neuropsychology, the best known may be cerebral specialization: the left and right hemispheres play different roles in language and other higher-order functions. This chapter discusses when and how and by whom the differences were found. It begins with an account of Gall's cortical localization theory, which set the stage. It then describes the discoveries themselves, reviews how the differences were explained, and concludes with a summary of further developments.

Introduction

In the long history of neuropsychology, a key advance and, today, perhaps the best known was the discovery that the cerebral hemispheres play different roles in higher-order functions. How and when were the differences found, and who found them?

Gall's Localization Theory

The stage was set in the early 1800s by Franz Joseph Gall (Fig. 1). In his localization theory, or *organology*, he proposed that the mind has 27 discrete, self-contained faculties, or modules, in two categories: *Intellectual*, ranging from speech, memory of words, and music, to sense of place, space, and persons, and *Moral*, encompassing passions and feelings, such as courage and love of family; that each faculty has a corresponding organ and location in the brain; that the organs come in pairs, one in the left hemisphere, one in the right; that their size reflects faculty strength; and that strengths and weaknesses appear as en-

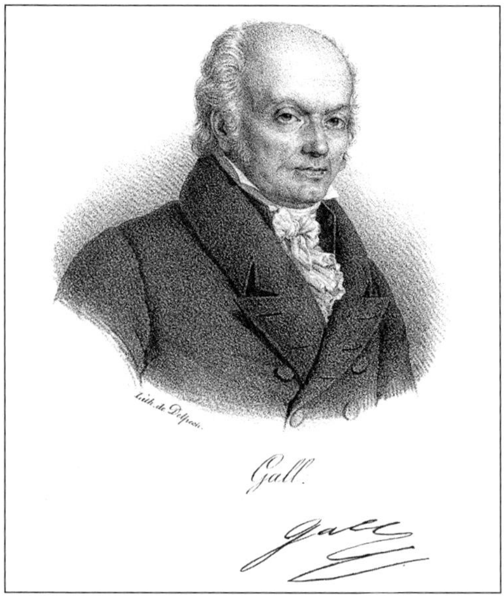

Fig. 1. Franz Joseph Gall (1758–1828). Oxford Science Archive / Heritage image. Reprinted with kind permission.

largements and depressions on the brain's surface and overlying skull, allowing their measurement by inspection ([1], p 71 ff.).

To map the brain, Gall examined heads of living persons along with skulls, plaster casts, and portraits, focusing on persons at the extremes. For example, he located the speech organ in the anterior half of the supra-orbital frontal gyri after finding an enlargement there in orators and writers and a depression in a lunatic unable to speak; for music, he looked for similarly differentiating features in persons with and without musical ability, the former including musicians, composers, and a 5-year-old child who could remember "whole concerts" heard "at most twice" ([2], p 63). Gall also studied persons with "accidental (brain) mutilations." In one, a soldier injured by a fencing foil that penetrated just below his left eye into the site of the speech organ, "nothing is lost … but the faculty of speaking" ([2], p 23). Organology, or phrenology, the name favored by Gall's associate, Johann Spurzheim, won both praise and scorn, the latter mostly from scientists (anatomists and physiologists), who criticized it for overstatements, reliance on anecdote and uncontrolled clinical reports, and for proposing that the organs could be measured by inspection when, as the anatomist Sewall [3] stated in 1837, "the frontal sinuses and temporal muscles alone" put the majority "beyond the reach of observation" (p 51). Gall's most resolute critic, Pierre Flourens [4], claimed from animal experiments that the faculties are co-extensive, not discrete, and that the brain and mind function wholistically. In 1838, François Magendie [5] summed it up: phrenology was "a *pseudo-science* of the present day" (p 150).

It endured nonetheless. Supporters liked its simplicity, grandness of scale (ever grander as the list of faculties grew), and promise of understanding the self (for which many were eager to pay) – in 1911, Bierce [6] called phrenology "picking the pocket through the scalp" (p 98). Most importantly, some physicians, prominently Bouillaud [7], believed that Gall was right at least about speech: they too had seen persons made speechless from stroke or "accidental mutilations" of the anterior lobes.

The Brain as a Double Organ: Localization without Lateralization

At the time, lateralization, or cerebral specialization, was not under debate. Xavier Bichat [8], seeing that all paired structures in the brain "resemble each other on every side," declared what came to be known as the *law of symmetry*: "two parts essentially alike in their structure cannot be different in their mode of acting" (pp 8, 14). Gall, likewise, envisioned the organs in each pair as anatomically and functionally identical, and overlooked the soldier's injury being on the left.

Not everyone saw the hemispheres that way. Vicq d'Azyr [9] and Malgaigne [10] were among those who remarked on their *asymmetrical* appearance. For Malgaigne, it meant that "if the phrenological organs are situated in these convolutions, the necessary conclusion will be that these organs are not the same in the 2 hemispheres" (p 371). But these were minority views, and the law of symmetry remained a core physiological principle.

Left-Hemisphere Specialization

It was in the 1860s when Paul Broca came on the scene (Fig. 2). By then, despite the critics, some physicians, like Bouillaud [11], remained steadfast in support of the principle, at least about speech and the anterior lobes. Broca [12] himself, while doubting the feasibility of "constructing a detailed system of localization" like Gall's, credited Gall with the "incontestable merit of proclaiming the great principle of cerebral localization" (p 191). That he also accepted the law of symmetry becomes clear in his reports on his soon-to-be-famous patient, Louis Victor Leborgne (whose full name we finally know, thanks to Cezary Domanski [13]).

Speech and the Frontal Lobe

Leborgne was a 51-year-old patient at the Bicêtre, a hospital on the outskirts of Paris, where Broca was on staff. He had been epileptic since his youth, and in 1850, following a series of strokes, became paralyzed on the right side, losing his ability to speak. In the hospital, he became known as "Tan" because, with one exception to be noted later, it was the only articulate sound he could make. Broca called the condition *aphemia*; the term we have come to use, *aphasia*, was Armand Trousseau's [14] (see Ryalls [15]). In 1861, when gangrene set in, Leborgne was treated by Broca but died soon after. Upon examining his brain, Broca found softening throughout the left frontal lobe apparently centered around F3, the posterior part of the third, or inferior, frontal convolution.

Broca's three reports [16–18] on Leborgne and a second speechless patient, Lezare Lelong, focused on the frontal location, but as evidence mounted, so did his appreciation for

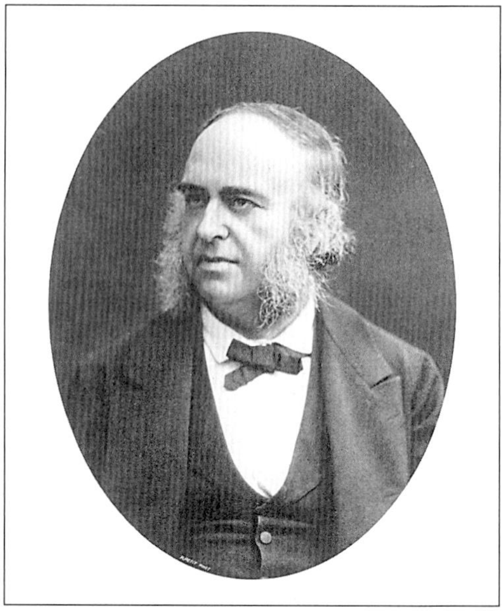

Fig. 2. Paul Broca (1824–1880). Wellcome Library. Public Domain.

the "remarkable fact" ([19], p 202) that the damage was always on the left. By 1863, he had ten such cases, and, finally, in 1865 [20], with still more, he famously declared, "we speak with the left hemisphere" ("nous parlons avec l'hémisphère gauche"), with F3 at the center (p 384).

More evidence soon came in support, either of speech loss after left-anterior injury or no loss after injury on the right. But as Broca [21] knew, "in pathology and especially in cerebral pathology, there is hardly any rule without exception" (p 385), and here the most challenging were reports of persons who became aphasic after injury to F3 on the *right*. Broca [20] acknowledged "the existence of a small number [*petit nombre*]" who "speak with the right hemisphere" (pp 385–386) and analogized them to another exceptional group, left-handers. Many assumed he meant it was left-handers who "speak with the right," but Broca rejected any necessary "coincidence" between the groups (p 387). Among other reasons, the numbers did not match, and Broca cited reports estimating the incidence of left-handedness at 1 in 10 but only 1 in 20 for right-hemisphere speech. The evidence for lateralization converted most but not all believers in the law of symmetry. Bastian [22], for one, said it was "only fair" to suppose that the hemispheres "should be endowed with like functions," since they, like the sense organs, "may be said to have a bilateral symmetry." He therefore was "strongly inclined still to believe in (their) similarity of function, … notwithstanding all that has been said of late in opposition to this doctrine" (p 455). In years past, the doctrine may have dissuaded some, like Bouillaud [7], from even looking for differences. There were 29 patients in his report linking aphasia to anterior-lobe lesions. From the list, Benton [23] determined that 25 had unilateral lesions, 11 left, 14 right, and that 8 (73%) of the former were aphasic, only 4 (25%) of the latter.

If Bouillaud fell victim to conventional wisdom, it was only in the sense that he failed to compare his left- and right-side cases or chose not to mention the difference. Marc Dax, in a paper written in 1836, actually proposed that the left hemisphere was the speech side after observing that aphasic patients more often have right than left hemiplegia. Dax prepared his paper for a medical society meeting but, evidently, never delivered it, and it remained unknown and unheralded until his son, Gustave, published it in 1865, along with his own report on the same subject ([24, 25]; for reviews, see Finger and Roe [26]; Joynt and Benton [27]).

What Was the Underlying Deficit?

Leborgne could not speak, but what was the underlying deficit? To understand Broca's answer, we must consider the state of theory and evidence on another issue – the motor excitability of the cerebral cortex. In the 1860s, this was still unknown. No one, that is, had distinguished between an anterior "motor" region and a posterior "somatosensory" region, approximately encompassing, respectively, the pre- and post-central gyri. That revelation came later, most importantly in 1870 from Fritsch and Hitzig's [28] experiments on dogs, and, in 1873, from Ferrier's [29] experiments on monkeys. Until then, the cortex was seen as purely for mental acts, with the "motor" centers lying below in the corpus striatum and other basal ganglia. In 1864, it was how John Hughlings-Jackson explained the frequent co-occurrence of right-hemiplegia with speech loss:

> The seat of the faculty of (speech) is near the upper part of the motor tract – the corpus striatum; so that, from mere relation of contiguity, (speech and motor functions) often suffer together ([30], p 39).

Broca [17] saw Leborgne's symptoms the same way. His lips and tongue were not paralyzed because he could use them for other acts, but he could not remember how to use them for speech. In declaring that we speak with the left hemisphere and in locating its seat in F3, Broca meant it was where memories were stored for performing linguistic-articulatory acts. Leborgne's aphasia, therefore, was a memory disorder. What was a motor disorder was his hemiplegia, signifying that his lesion extended into the corpus striatum, "the motor organ nearest the anterior lobes" (p 347).

The Left Hemisphere Is Not the Seat of All Language Functions

Broca [17] did not credit the left hemisphere with all language functions: the patient has "generally lost only the ability to reproduce the articulate sounds of the language", he still understands "what is said to him and, consequently, understands the relation between ideas and words." Leborgne, for one, seemed to understand "nearly (everything) said to him" (p 345). The "faculty of creating those relations (thus) belongs simultaneously to (both) hemispheres … but the faculty of expressing them by coordinated movements … would appear to belong only to one," "nearly always … the left" ([20], p 386).

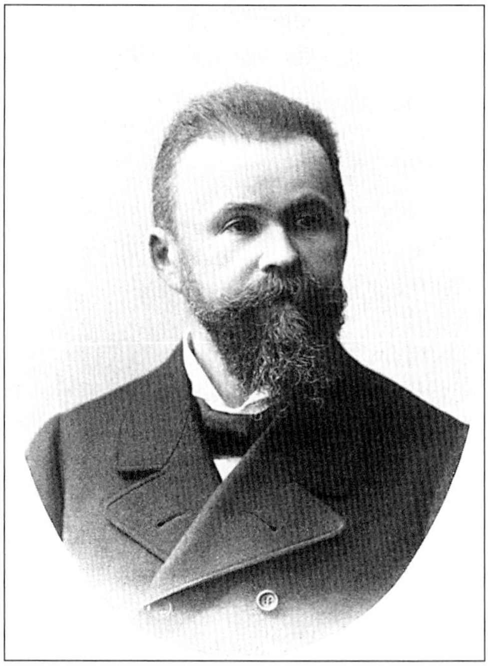

Fig. 3. Carl Wernicke (1848–1905). From *Galerie Hervorragender Ärzte und Naturforscher.* J.F. Lehmanns Verlag, 1893. Public Domain.

Comprehension and the Temporal Lobe

Broca was correct to link speech loss (later called motor, or non-fluent, aphasia) to left-hemisphere dysfunction, but he was mistaken if, in stating that comprehension belongs "simultaneously" to both hemispheres, he meant "equally." Further studies of persons with comprehension deficits showed that here too the left hemisphere had a special role (e.g., Bastian [31]; Broadbent [32]).

The most revealing accounts came in 1874 from Carl Wernicke (Fig. 3, [33]), then a 26-year-old medical student. His first patient, Suzanne Adam, after falling ill from an unknown cause, could "comprehend absolutely nothing … said to her." Her speech, though fluent, was confused, with "meaningless, garbled words" and paraphasias, although the overall meaning was "graspable in a general way" (quoted in translation in Eggert [34], p 120). Wernicke traced the symptoms to a posterior lesion in the superior temporal lobe on the left side.

Dementia or Aphasia?

In the past, as Wernicke noted, persons with fluent but confused, unintelligible speech were often diagnosed as demented or psychotic, especially those without paralysis or other physical signs of brain injury. Adam herself initially was diagnosed with dementia and placed in a psychiatric ward. Clarification of the symptoms would be important for diagnosis and nosology as it came to be understood that, at least in some cases, like Adam's, the symptoms, in the absence of general dementia, were neurological and that the patients had another kind of aphasia, later to be called sensory, or fluent, aphasia.

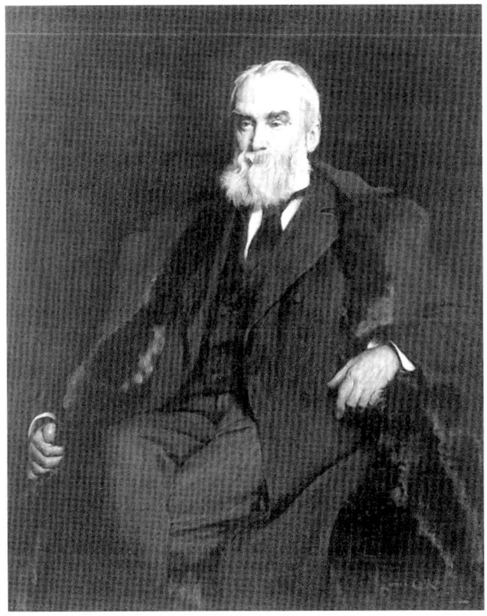

Fig. 4. John Hughlings-Jackson (1835–1911). Wellcome Library. Public Domain.

Cerebral Dominance

The discoveries of the left hemisphere's role in speech and comprehension were followed by reports linking it to other language skills, including Dejerine's report in 1892 [35] on reading and writing. All such evidence eventually fostered the concept of "cerebral dominance," implying that the left hemisphere was "dominant" not just for language but for all higher-order functions, including reasoning and abstract problem-solving, with the right hemisphere, to use Benton's [36] phrase, as the "for the most part silent partner" (p 7), able to do some of the same things but not as well. In 1900, Liepmann [37]) proposed that the left hemisphere also was responsible for planning and coordinating sequences of skilled movements, or praxis. Given their differences in status, the two sides began to be called "major" and "minor."

Right-Hemisphere Specialization

"Objects, Places, Persons, &c."
Along with language disorders being so obvious and debilitating, this elevated view of the left hemisphere may help explain why it took longer to appreciate that the right had powers of its own. A breakthrough came in 1874 [38] when Hughlings-Jackson (Fig. 4) reported that persons with right hemisphere injuries, but now *posterior*, had deficits in "*recognition* of objects, places, persons, &c." (p 70). Note the similarity in names to Gall's faculties of "place," "space," and "person." Gall, of course, saw the faculties and their corresponding organs, like those for language, as identical pairs, one to each side.

Hughlings-Jackson's second report, in 1876 [39], was especially compelling. His patient Eliza T., 2 months after complaining of headache and "neuralgia," began making odd mistakes, such as putting her clothes on the wrong side and losing her way in a park she had visited for decades. After being admitted to hospital, more symptoms appeared: an inability to name common objects and mistaking the people around her, for example, calling all the nurses "Annie" (her daughter's name). She died soon after, and the autopsy showed a tumor in her right temporo-occipital cortex. Hughlings-Jackson called her combination of symptoms – visual disorientation, facial agnosia, and dyspraxia for dressing – "imperception" and proposed that it was as characteristic of posterior right-hemisphere disease as aphasia was of disease of the anterior left.

Further reports came in support. Two examples will serve. In 1895, Dunn [40] described a man with defects in topographical orientation following a right-hemisphere stroke. Dunn posited a "geographical centre" in the right hemisphere for recording "optical images of locality, analogous to (Broca's region for) speech on the left ..." (p 54). In 1905, Lenz [41] described 8 patients with homonymous hemianopia with visual disorientation. Finding that 7 had a left-field defect, Lenz suggested that "the right occipital lobe is perhaps more strongly related to orientation ..." (quoted in translation in Benton [36], p 11).

Emotion

In 1881, a right-hemisphere role for emotion was proposed as well. Luys [42] compared patients with opposite-side lesions, their locations in most cases indicated by the side of hemiplegia and confirmed by autopsy. Whereas "ordinary" right-hemiplegics (with left-side lesions) are "apathetic," "silent," and "stricken with hebetude," "emotional" left-hemiplegics show "an abnormal impressionability ... respond[ing to questions] in a limping voice, broken up by a kind of sobbing." Other times, "they are boisterous and loquacious" (pp 379–380). Leborgne, whom Luys presumably would have called "ordinary," partly fit the pattern: silent save for his monosyllabic "tan" but, when angry, able to utter a multisyllabic curse – *Sacré nom de Dieu!* (Broca [17], p 344). (This was the exception I noted earlier.) To explain symptoms like these, Luys proposed an emotion center in the right hemisphere to complement the intellectual center in the left.

Music

Still other evidence pointed to a right-hemisphere role for music. Persons made speechless by left-hemisphere injury could still sing or carry a tune, abilities presumably mediated by the intact right hemisphere. Hughlings-Jackson [38] found 3 such persons among 28 with aphasia; Bouillaud [11] found one more, a man who composed and sang without "even a minor mistake [in articulating] the appropriate sounds" (quoted in translation in Della Rocca [43], p 140); and in possibly the earliest report, from 1745, van Dalin [44] described a man who, after a stroke with loss of speech and right-side paralysis, could "sing" and "whistle hymns ... learned before he became ill ... so purely and explicitly like any other normal person" (quoted in translation in Johnson et al. [45], p 18). All this evidence was only indirect. Direct evidence came from patients with right-hemisphere lesions who showed the symptoms in reverse: they could still speak but not carry a tune, and their speech lacked normal "song," or prosody. August Knoblauch [46] called the condition "amusia" but, envisioning the motor and auditory centers for tones as being close to those for speech and comprehension, localized music in the left hemisphere, not the right (see Johnson and Graziano [47], p 112).

Localization of Symptoms or Localization of Function?

Along with his reports on imperception, Hughlings-Jackson [38] made another signal contribution. He identified what he saw as a common error in interpreting clinical data: speech loss following F3 damage on the left was widely taken to mean that speech was *located* there. The error lay in equating localization of *symptoms* with localization of *function*:

> Whilst I believe that the hinder part of the left third frontal convolution is the part most often damaged (when speech is lost), I do not localize speech in any such small part of the brain. To locate the damage which destroys speech and to locate speech are two different things ([30], p 81).

Hughlings-Jackson instead saw speech, and language more generally, as a dynamic process involving the integrated functioning of the whole brain, such that the more complex the task, the more regions involved, each contributing in its own way. The question was not, where is language located, it was, what is each region's contribution? His answer was that language is represented in both hemispheres at different functional levels: Emotional utterances (the lowest level) were the least lateralized, or most bilateral, which explained the preservation of "emotional speech," such as oaths and other "automatic," "involuntary" phrases in persons with aphasia, persons like Leborgne. Comprehension was more lateralized, and "propositional speech" (the highest level), together with the background of conceptual thought it requires, depended wholly on the left hemisphere.

Explanations of Hemispheric Specialization

How could cerebral specialization be explained? For Broca [20], the challenge was significant because, in declaring that we speak with the left hemisphere, he noted that, except for certain "secondary convolutions," the hemispheres were "perfectly alike" (p 381). (Malgaigne [10], we recall, saw things differently.) How, then, could *asymmetrical* control for speech be reconciled with the "general truths [the law of symmetry] it seems to contradict" (pp 381–382)?

Broca saw a clue in something Leurat and Gratiolet [48] found in the brains of human fetuses: frontal convolutions appear earlier on the left. Could that dispose the left hemisphere to take the lead in complex acts like speech and language? Further reports, however, were mixed, some finding earlier development on the left (e.g., [49], others on the right, e.g., [50], and still others, no differences [51]). The discrepancies were never resolved. As the author of one of the reports later remarked, "the question which side is first developed seems still doubtful" ([52], p 293).

Could the difference instead lie in the number of convolutions? In the adult brain, Broca, in an apparent change from his prior [20] position, reported finding "notably more" on the left (quoted in Bateman [53], p 380). He also found the left frontal lobe to be heavier ([54]). Asked whether F3 made the difference, he said he was inclined to this view but was reluctant to say more given the difficulty in surgically isolating this structure (reported in [55]).

Size was considered too. Cunningham [56] measured the upward angle of the Sylvian fissure's posterior ramus in human fetuses. Finding it smaller on the left, he concluded that the region it bounded ventrally, containing the planum temporale, part of what by then was being called Wernicke's area, was larger on that side. But seeing the same in great apes – animals with no known language – he questioned whether it is "in any way associated with … localization of the active speech centre …" (p 293). He presumably meant "*comprehension* centre."

What about the right hemisphere? For the temporal and occipital lobes, Gratiolet found earlier convolutional development on the right, the reverse of that for the frontal lobes. For the occipital lobe, Broca reported the same for number: "the right is richer in convolutions" (in [53] but, with his focus on speech, would have had no reason to see it as significant. Hughlings-Jackson [38] had very good reason: "These anatomical facts, I submit, support the view … that the hinder part of the brain on the right side, is the chief seat … in the *recognition* of objects, places, persons, &c." (p 70).

The Role of the Corpus Callosum

By the 1920s, with the discovery and further documentation of lateral differences in function along with reports of possible clues to their anatomical origins, cerebral specialization had become a bedrock principle of neuropsychology, although the terms "major" and "minor" persisted, implying that left-hemisphere functions were still seen as more important.

The discovery rekindled the interest in an old question about the corpus callosum. Before Broca, it was regarded as a bridge between functionally symmetrical hemispheres. Thus Gall [57], recognizing that each pair of organs must be "united for mutual influence and the attainment of a common end," named the "transverse layers of fibers (commissures)" as the link (p 600). This was a major advancement from the still older view of Vesalius [58] that its role was purely mechanical: to connect the two halves of the brain, thereby "preserv(ing) the patency of the ventricular cavities and support(ing) the fornix" (p 578; for review, see Harris [59].

In the new era of cerebral specialization, the corpus callosum could be seen as connecting functionally asymmetric hemispheres, allowing their differences to merge in the service of mind. The new era also raised new questions: What if a lesion destroyed the left visual cortex and the splenium of the corpus callosum, preventing information sent to the right visual cortex from reaching the angular gyrus of the left hemisphere? Or, after research showed a region of cortex to be motorically excitable, what if an anterior callosal lesion prevented a verbal command to use the left hand from reaching that region of the right hemisphere? It was these questions that inspired analyses of disorders of reading (Dejerine [35]) and praxis (Liepmann [37]).

Further Developments

Since the 1950s, and at an accelerating pace, have come ever deeper analyses of cerebral specialization stemming from advances in virtually every facet of neuropsychological science: the development and adoption of standardized tests of the aphasias, agnosias, and other neuro-cognitive as well as neuro-affective disorders; the incorporation of theory and research in cognitive science, including the study of memory, perception, attention, problem-solving, and executive control; large-scale studies, many of war veterans, comparing left- and right-hemisphere injuries; and, using such new electrophysiological and imaging methods as ERP, PET, MRI, fMRI, MEG, and SPECT, vast improvements in measuring structure and function in clinical and non-clinical populations, and with DTI (diffusion tensor imaging), in providing new details on connectivity through in vivo delineation of white-matter tracts. Along with these advances have come studies of the development of cerebral specialization; of the corpus callosum and the effects of its surgical separation; of the effects of side, time, and type of injury on function; and of the relation between cerebral specialization and a host of variables, including sex, handedness (degree as well as direction), intelligence, culture, literacy, and special talents and disabilities. Still other studies are focusing on cerebral specialization in other species; its embryological, anatomical, hormonal, genetic, and evolutionary foundations; and, ultimately, its benefits for the individual and the species. The outcome is that much progress has been made and many lessons learned. To name just a few examples: Broca was correct: a "small number" of persons do "speak with the right hemisphere," and there is indeed no necessary coincidence between them and left-handers, the majority of whom, like nearly all right-handers, speak with the left (Harris [60]); Broca's *region*, however, is found to have a broader range of language-related functions than speech-production [61]. Developmental studies also reveal hemispheric differences in motor and cognitive functions in infancy and even well before birth (e.g., [62, 63]), and methods such as DTI are revealing promising clues to the origins of cerebral specialization in the form of hemispheric differences in macro- and microscopic structural organization (e.g., [62]; see also [64]). New research also suggests an important benefit of a lateralized brain: greater processing efficiency [65], which makes more understandable why cerebral specialization is increasingly found to be a species-wide characteristic in vertebrates [66] as well as invertebrates [67]. Along with these examples, more general descriptions of cerebral specialization are being sought; one sees the left as specialized for well-learned action sequences, the right for detecting and responding to unexpected, behaviorally relevant stimuli in the environment [68]. And as a last and especially telling example, "faculties" are no longer regarded as complete in themselves and wholly lateralized to either side. Consider language and music: as noted by Patel [69], although languages have nouns and verbs, grammatical categories with no analogues in music, they have other features in common and are served by both hemispheres, each taking the lead for certain ones. As summarized by Peretz et al. [70], the left leads for pitch (tone) intervals, rhythm and timing (temporal order), sequencing, and perception of duration; the right for tonal patterns, melody, timbre, and emotion. And instead of modularity, with each feature, or function, uniquely associated with an anatomically distinct region, they are organized into cortical as well as sub-cortical neural networks (a so-called distributive-processing model), some working in parallel, others overlapping. Progress has not always been fast or smooth: for instance, the terms "major," "minor," and "cerebral dominance" in its original sense were not abandoned until the 1970s; and we still await definitive explanations of cerebral specialization. Some past lessons also may need re-emphasis lest they be forgotten. For one, despite Wernicke's warning against diagnosing fluent aphasia as psychosis, the error evidently occurs often enough to warrant mention in the psychiatric literature (e.g., [71, 72]). For another, the power of neuroimaging to pinpoint damage in injured brains and to identify activated regions under different cognitive and emotional conditions runs the risk of "over-localizing" and thus neglecting Hughlings-Jackson's maxim about localizing symptoms versus localizing functions. These matters aside, the study of cerebral specialization has come a long way since its beginning, and, looking back, we can thank our predecessors for starting us on a challenging but rewarding scientific journey. Like all such journeys, it is far from over.

References

1 Gall FJ: Anatomie et Physiologie du Système Nerveux en Général, et du Cerveau en Particulier: Quatrième Volume. Physiologie du Cerveau en Particulier. Paris, Chez N. Maze, Libraire, 1819.
2 Gall FJ: On the Origin of the Moral Qualities and Intellectual Faculties of Man, and the Conditions of Their Manifestation. In 6 Volumes, Trans. from the French by W. Lewis. Boston, Marsh, Capen & Lyon, 1835.
3 Sewall T: An examination of phrenology; in two lectures, delivered to the students of the Columbian College, District of Columbia. Washington City [Washington, D.C.], B. Homans, 1837.
4 Flourens MJP: Recherches expérimentales sur les propriétes et les fonctions du système nerveux dans les animaux vertébrés. Paris, Crevot, 1824.
5 Magendie F: (1838). An Elementary Treatise on Human Physiology. Translation of Précis Elémentaire de Physiologie, ed 5. By John Revere. New York, Harper & Brothers, 1855.
6 Bierce A: The Devil's Dictionary. New York, Dover Publications, 1958. Republication of the Work Originally Published in 1911 by Neale Publishing Company, Washington, DC, 1911.
7 Bouillaud JB: Recherches cliniques propres a démonstrer que la perte de la parole correspond à la lesion des lobules anterieurs du cerveau, et confirmer l'opinion de M. Gall, sur le siège de l'organe du langage articulé. Archives Générales de Médecine 1825;8:25–45.
8 Bichat X: Physiological Researches Upon Life and Death. First English trans., 1809, by Tobias Watkins, of the Second Paris Edition, 1805, of Recherches physiologique sur la vie et la mort. Philadelphia, Smith & Maxwell, 1805/1809.

9 Vicq d'Azyr F: Traité d'anatomie et physiologie avec des planches coloriees représentant au natural les divers organes de l'homme et des animaux (vol. 1). Paris, F.A. Didot l'aine, 1786.
10 Malgaigne J-F: Traité d'anatomie Chirurgicale et de Chirurgie Expérimentale, ed 2. Two volumes. Paris, J.-B. Balliere et Fils, 1859.
11 Bouillaud JB: Discussion sur la faculté du langage articulé. Réplique au discours de M. le professeur Trousseau; nouveaux faits à l'appui de notre doctrine. Bulletin de l'Académie Impériale de médecine 1865;30:724–781.
12 Broca P: Sur le volume et la forme du cerveau suivant les individus et suivant les races. Bulletins de la Société d'Anthropologie de Paris 1861;2:139–207.
13 Domanski CW: Mysterious "Monsieur Leborgne": the mystery of the famous patient in the history of neuropsychology is explained. J Hist Neurosci 2013;22:47–52.
14 Trousseau A: De l'aphasie, maladie décrite recemment sous le nom impropre d'aphémie. Gazette des Hôpitaux, 1864, 30, January 12.
15 Ryalls J: Where does the term "aphasia" come from? Brain Lang 1984;21:358–363.
16 Broca P: Perte de la parole, ramollissement chronique et destruction partielle du lobe anterieur gauche du cerveau. Bulletins de la Société d'Anthropologie de Paris 1861;2:235–238.
17 Broca P: Remarques sur le siège de la faculté du langage articulé, suiviés d'une observation d'aphemie (perte de la parole). Bulletins de la Société Anatomique de Paris 1861;6:330–357.
18 Broca P: Nouvelle observation d'aphemie produite par une lesion de la moitie posterieure des deuxieme et troisieme circonvolutions frontales gauches. Bulletins de la Société d'Anthropologie de Paris 1861;2:139–207.
19 Broca P: Localisation des fonctions cérébrales. Siège de la faculté du langage articulé. Bulletins de la Société d'Anthropologie de Paris 1863;4:200–204.
20 Broca P: Sur le siège de la faculté du langage articulé. Bulletins de la Société d'Anthropologie de Paris 1865;6: 377–393.
21 Broca P: Remarques sur le siège, le diagnostic et la nature de l'aphémie. Bulletins de la Société Anatomique de Paris 1863;8:379–383, 393–399.
22 Bastian HC: Note on the localisation of function in the cerebral hemispheres. J Ment Sci 1869;14:454–460.
23 Benton AL: Hemispheric dominance before Broca. Neuropsychologia 1984;22:807–811.
24 Dax G: Sur le même sujet. Gazette Hebdomadaires de Médecine et de Chirurgie (Paris), April 28, 2nd series, 1865;2:260–262.
25 Dax M: Lésions de la moitié gauche de l'encephale coincidant avec l'oubli des signes de la pensée (lu à Montpellier en 1836). Gazette Hebdomadaires de Médecine et de Chirurgie (Paris), April 28, 2nd series, 1865;2:259–260.
26 Finger S, Roe D: Does Gustave Dax deserve to be forgotten? The temporal lobe theory and other contributions of an overlooked figure in the history of language and cerebral dominance. Brain Lang 1999;69:16–30.
27 Joynt RJ, Benton AL. The memoir of Marc Dax on aphasia. Neurology 1964;14:851–854.
28 Fritsch G, Hitzig E: Ueber die elektrische Erregbarkeit des Grosshirns. Archiv fuer Anatomie, Physiologie, und Wissenschaftl. Medizin 1870; 300–332. English translation in G. von Bonin (Ed. and trans.), Some papers on the cerebral cortex (pp 73–96). Springfield, IL, Charles C. Thomas, 1960.
29 Ferrier D: Experimental researches in cerebral physiology and pathology. J Anat Physiol 1873;8:152–155.
30 Hughlings-Jackson J: Loss of speech: its association with valvular disease of the heart and with hemiplegia on the right side. – Defects of smell. – Defects of speech in chorea. – Arterial lesions in epilepsy. Clinical Lectures and Reports by the Medical and Surgical Staff of the London Hospital 1864;1:388–471. (Reprinted in Brain 1915;38: 28–42.)
31 Bastian HC: On the various forms of loss of speech in cerebral disease. Br Foreign Med Chir Rev 1869;43:209–236.
32 Broadbent WH: On the cerebral mechanism of speech and thought. Med Chir Trans 1872;55:145–194.
33 Wernicke C: Der Aphasiche Symtomencomplex. Eine Psychologische Studie auf Anatomischer Basis. Breslau, M. Cohn and Weigart, 1874.
34 Eggert GH: (Ed. and Trans.). Wernicke's Works on Aphasia: A Sourcebook and Review (Early Sources in Aphasia and Related Disorders, vol I). The Hague, Mouton Publishers, 1977.
35 Dejerine JJ: Contribution a l'étude anatamo-pathologique et clinique des différentes variétés de cécité verbale. Comtes Rendus des Séances de la Société de Biologie 1892;4:61–90.
36 Benton AL: The "minor" hemisphere. J Hist Med Allied Sci 1972;27:5–14.
37 Liepmann H: Das Krankheitsbild der Apraxie (motorischen Asymbolie) auf Grund eines Falles von einseitiger Apraxie. Monatsschr Psychiatr Neurol 1900;8: 15–44; 102–132; 182–197.
38 Hughlings-Jackson J: On the nature of the duality of the brain. Med Press Circ 1874;1:19–25, 41–49, 63–70. (Reprinted in Brain 1915;38:80–103.)
39 Hughlings-Jackson J: Case of large cerebral tumour without optic neuritis and with left hemiplegia and imperception. Royal London Ophthalmic Hospital Reports 1876;8:434–444. Reprinted in Taylor J (ed): Selected writings of John Hughlings Jackson, vol 2. New York, Basic Books, 1958, pp 146–152.
40 Dunn TD: Double hemiplegia with double hemianopsia and loss of geographical centre. Trans Coll Phys Phila 1895;17:45–56.
41 Lenz GK: Beiträge zur Hemianopsie. Stuttgart, Germany, Hoffmannsche Buchdruckerei, 1905.
42 Luys J: Recherches nouvelles sur les hémiplégies émotives. Encéphale. J Mal Ment Nerve 1881;1:378–398.
43 Della Rocca M: The "other" localization: XIX century French neurophysiological models for the seat of the musical faculty in the brain. Rev Int Filosofia Psicol 2013;4:134–142.
44 van Dalin O: Beräattelse om en dumbe, som kan siumga (On a mute who can sing). Kungliga Svenska Vetenskap Academiens nya Handlingar. Stockholm, Sweden, 1745, vol 6, pp 114–115.

45 Johnson JK, Graziano AB, Hayward J: Historical perspectives on the study of music in neurology; in Rose FC (ed): Neurology of Music. London, Imperial College Press, 2010, pp 17–30.
46 Knoblauch A: Ueber Störungen der musikalischen Leistungfähigkeit infolge von Gehirnläsionen [On disorders of musical ability as a result of brain lesions]. Deutsches Archiv für Klinische Medicin 1888;43:331–352.
47 Johnson JK, Graziano AB: August Knoblauch and amusia: a nineteenth-century cognitive model of music. Brain Cogn 2003;51:102–114.
48 Leurat F, Gratiolet P: (written by P. Gratiolet). Anatomie Comparée du Système Nerveux, Consideré des ses Rapports Avec l'Intelligence (vol. 2). Paris, J. B. Balliere et Fils, 1857.
49 Ireland WW: Notes on left-handedness. Brain 1880;3: 207–214.
50 Parrot MJ: Sur le developpement du cerveau chez les enfants du premier age. Archives de Physiologie Normale et Pathologique (2nd Series) 1879;6:505–521.
51 Ecker A: Zur Entwicklungsgeschichte der Furchen und Windungen der Grosshirn-Hemisphären im Foetus des Menschen. Archiv für Anthropologie 1868;3:212–223.
52 Ireland WW: The Blot Upon the Brain: Studies in History and Psychology. New York, G. P. Putnam's Sons, 1886.
53 Bateman F: Aphasia or loss of speech in cerebral disease. J Ment Sci 1869;15:102–119; 367–392.
54 Broca P: Sur le poids relatifs du deux hémisphères cérébraux et de leur lobes rontaux. Bulletins de la Société d'Anthropologie de Paris 1875;10:534–535.
55 Assézat J: Recording of discussion of P. Broca, Sur le poids relativ des deux hémisphère cérébraux et de leurs lobes frontaux. Bulletins de la Société Anatomique de Paris 1875;10:535–536.
56 Cunningham DJ: Right-handedness and left-brainedness. The Huxley lecture for 1902. J R Anthropol Inst Great Br Ireland 1902;32:273–296.
57 Gall FJ, Spurzheim G: Anatomie et physiologie du système nerveux en général, et du cerveau en particulier: premier volume. Anatomie et physiologie du système nerveux en général, et anatomie du cerveau en particulier. Paris, F. Schoell, 1810.
58 Vesalius A: (1543). De Humani Corporis Fabrica Libra Septum. Translated Excerpts in E. Clarke & C. D. O'Malley, The Human Brain and Spinal Cord: A Historical Study Illustrated by Writings from Antiquity to the Twentieth Century (pp 578–580). Berkeley, The University of California Press, 1968.
59 Harris LJ: The corpus callosum and the question of hemispheric communication: an historical survey of theory and research; in Kitterle F (ed): Advances in Cerebral Laterality Research: Hemispheric Communication: Mechanisms and Models. New York, Erlbaum, 1995, pp 1–60.
60 Harris LJ: Right-handers speak with the left hemisphere, left-handers with the right: the rise and fall of a neuropsychological hypothesis; in Barr WB, Bieliauskas LA (eds): The Oxford Handbook of History of Clinical Neuropsychology. Oxford Handbooks Online. Oxford, Oxford University Press, 2016.
61 Nishitani N, Schurmann M, Amunts K, Hari R: Broca's region: from action to language. Physiology 2005;20: 60–69.
62 Dubois J, Hertz-Pannier L, Cachia A, Mangin JF, Le Bihan D, Dehaene-Lambertz G: Structural asymmetries in the infant language and sensori-motor networks. Cerebral Cortex 2009;19:414–423.
63 McCartney G, Hepper P: Development of lateralized behaviour in the human fetus from 12 to 27 weeks' gestation. Dev Med Child Neurol 1999;41:83–86.
64 Mori S, Oishi K, Faria AV: White matter atlases based on diffusion tensor imaging. Curr Opin Neurol 2009;22: 362–369.
65 Rogers LJ, Zucca P, Vallortigara C: Advantages of having a lateralized brain. Proc Biol Sci 2004;271(suppl 6): S420–S422.
66 Rogers LJ, Vallortigara C, Andrews RJ: Divided Brains: The Biology and Behaviour of Brain Asymmetries. Cambridge, Cambridge University Press, 2013.
67 Frasnelli E: Brain and behavioral lateralization in invertebrates. Front Psychol 2013;4:939.
68 MacNeilage PF, Rogers LJ, Vallortigara G: Origins of the left & right brain. Sci Am 2009;301:60–67.
69 Patel AD: Language, music, syntax and the brain. Nat Neurosci 2003;6:674–681.
70 Peretz I, Vuvan D, Lagrois MÉ, Armony JL: Neural overlap in processing music and speech. Philos Trans R Soc Lond B Biol Sci 2015;370:20140090.
71 Kaplan HI, Sadock BJ, Grebb JA: Kaplan and Sadock's Synopsis of Psychiatry: Behavioral Sciences, Clinical Psychiatry, ed 7. Baltimore, Williams & Wilkins, 1994.
72 Lane ZP, Singer A, Roffwarg DE, Messias E: Differentiating psychosis versus fluent aphasia. Clin Schizophr Relat Psychoses 2011;4:258–261.

Lauren Julius Harris
Department of Psychology, Michigan State University
316 Physics Road
East Lansing, MI 48824 (USA)
E-Mail HarrisL@MSU.edu

Bogousslavsky J, Boller F, Iwata M (eds): A History of Neuropsychology.
Front Neurol Neurosci. Basel, Karger, 2019, vol 44, pp 15–22 (DOI: 10.1159/000494946)

The Introduction of Emotions and Behavior in the Assessment of Neurological Patients

Melanie Genetti Gatfield[a] Françoise Colombo[a] Jean-Marie Annoni[b, c]

[a]Neuropsychology and Aphasiology Unit, Fribourg Hospital, Fribourg, Switzerland; [b]Neurology Unit, Fribourg Hospital, Fribourg, Switzerland; [c]Laboratory for Cognitive and Neurological Sciences, Department of Medicine, University of Fribourg, Fribourg, Switzerland

Abstract

In neurology and neuropsychology, behavior refers to the way human beings act and make decisions in contact with their environment. Behavioral impairment is therefore defined as a pathology, following brain lesion, that impacts the interactions between the brain-lesioned individual and his/her surrounding social world. First descriptions of behavioral disorders, including neuroanatomical correlates, date back to the mid-19th century. However, attempts towards their systematic identification and analysis only began at the turn of the 19th to 20th century. In this chapter, we shall span 3 main themes by introducing the first case reports based on thorough clinical descriptions, dating back to the 19th century. We then examine the emergence of checklist questionnaires and their application to large cohorts of individuals starting after World War II. Finally, we outline how, over the last 3 decades, the pace has significantly accelerated in the pursuit of defining the fine-grained processes underlying behavioral functioning, as well as the development of new and more complex measures, along with the emergence of the social cognition and social brain concepts. As the assessment tools have expanded and become more specific, an increasing complexity of mechanisms underlying behavior has begun to emerge.

Introduction

Starting in the 19th century, human behavior has been the subject of abundant studies and to a range of definitions. In neurology and neuropsychology, behavior refers to the way human beings act and make decisions in contact with their environment. Neurobehavioral impairment (for simplicity purposes, we shall only use the term "behavioral" in the following) is therefore defined as a pathology, following brain lesion, that impacts the interactions between the individual and his/her surrounding social world.

Inherent to the nature of clinical examination, behavioral assessment belongs nowadays formally to guidelines and recommendations for most neurological diseases. For example, the fifth major revision of the Diagnostic and Statistical Manual of Mental Disorders (DSM-5) has not only included behavior change as a criterion in the diagnosis of neurocognitive impairment, but has also determined social cognition as one of the cognitive domains to be assessed [1].

First descriptions of behavioral disorders including neuroanatomical correlates date back to the mid-19th century [2]. However, attempts towards their systematic identification and analysis only began around the turn of the 19th to 20th century. Some authors have argued that interest in the neural basis of behavior and moral reasoning might have been delayed due to the particular taboos existing at that time [3]. In an editorial about the frontal lobe and behavior, Mesulam discussed the difficulties encountered in behavioral assessments [4]. He first denoted the variety and complexity of behavioral deficits. Despite certain shared features, the panel of behavioral changes observable after brain lesions thus remains difficult to explain; despite numerous studies in the field over the last decades, a unified, widely accepted model is still lacking. Second, behavioral changes are generally difficult to quantify by standard testing. They are not always evident – and can be overlooked due to well-preserved performance on routine examination. Moreover, behavioral deficits evolve (acute vs. chronic stages), can fluctuate under certain circumstances, and may be contained in the examination room (e.g., due to external control). Finally, any occurring changes must be evaluated against the background of pre-morbid personality traits "rather than in reference to any set of absolute behavioral standards" [4].

Behavioral impairments have been associated with lesions to cortical and sub-cortical structures across a wide array of etiologies, including trauma, tumors, surgical interventions (e.g., lobectomy, lobotomy), strokes, infections (e.g., syphilitic), and dementia. Striking behavioral disorders are associated with the broad, yet somewhat poorly defined concept that has been named the "frontal syndrome" [5]. Typically, despite behavioral deficits, patients with a "frontal syndrome" can perform quite well on classical cognitive tasks. In this chapter, we shall outline how, over the past 150 years, behavioral measurements have been developing hand-in-hand with attempts to unravel the mysteries of the frontal lobe. Of note, we thus intentionally focus on semiology consecutive to frontal lobe damage to discuss the introduction of behavioral assessment in neurological patients. Overall, we shall span 3 main themes by introducing (1) the first case reports based on thorough clinical descriptions, dating back to the 19th century. We then examine (2) the emergence of checklist questionnaires and their application to large cohorts of individuals starting after World War II. Finally, we outline (3) how, over the last 3 decades, the pace has significantly accelerated in the pursuit of defining and measuring the fine-grained processes underlying behavioral functioning, as well as the development of new and more complex measures, along with the emergence of the social cognition concept.

From Descriptive Single Case Reports to First Neuroanatomical Correlates

The original case of Phineas Gage, a 25-year-old railroad foreman who was caught in a dramatic explosion that resulted in a 3 cm-thick tamping iron penetrating his left cheek, skull, and brain, remains the classic introduction to the field of behavioral disorders [2, 3]. Gage survived and recovered without any motor or cognitive impairment. However, "he was no longer Gage," according to his friends [2]. Formerly, a responsible and socially well-adapted individual, he became irreverent and capricious, could not hold a job and died 12 years later under the custody of his family. Harlow published a very comprehensive description of the behavioral changes occurring after Gage's accident, which included a several-year-long follow-up of the patient and testimony of relatives and friends [2]. He also presumed that these behavioral modifications were associated with lesions to a particular region of the frontal cortex, making it one of the earliest correlations between behavioral disorders and neuroanatomy.

In addition to medical records, behavioral changes have occasionally become the object of public perception through artistic acknowledgment and penal proceedings. Contemporary to Phineas Gage, Eadweard Muybridge, a bookseller established in San Francisco, survived a stagecoach accident in 1860 [6]. Again, this patient recovered physically and intellectually but his personality transformed dramatically. He changed the spelling of his name dozens of times and was even charged with the murder of a man suspected of having an affair with his wife. Yet, this lesion triggered a new artistic expression and reoriented his career: He became a pioneering photographer and developed the "zoopraxiscope," a precursor of motion pictures. Based on visual symptoms and the loss of smell and taste, Eadweard Muybridge's brain lesion is assumed to have occurred in the orbitofrontal cortex.

These 2 case reports of trauma established the relationship between lesions to a specific brain area and acquired behavioral deficits that spared intellectual abilities. A few decades later and with the development of neurosurgical procedures, neuroanatomical correlates became accessible to more specific investigation and further underscored the relevance of behavior assessment. One of the sessions at the 2nd International Neurological Congress in London (1935) was thus dedicated to the functions of the frontal lobe [7], and included the well-documented follow-up of patient Joe A., the first bilateral frontal lobectomy case with long survival [8]. Intellectual performance in this patient was assessed using psychometric testing, whereas behavioral status remained at the descriptive level, relying (as for almost all cases of that era) mainly on the neurologist's observations and heteroanamnesis. Following the resection, Joe A. became logorrheic, self-absorbed, puerile and distractible, with perseverations and sudden mood changes. Whilst Brickner showed severe deterioration in Joe A.'s behavior after surgery, Hebb and Penfield reported a 27-year-old patient who improved after partial bilateral frontal lobectomy [9, 10]. Following a traumatic brain injury to the frontal poles at the age of 16 years, K. M. suffered from severe epileptic seizures. During interictal states, he was described as "childish, violent, stubborn and destructive" by his relatives and the whole neighborhood. After operation, he became "normal in every way" [9]. The 6-year follow-up showed that he had been independent in his daily life activities and successful in finding jobs since his discharge from the army. Although he frequently changed jobs, he was able to save for the future. Here, K. M.'s post-surgical behavioral improvement was evaluated through information given by his parents and his brother, as well as through the "independent testimony of 3 residents of the village," namely a taxi driver, a storekeeper, and a waitress.

Two decades later, Luria et al. [11] went a step further and published a seminal detailed experimental analysis about the impairment in behavioral regulation after the removal of part of a left frontal meningioma. Patient Zav underwent a full test battery addressing different modalities (verbal, non-verbal, symbolic instructions) and assessing various levels of behavioral regulation (apprehension of instructions, evaluation of errors). This study also introduced the innovative concept of "orienting reaction," that is, an autonomic signal based on previously registered feedbacks produced by the outcomes of actions, which is assumed to be disturbed in patient Zav. The recording of vascular and galvanic skin responses (GSR) indeed showed the absence of activation during tasks and reinforced the hypothesis of a lack of error utilization underlying behavioral regulation and decision-making impairments. As described below, this pioneering approach was made popular 30 years later with the "somatic marker hypothesis" [12, 13].

Advances in neurosurgery and the London congress also led to the rise of lobotomy. Initiated by Swiss psychiatrist Gottlieb Burckhardt as early as 1888 and later extensively implemented by Egas Moniz and Walter Freeman, the controversial "psychosurgery" consisted mainly of frontal lobotomy, that is, the (minimal-to-extensive) deletion of the fibers connecting the frontal areas with the rest of the brain, to decrease symptoms of mental illness [14, 15]. Post-surgery patients typically showed apathy, loss of initiative, and a decrease in social interactions. Not only were these behavioral characteristics just outlined and their follow-up was brief, but they were also certainly biased by pre-existing mental disorders.

War Times, Questionnaires, and Group Studies

World War I sadly supplied much data for the understanding of personality changes due to brain trauma [16]. However, World War II triggered more systematic and larger-scale assessments: Interviews and questionnaires with features amenable to quantification and scoring thus resulted in first group studies.

Large cohort studies with patients based on war records were carried out retrospectively. For instance, Lishman examined psychiatric and behavioral disabilities after head injury from the Oxford collection of head injury records, compiled during World War II [17]. A detailed follow-up was available up to 5 years after the acute stage for most patients, much of this material consisting of questionnaires listing a wide range of symptoms. In Lishman's study, altered behavior was part of the category "psychiatric disability" defined "as disturbance in any area of mental life, as reflected by impaired intellectual function, disorder of affect, disorder of behavior, somatic complaints without demonstrable physical basis, and/

or formal psychiatric illness." Affective disorders consisted of depression (episodic or continuous), emotional lability, morbid anxiety and phobias, irritability, overt aggression, apathy, loss of initiative and euphoria, whereas behavioral disorders involved crime or misdemeanours, sexual disturbance, lack of judgment, reliability, consideration for others, childish or facile behavior, restlessness, impulsiveness, and disinhibition. Likewise, Grafman et al. [18] retrospectively investigated the presence of aggressive and violent behavior in veterans who suffered a penetrating brain injury during their service in Vietnam. Besides an open question asked by the neurologist ("Have you ever had any violent behavior against persons or things? We all lose our temper now and then, but have you ever beaten someone up or torn up a room?"), the veteran and family members completed questionnaires. It included the Beck Depression Inventory [19], the Katz Adjustment Scale (relatives' judgment of the subject's competency across a variety of social and behavioral domains) [20], and the VHIS Family Questionnaire (addressing the relatives' ability to cope with the subject's behavior). Finally, the examiner filled in the Neurobehavioral Rating Scale, an inventory sensitive to aberrant behavior [21]. Overall, questionnaires were quantitative, interrogated patients and relatives, and therefore led to more systematic assessments. This set-up allowed the evaluation of behavioral deficits on large cohorts of individuals, as well as conducting follow-up investigations to shed light on the long-term outcome of patients.

1980–1990s, Innovations and Emergence of Social Cognition

A key factor in the 1980s is a change of perspective: it was realized that certain symptoms occurring in real life cannot be pinpointed with classical "laboratory" tests nor in the examination room. In other words, formal neurological/neuropsychological assessments can (1) miss certain behavioral impairments, and can (2) exert external constraints and conditions that differ sufficiently from daily life as to impact test results. This notion introduces the concept of "ecological validity." Moreover, coming back to our neurological definition of behavior, the last decade of the 20th century has seen the emergence of a specific field dedicated to the study of cognitive processes required in social behavior, referred to as "social cognition."

This new perspective is illustrated, for example, by the characterization of "imitation and utilization behavior," a disturbed response to external stimuli which belongs to the "dependency syndrome" [22]. Lhermitte [23] thus established fairly unusual and innovative methodology to study the presence of this phenomenon in patients with cerebral lesions. In stark contrast to classical examination settings, the examiner remains neutral and indifferent to the patient during the whole examination, and then makes a series of gestures, such as body, symbolic and gymnastic gestures, gestures involving objects, and pronounces short sentences, sings, writes and draws. The patient is told not to copy the examiner, who then repeats his sequence of gestures. The patient's behavior is observed and evaluated. To better understand the impact of the environment on the dependency syndrome, the study went a step further by taking the patients outside the examination room, filming and photographing all steps [23]. The patient was thus put in situations of everyday life (e.g., doctor's office, garden, gift shop). Although creative, less structured and probably more ecological, this methodology obviously poses ethical issues with respect to the patient and his family.

The discrepancy between good performance in classical tests in the examination room and successive failures in daily life observed in some patients has led scientists to address those mechanisms which are impaired and cause emotional and behavioral changes. Before the availability of dedicated tests, such investigations made use of personality trait inventories [5, 24] and tools from developmental psychology [5, 25, 26]. In these studies, tasks targeted different components of social behavior, namely self vs. others perspective, social knowledge, and moral reasoning. All of them consisted of standardized verbal presentations of moral dilemmas or social situations that required verbal responses. Inspired by these studies, new paradigms have been designed, in particular to evaluate "pseudopsychopathy" [16], later called "acquired sociopathy" [13]. This term refers to individuals developing high levels of aggression and antisocial behavior with reduced empathy and guilt after acquired lesion to the orbitofrontal cortex. This is, for example, the case of patient EVR who underwent a resection of a large orbitofrontal meningioma compressing both frontal lobes [5]. Previously, a sensible and successful fellow, EVR changed dramatically after surgery; he separated from his family, became unable to hold a job and made unreasonable decisions. The integrity of his knowledge of normal patterns of social behavior and its application were measured. Despite his ability to reason appropriately about moral problems that were presented to him, and a performance in social cognition tasks that lay in the range of (or even excelled) healthy controls, he was unable to apply such reasoning in real-life situations [5, 13]. Of note, despite their social nature, these tasks do not seem to sufficiently match real-life situations for several reasons (e.g., verbal tasks vs. multimodal inputs, observer vs. protagonist in real life), thus suggesting that a decision-making disorder lies at the core of the impairment. The social knowledge and access to it was preserved, yet EVR failed to apply the appropriate choice-making strategy. These observations were further developed in the "somatic marker hypothesis" [13], which denotes the covert influence of a somatic process on decision-making, as suggested by Luria thirty years before [11]. To validate this hypothesis, "reversal learning" tasks were developed, such as the Iowa Gambling Task that mimics real-life decisions by including uncertainty, rewards, and penalties [12]. The subjects (players) are presented with 4 decks of cards, a loan of a certain amount of facsimile U.S. dollar bills and asked to play. They are also instructed to lose the least amount of money and win the most. There are 2 advantageous and 2 disadvantageous decks, the latter leading to an overall loss. Simultaneously, physiological data such as GSR are recorded. The reference study showed first that healthy controls chose advantageous decks whereas patients with prefrontal lesions did not [12]. Second, healthy controls generated anticipatory GSR (i.e., autonomic response) before being explicitly aware of a risky choice, whilst patients did not, even with knowledge of their risky choice.

GSR measures were utilized in combination with other modality tasks, for example, by Blair and Cipolotti [27]. Patient JS, who developed acquired sociopathy following a trauma that lesioned the orbitofrontal cortex bilaterally, has been assessed in much detail with a series of twelve tests embracing 3 types of processing, namely (1) reversal learning, (2) expression recognition and emotional responding, and (3) social cognition. Together with simultaneous GSR recordings, salient facial and environmental stimuli as well as visual and auditory inputs were applied during expression and emotional tasks. Moreover, different levels of social cognition were investigated. These measures included emotion attribution, theory of mind (i.e., the ability to attribute mental states to oneself and to others), moral/conventional distinction, and social situation tasks. JS performed well on the reversal learning tasks but was severely impaired on expression recognition and emotional responding tasks despite intact face processing. Autonomic responses (i.e., GSR) were preserved for auditory but not for visual stimuli. Finally, although showing no impairment on the theory of mind task, he failed almost all the social cognition tasks. JS's results were significantly different from those of a dysexecutive patient without aberrant behavior as well as from a group of individuals with developmental psychopathy. This study therefore showed that autonomic measures can contribute, but are not sufficient to disentangle the complex processes underlying acquired sociopathy. More generally, it revealed that the more various and "composite" the measures are, the broader the resulting behavioral spectrum is.

Conclusions

We have discussed the introduction of assessment of emotions and behavior in neurological patients along with the understanding of frontal lobe functions. From observational and descriptive reports, behavioral measures have moved to auto- and hetero-evaluation questionnaires. It has then evolved to tasks where patients are more actively involved, resembling daily life situations. Not unexpectedly, as the assessment tools have expanded and become more specific, an increasing complexity of mechanisms underlying behavior has begun to emerge.

Behavioral assessment is nevertheless of importance since impairments are strongly related to poor outcome. Together with the interaction of pre-morbid factors such as personality and cognitive deficits, behavioral deficits diminish independent social behavior and increase social handicap [28]. However, measuring behavior directly faces the normality issue. In analogy to Mesulam questioning the existence of standards regarding behavior [4], this raises the necessity to consider an individual's behavior in its entirety, which includes pre-morbid functioning, interindividual and cultural differences. Finally, as an encouraging perspective, it is worth noting that behavioral disorders can benefit from neurorehabilitation: both individual and group training programs have shown successful results [29, 30].

Acknowledgements

The authors would like to thank Ian Gatfield for language editing and proofreading.

References

1 American Psychiatric Association and American Psychiatric Association DSM-5 Task Force, Diagnostic and Statistical Manual of Mental Disorders: DSM-5, ed 5. Washington, DC, American Psychiatric Publishing, 2013.
2 Harlow JM: Recovery from the passage of an iron bar through the head. Publ Mass Med Soc 1868;2:327–347.
3 Damasio H, et al: The return of Phineas Gage: clues about the brain from the skull of a famous patient. Science 1994;264:1102–1105.
4 Mesulam MM: Frontal cortex and behavior. Ann Neurol 1986;19:320–325.
5 Eslinger PJ, Damasio AR: Severe disturbance of higher cognition after bilateral frontal lobe ablation: patient EVR. Neurology 1985;35:1731–1741.
6 Manjila S, et al: Understanding Edward Muybridge: historical review of behavioral alterations after a 19th-century head injury and their multifactorial influence on human life and culture. Neurosurg Focus 2015;39:E4.
7 International neurological congress in London. Later proceedings. Br J Med 1935;2:269–272.
8 Brickner RM: Brain of patient A. after bilateral frontal lobectomy; status of frontal-lobe problem. AMA Arch Neurol Psychiatry 1952;68:293–313.
9 Hebb DO: Man's frontal lobes. AMA Arch Neurol Psychiatry 1945;54:10–24.
10 Hebb DO, Penfield W: Human Behavior after extensive bilateral removal from the frontal lobes. Arch Neur Psych 1940;44:421–438.
11 Luria AR, Pribram KH, Homskaya ED: An experimental analysis of the behavioral disturbance produced by a left frontal arachnoidal endothelioma (meningioma). Neuropsychologia 1964;2:257–280.
12 Bechara A, et al: Deciding advantageously before knowing the advantageous strategy. Science 1997;275:1293–1235.
13 Saver JL, Damasio AR: Preserved access and processing of social knowledge in a patient with acquired sociopathy due to ventromedial frontal damage. Neuropsychologia 1991;29:1241–129.
14 Manjila S, et al: Modern psychosurgery before Egas Moniz: a tribute to Gottlieb Burckhardt. Neurosurg Focus 2008;25:E9.
15 Freeman W: Psychosurgery. J Natl Med Assoc 1950;42: 206–209.
16 Blumer D, Benson DF: Personality Changes with Frontal and Temporal Lobe Lesions, in Psychiatric Aspects of Neurological Disease, D.F. Benson and D. Blumer, Editors. New York, Grune and Stratton, 1975.
17 Lishman WA: Brain damage in relation to psychiatric disability after head injury. Br J Psychiatry 1968;114: 373–410.
18 Grafman J, et al: Frontal lobe injuries, violence, and aggression: a report of the Vietnam head injury study. Neurology 1996;46:1231–1238.
19 Beck AT: Beck Depression Inventory Manual. San Antonio, TX, The Psychological Corporation, 1987.
20 Katz M, Lyerly S: Methods for measuring adjustment and social behavior in the community. 1. Rationale, description, discriminative validity and scale development. Psychol Rep 1963;13:503–535.
21 Levin HS, et al: The neurobehavioural rating scale: assessment of the behavioural sequelae of head injury by the clinician. J Neurol Neurosurg Psychiatry 1987;50: 183–193.
22 Lhermitte F, Pillon B, Serdaru M: Human autonomy and the frontal lobes. Part I: Imitation and utilization behavior: a neuropsychological study of 75 patients. Ann Neurol 1986;19:326–334.
23 Lhermitte F: Human autonomy and the frontal lobes. Part II: Patient behavior in complex and social situations: the "environmental dependency syndrome". Ann Neurol 1986;19:335–343.
24 Eslinger PJ, et al: Developmental consequences of childhood frontal lobe damage. Arch Neurol 1992;49:764–769.
25 Price BH, et al: The comportmental learning disabilities of early frontal lobe damage. Brain 1990;113(pt 5): 1383–1393.
26 Anderson SW, et al: Impairment of social and moral behavior related to early damage in human prefrontal cortex. Nat Neurosci 1999;2:1032–1037.
27 Blair RJ, Cipolotti L: Impaired social response reversal. A case of 'acquired sociopathy'. Brain 2000;123(pt 6): 1122–1141.
28 Wood RL, Alderman N, Williams C: Assessment of neurobehavioural disability: a review of existing measures and recommendations for a comprehensive assessment tool. Brain Injury 2008;22:905–918.
29 Ruffieux N, et al: Successful neuropsychological rehabilitation in a patient with cerebellar cognitive affective syndrome. Appl Neuropsychol Child 2017;6:180–188.
30 Aboulafia-Brakha T, et al: Feasibility and initial efficacy of a cognitive-behavioural group programme for managing anger and aggressiveness after traumatic brain injury. Neuropsychol Rehabil 2013;23:216–233.

Jean-Marie Annoni
Neurology Unit, Fribourg Hospital
Chemin des Pensionnats 2-6
CH–1700 Fribourg (Switzerland)
E-Mail Jean-Marie.Annoni@h-fr.ch

Bogousslavsky J, Boller F, Iwata M (eds): A History of Neuropsychology.
Front Neurol Neurosci. Basel, Karger, 2019, vol 44, pp 23–29 (DOI: 10.1159/000494948)

Anatomical Error of Pierre Marie's "Zone Lenticulaire"

Makoto Iwata
Tokyo Women's Medical University, Tokyo, Japan

Abstract
In a series of papers which appeared in 1906, Pierre Marie advanced a new concept of aphasiology against the classical view based on functional localization of cerebral cortex. He denied the role of Broca's area in language function and proposed as the center for articulation "zone lenticulaire," the lesion of which causes anarthria. But his illustration of "zone lenticulaire" which appears repeatedly in his papers dealing with aphasia, is anatomically incorrect since the most important portions of Broca's area, opercular part and triangular part of the inferior frontal gyrus are missing in his illustration. The detailed anatomical investigation of Marie's illustrations reveals that he repeated the same errors in identifying rolandic and frontal opercula. But the similar mistake of identifying these opercula is also seen in Dejerine's "Anatomie des Centres Nerveux."

Pierre Marie's "Zone Lenticulaire"

In 1906, Pierre Marie published a series of three papers criticizing the classical view of aphasiology [1–3]. In these papers, he proposed a new concept of his own which was against the theory of functional localization of the cerebral cortex. According to him, aphasia was a single pathological condition of intelligence impairment caused by the lesion of the Wernicke area and the so-called Broca's aphasia was a syndrome consisting of intelligence disturbance due to a lesion of Wernicke area combined with anarthria caused by a lesion located in the "zone lenticulaire." Thus, he denied the role of Broca's area the lesion of which was thought to be responsible for expressive type of aphasia crowned by the name of Broca.

The cardinal theoretical base of his new concept of aphasiology was based on 2 anatomo-pathological findings; first, lesions of the Broca's area did not necessarily cause Bro-

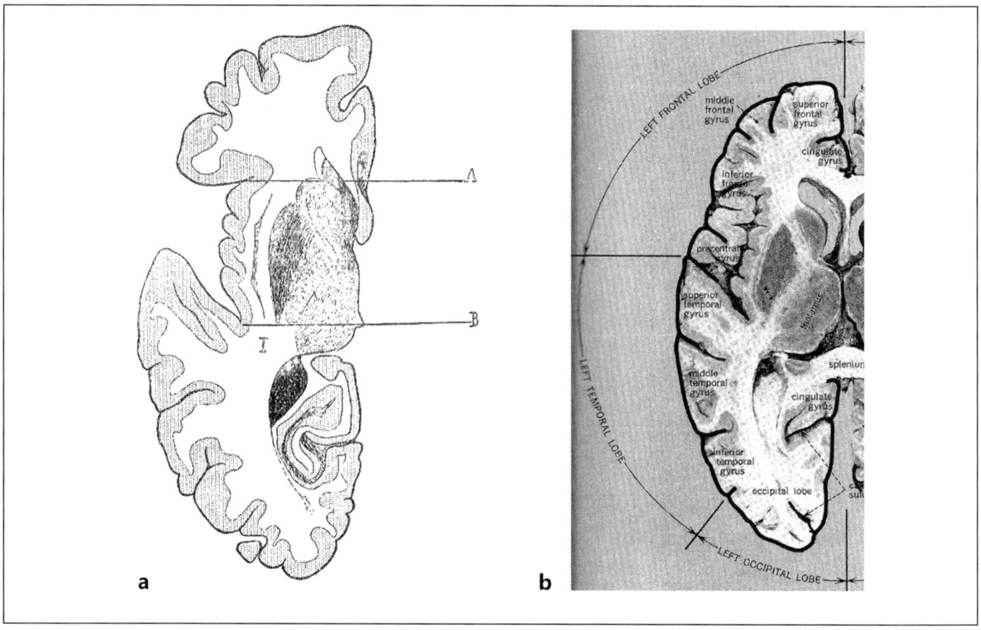

Fig. 1. a Pierre Marie's illustration showing "zone lenticulaire" (from Marie [1–3]), **b** the corresponding horizontal brain slice (modified from Matsui [4]).

ca's aphasia and second, there were reports of patients showing Broca's aphasia without any destructive lesion of the Broca's area. To explain the second point, he showed the famous illustration of "zone lenticulaire" which was the site of anarthria, and also showed cases of Broca's aphasia with lesion situated in this zone. He also described a case of small hemorrhagic lesion in this zone which had caused only anarthria without true aphasia. According to him, a lesion within the "zone lenticulaire" caused the patient severe anarthria but he did not show aphasia because his Wernicke's area was intactly preserved, only the lesion of which was thought to produce aphasia.

All of these 3 papers of Pierre Marie showed the famous illustration of "zone lenticulaire," the lesion of which was responsible for producing anarthria (Fig. 1). However, from the view point of a neuropathologist accustomed to the horizontal sections of autopsied brain [4], his "zone lenticulaire" seems to be very unnatural, because he had shown a big blank space at the level of Sylvian fissure between the frontal lobe and the temporal lobe outside of insula. Actual horizontal slice of human brain at this level usually does not show such vacant space as shown in Marie's illustration, on the contrary this space is filled with pieces of cortices corresponding to the opercular part and triangular part of the inferior frontal gyrus [4]. Broca's area consists of Brodmann's Area 44 and Area 45, the former is located on the opercular part and the latter on the triangular part of the inferior frontal gyrus. Therefore, both of these cortices of Broca's area are totally missing from the Marie's illustration of "zone lenticulaire."

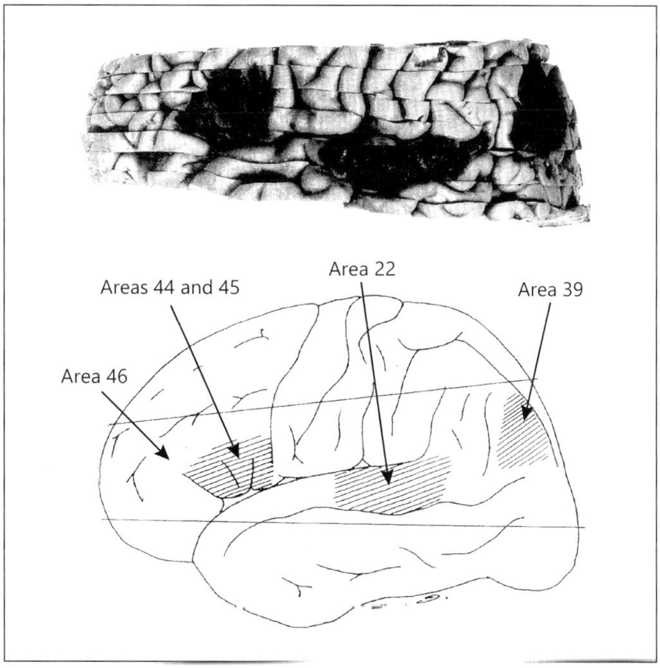

Fig. 2. Piled up horizontally cut slices of the left hemisphere of a normal brain between 2 horizontal lines shown below. Cortical surface of the 3 language areas are marked with Indian ink (modified from Iwata [5]).

Confirmation of the Missing Portions from the Brain Slice

To confirm the anatomical localization of Broca's area, Brodmann's Areas 44 and 45 in the horizontal slices of brain, I made serial horizontal sections of neurologically normal autopsied brain which was marked in advance on the cortical surface of areas 44 and 45 and other language areas (Area 22 corresponding to the Wernicke's area and Area 39 of the angular gyrus) with Indian ink (Fig. 2) [5]. Figure 3 shows the horizontally cut slice of thus marked normal brain at the same level of Sylvian fissure as the illustration of Pierre Marie showing the "zone lenticulaire" (Fig. 1). Comparing the Marie's figure and the real brain slice, it is quite evident that both opercular and triangular parts of the inferior frontal gyrus corresponding to Area 44 and Area 45 of Brodmann, which are the most important areas in discussing the anatomo-pathological investigations of aphasia, are completely missing from the illustration of Pierre Marie [6].

Since the opercular part of the inferior frontal gyrus (Area 44) is separated from the inferior tip of the precentral gyrus only by a shallow precentral sulcus, both of these 2 cortices form a continuous cortical area which is clearly separated from the superior temporal gyrus by the posterior ramus of the Sylvian fissure and also separated from the triangular part of the inferior frontal gyrus by the deep ascending ramus of Sylvian fissure. Another portion of the Broca's area, triangular part of the inferior frontal gyrus corresponding to Area 45 is separated posteriorly by the ascending ramus and anteriorly by the horizontal ramus of the Sylvian fissure. Consequently, the two cortical areas consisting of

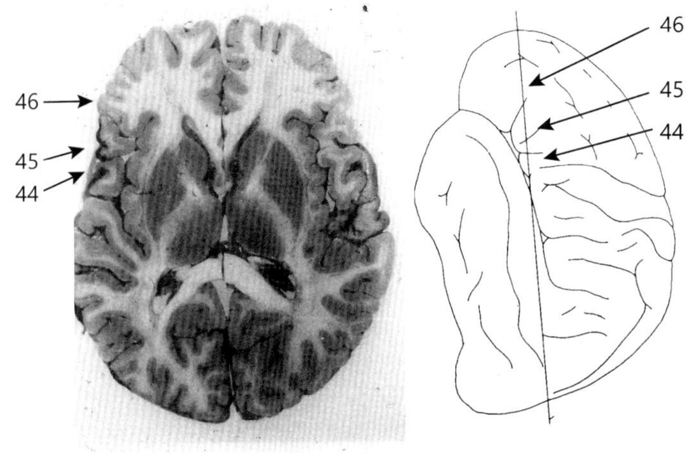

Fig. 3. Horizontally cut brain slice at the same level as Marie's illustration (Fig. 1) showing Areas 44 and 45 (cortical surface of which are marked with Indian ink) and Area 46 (not marked). Slice level is shown on the right side.

the Broca's area, opercular part and the triangular part of the inferior frontal gyrus, are horizontally disconnected from other adjacent cortical areas and connected only vertically with the rest of the brain areas. As a consequence, these two cortical areas are usually completely detached from the rest of the horizontal slice through Sylvian fissure.

Pierre Marie's Error in Identifying the Cortical Areas

In his first paper [1], Pierre Marie showed a patient who did not show any language disturbance in spite of a destructive lesion of Broca's area, but the destructive lesion of the case of this patient is actually situated anterior to the horizontal ramus of Sylvian fissure (Fig. 4a), that is to say on Area 46 of Brodmann and we can never know whether Broca's area (Area 44 and 45) is affected or not, because these 2 cortical areas are completely missing from the illustration.

In his second paper [2], Marie showed an illustration of brain slice of Case Bal…, who clinically showed Broca's aphasia (Fig. 4b). According to Marie, the lesions of this patient affected the "zone lenticulaire" and the deep white matter of the Wernicke area together with the white matter of the temporal lobe. But again, since both opercular and triangular parts of Broca's area are missing from the illustration, we can never know whether these most important cortical areas are intact or not. In this paper [2], Marie cited the illustration of the brain slice of Bernheim's case with Broca's aphasia which appeared in Dejerine's book (Fig. 4c). Marie discussed the clinicopathological similarities between these two

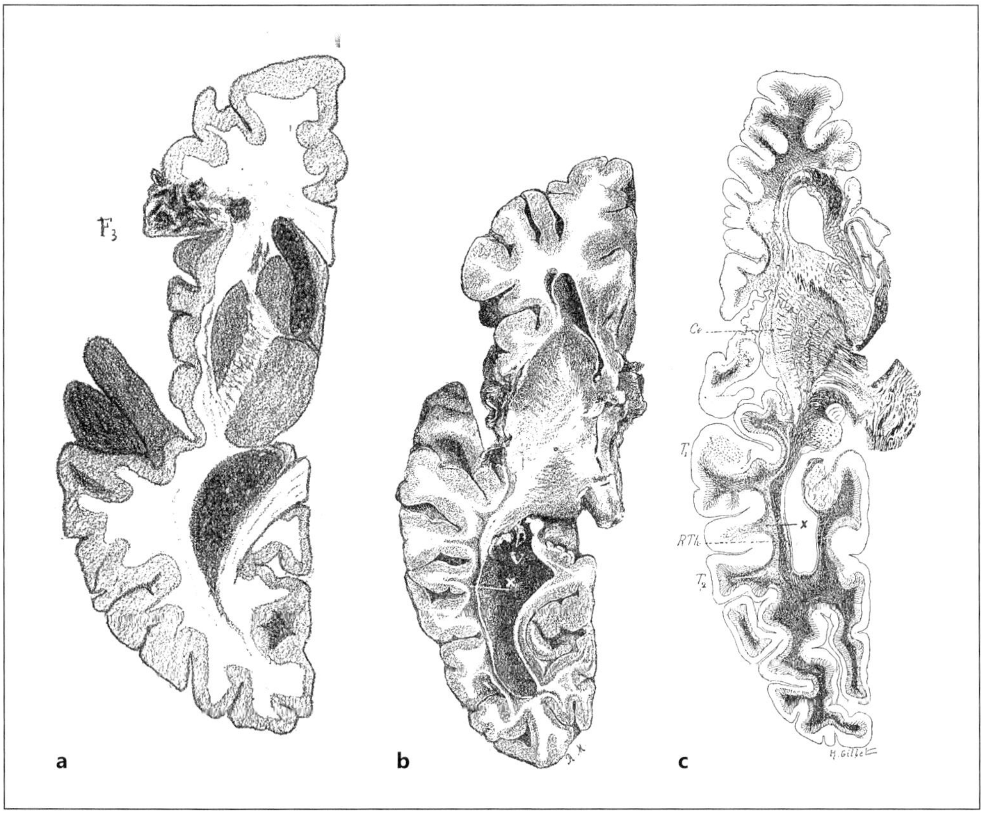

Fig. 4. a Marie's non-aphasic case with a destructive lesion which Marie thought had destroyed Broca's area but actually the lesion is located in Area 46. **b** Marie's case with Broca aphasia without lesion on the Broca's area. Areas 44 and 45 are missing. **c** Dejerine's case cited by Marie as a case of Broca aphasia without lesion on the Broca's area. Area 45 of the Broca's area is evidently affected. (**a** cited from [1], Band **c** cited from [2]).

cases, but the illustration of the Bernheim's patient cited in Marie's paper clearly shows that the opercular part of the inferior frontal gyrus corresponding to Area 44 is preserved but the triangular part of the same gyrus corresponding to Area 45 of the Broca's area is totally damaged and atrophied. Marie seemed to have repeatedly made errors in identifying the anatomical site of the Broca's area not only in his own cases, but also with the anatomo-pathological reports of other investigators [6].

Why Marie Did Not Notice the Missing Parts?

Then the question arises. Why Pierre Marie had repeatedly made this kind of simple error to identify the cortical areas? The answer is given by one of his last pupils form the United States. Percival Bailey, the famous neurosurgeon, entered Marie's clinic at the Salpêt-

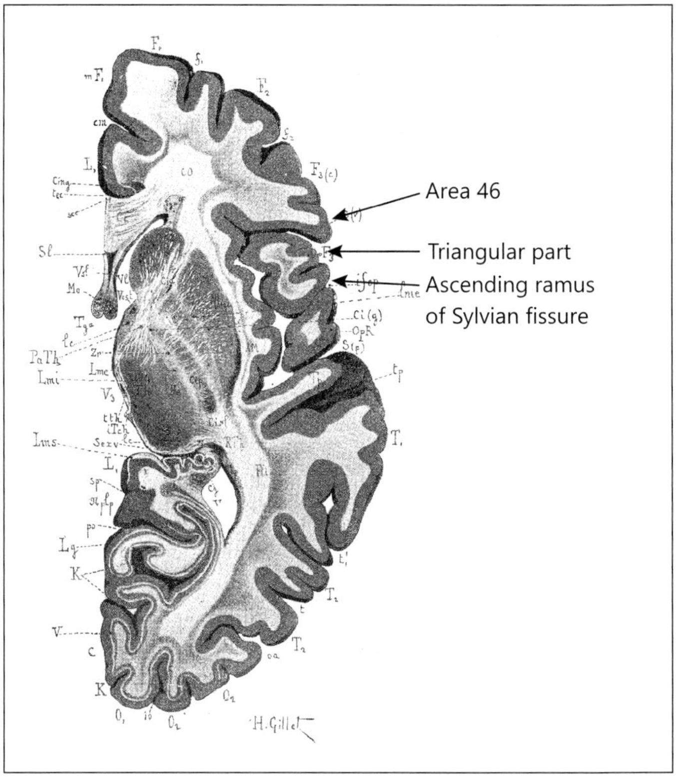

Fig. 5. Dejerine's error in identifying the triangular part of the inferior frontal gyrus (corrected anatomical names are given with arrows; modified from [8]).

rière in 1921 as foreign assistant. He wrote "Only rarely did he enter the wards and never the laboratory, for he was very sensitive to formalin and would look at fixed brains only through a window, and there dictate his description" [7]. Although the above-mentioned anatomo-pathological studies of patients with aphasia were done in the Hospice de Bicêtre, and not in the Salpêtrière, he was sure to use it to observe the already cut horizontal brain slices indirectly through a window, as Bailey described. As shown in the previous Figures 1 and 4, two most important pieces of the posterior part of the inferior frontal gyrus, opercular and triangular parts are liable to be dropped out from the entire horizontal slice at the level of Sylvian fissure because they are not connected with the rest of the brain. My speculation is that Pierre Marie, in his routine laboratory works, made his assistants to cut the brains, but they did not pay enough attention to these 2 small pieces of brain inevitably detached from the rest of the brain slice.

Dejerine's Error in Identifying Triangular Part

Similar error of identification of the easily detached small pieces of Broca's area was also seen in Figure 225 of Dejerine's "Anatomie de Centres Nerveux, Tome 1" [8]. The figure (Fig. 5) is a horizontal slice of normal brain and clearly shows two small pieces within the

Sylvian fissure. Dejerine identified the posterior piece as Rolandic operculum and the anterior piece as frontal operculum, and the deep fissure between these two pieces as frontal opercular incisure, but the truth is that this deep fissure is ascending ramus of Sylvian fissure and the anterior piece which Dejerine identified as frontal operculum is actually the triangular part of the inferior frontal gyrus. Due to this misidentification of the ascending ramus of Sylvian fissure, Dejerine noted erroneously the above-mentioned anterior piece of brain as the opercular part and the cerebral gyrus situated anterior to this fissure as the triangular part (cap de la troisième circonvolution), but his anatomical identification was incorrect (Fig. 5).

Consequently, as to the identification of triangular part of the inferior frontal gyrus including Area 45 of Brodmann in the horizontal brain slice, Dejerine shared the same error with Marie. As shown above, Marie showed in his first paper [1] a case of his own who had no language impairment in spite of a lesion on the Broca's area. The site of the lesion of this case was erroneously located on the triangular part by Marie, and the real site of the lesion was on the anterior part of the inferior frontal gyrus, probably Area 46 of Brodmann. Dejerine did not point out the misidentification of the site of the lesion of this case, since he had made the same error of identification of triangular part in the horizontal brain slice [8]. It seems rather very strange that both the experts in clinicopathological studies of aphasia had shared the same mistake. Marie's papers finally elicited the famous aphasia debate in 1908, but the problem of incorrect location of the Broca's area, especially of Area 45, was never discussed either by Marie or by Dejerine, because not only Marie but also Dejerine had made the same error in identifying Area 45 of the Broca's area in the horizontal brain slice.

References

1 Marie P: Révision de la question de l'aphasie. La troisième circonvolution frontale gauche ne joue aucun role spécial dans la function du langage. Semeine Médicale du 23 mai 1906. (Marie P: Travaux et Memoires, Tome 1, Paris, Masson et Cie, 1926, pp 3–30).
2 Marie P: Que fault-il penser des aphasies sous-corticales (apahsies pures)? Semaine Médicale du 17 octobre 1906. (Marie P: Travaux et Memoires, Tome 1, Paris, Masson et Cie, 1926, pp 31–64).
3 Marie P: L'apahsie de 1861 á 1866. Essai de critique historique sur la genèse de la doctrine de Broca. Semaine Médicale du 28 novembre 1906. (Marie P: Travaux et Memoires, Tome 1, Paris, Masson et Cie, 1926, pp 65–92).
4 Matsui T, Hirano A: An Atlas of the Human Brain for computerized Tomography. Tokyo-New York, Igaku-Shoin, 1978, p 153.
5 Iwata M: CT anatomy of aphasia. Progress in CT 1884;6: 133–137. (in Japanese)
6 Iwata M: CT anatomy of the frontal lobe, especially in relation with language function. Seishin-Igaku 1895;27: 619–624. (in Japanese)
7 Bailey P: Pierre Marie (1853–1940); in Haymaker W, Schiller F (eds): The Founders of Neurology, ed 2. Springfield, IL, C. C Thomas, 1970, pp 476–479.
8 Dejerine J: Anatomie des Centres Nerveux Tome 1. Paris, Rueff et Cie, 1895, pp 404–405.

Makoto Iwata
Tokyo Women's Medical University
4-46-19, Hikawadai, Nerima-ku
Tokyo 179-0084 (Japan)
E-Mail iwata.makoto@twmu.ac.jp

Bogousslavsky J, Boller F, Iwata M (eds): A History of Neuropsychology.
Front Neurol Neurosci. Basel, Karger, 2019, vol 44, pp 30–38 (DOI: 10.1159/000494950)

Gogi (Word Meaning) Aphasia and Its Relation with Semantic Dementia

Atsushi Yamadori

Tohoku University Graduate School of Medicine, Sendai, Japan

Abstract

In 1943, Tsuneo Imura, a neuropsychiatrist at Tokyo University, proposed a new aphasic syndrome and designated it as Gogi (word meaning) aphasia. According to Imura, it is characterized by (1) difficulty in comprehending spoken words despite good perception of sound, (2) disorders of expression due to loss of vocabulary and verbal paraphasia, (3) preserved ability of repetition, and (4) selective difficulty in reading and writing kanji (Japanese logographic character) with preserved ability of reading and writing kana (Japanese syllabic character). To be more specific, the difficulty in comprehending spoken words in Gogi aphasia is limited to substantive words as the name of the syndrome indicates, while comprehension of syntax remains unimpaired. Preserved repetition ability cannot be simply regarded as an automatic response, that is, echolalia, because the patient's attitude in repeating was quizzical, picking up the particular word he did not comprehend. Imura vaguely attributed the responsible lesion to the second and third temporal gyri on the left side. Although the general pattern of the syndrome can be placed in the category of transcortical sensory aphasia, its uniqueness as the syndrome still stands out. Another uniqueness of the syndrome is its characteristic pattern of dissociated kanji-kana difficulty in reading and writing. This linguistic symptomatology observed in Gogi aphasia was first introduced to the western academic world on a German neuropsychiatric journal by Panse and Shimoyama in 1955. Ever since, the existence of Gogi aphasia as an independent syndrome among disorders of spoken language has gradually gained international recognition. But whether the pattern of the kanji-kana dissociation described by Imura is an integral part of the syndrome remains unsettled. A recently proposed concept of semantic dementia suggests symptomatic continuation of word meaning loss with non-linguistic semantic memory loss.

In 1943 Tsuneo Imura, a neuropsychiatrist at Tokyo University, reported a new aphasic syndrome which he proposed to be called "Gogi aphasia" in an article published in Japanese [1]. "Go" of "gogi" means word, and "gi" means meaning. He admitted that the syndrome belongs to a broad category of transcortical sensory aphasia but claimed it has a unique characteristic and should be treated as a syndrome. The proposal remained unnoticed outside Japan until 1955 when Imura's contribution to Japanese aphasiology was introduced along with his concept of "semantische Aphasie" in a German journal as a 2-part article by Panse and Shimoyama [2, 3]. The first part of this article was later translated into English [4]. In 1975, Sasanuma and Monoi [5] published a detailed linguistic study of a case with Gogi aphasia emphasizing the uniqueness of the syndrome because its symptomatology is inherently correlated with the complicated writing system of Japanese. In the article, Imura's original concept of Gogi aphasia and its later impact on Japanese aphasiology were summarized briefly.

A Brief Introduction of the Japanese Script System

Since the symptom of Gogi aphasia is believed to be closely associated with a peculiar difficulty in reading and writing, a brief introduction of the Japanese script system might be necessary before describing the syndrome. In short, Japanese script is a hybrid of two different types of characters. Kan-ji was originally imported from China and literally means Han-letter. The Japanese applied these Han-letters to corresponding Japanese names with the similar concept as well as to Japanese syllables with similar Chinese sounds. This effort resulted in the complicated use of kanji for both names of concept and notification of pronunciation. Since Japanese system of syllables are quite different from Chinese, kana characters for Japanese syllables simplifying kanji form slowly developed. Kana has one letter-one syllable regularity, and the number is rather small, that is, 46. A kanji has multiple readings with no regularity. Also, its inventory is huge. For instance, the Japanese Government recommends using no more than 2,136 kanji in newspapers or laws to curb the kanji numbers in daily use. In usual Japanese script, semantic part is written by kanji and morphemic part (grammatical part) is written by kana.

The Syndrome of Gogi Aphasia

According to Imura, Gogi aphasia is characterized by 4 features [1]:

The first is difficulty in comprehending the meaning of a sentence spoken to. Although a typical patient could grasp the sound of the sentence correctly, he does not understand what they mean. He would repeat the sentence either automatically or intentionally to grasp the meaning. The most difficult part of a sentence to comprehend is substantive words that have restrictive meaning such as names of object or content.

Second, in spontaneous speech the patient would show word amnesia, verbal paraphasia, and a kind of paragrammatism. The anomia is most prominent for names of concrete things and proper names. Unlike amnesic aphasia, the patient would show difficulty in recognition of the name even if the correct one is produced. Generally, speech is fluent and articulation clear. But sentences produced are incoherent and incomplete. No difficulty is seen in the use of grammatical words.

Third, ability to repeat spoken language is sufficiently preserved. The way the patient repeats cannot be considered as automatic echolalia. It implies his intention for comprehension.

Fourth, there is a unique difficulty in oral reading and writing. Imura summarized this difficulty as "oral reading without comprehension" and "writing without comprehension." The difficulty manifests itself as a dissociated ability to handle kanji and kana. Kana can be read or written rather easily without comprehension, while kanji is difficult in both comprehension and writing.

Overall, Imura considered this symptom complex belongs to the category of transcortical sensory aphasia in Wernicke-Lichtheim diagram, but nonetheless emphasized its uniqueness because the difficulty is most conspicuous in comprehension of the meaning of substantive words rather than comprehension of spoken language in general and insisted it should be treated as a separate aphasic syndrome.

An Illustrative Case

In the 1943 paper, he wrote he had experienced 4 cases of Gogi aphasia. But only 3 cases were concretely described. He himself claimed that out of 4 cases, 3 cases showed a typical pattern of Gogi aphasia [1]. Of these 3, one illustrative case is quoted below which was originally described in 1940 [6].

Case E. is a 57-year-old businessman. He had been forgetful the previous year, and recently started having difficulty in reading. He also became obstinate and short tempered. No physical neurological signs were found on admission.

Comprehension of Spoken Language

He did not understand the examiner's questions. For example, when asked to tell his address, he responded, "What is address?"

When asked whether he travels by airplane, he responded, "What is airplane?"

When asked to tell his hobby, he said, "What is hobby?"

When asked to choose a brush from a group of 10 pictures, he responded, "What is brush?"

When asked to choose a picture of a comb, he said, "What is comb?"

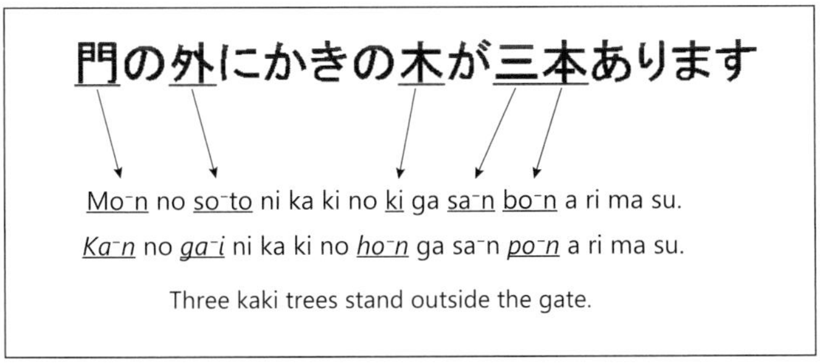

Fig. 1. Reading performance of Imura's case E. The first row of the table shows a sentence from a contemporary primary school textbook which is written in mixed kanji and kana characters. Underlined characters are kanji. Others are kana. The second row shows its pronunciation in romanized letters (romaji). Each kana pronunciation is shown separately for the purpose of easy correspondence. Underlined parts correspond to kanji portion. The third row is reading by the patient. Errors are shown in italics and underlines. For details, see text. The fourth row is an English translation of the text [13].

Naming of Objects

Very Difficult. He seemed to know the concept of an object that was shown but could not recall an appropriate name. For example, when asked to give the name of a matchbox, he responded, "this is not tobacco. Make a fire. Tobacco."

Repetition

Almost always correct. Non-sense words could also be correctly repeated.

Oral Reading

Reading aloud kana words and sentences was on the whole correct, but reading aloud kanji words was severely impaired. As mentioned, a kanji has more than two ways of reading but only one of them is appropriate when it is embedded in a particular kanji-kana mixed sentence. The patient simply misread the kanji part of a sentence, either producing a correct but inappropriate name for the sentence, or confusing it with another kanji similar in form.

To make the point easy to understand for non-Japanese readers, an example of his reading errors is illustrated in Figures 1 and 2. In this reading of a sentence: "Three kaki trees stand outside the gate," his errors were restricted to kanji characters (Fig. 1). He erroneously read the first kanji meaning gate for "ka-n," which is a name for other characters similar in form (Fig. 2). The second kanji meaning outside he read as "ga-i," which is wrong in this sentence but is one of the correct readings of the character (Fig. 3). The third kanji meaning tree should be read as "ki," but he misread it as "ho-n," probably confusing it with the visually similar fifth character (Fig. 2). The fourth kanji meaning three he read correctly as "sa-n." The fifth kanji is usually used as postposition for numbers when counting long objects such as trees or sticks. His reading "po-n" is not acceptable in this context but one of its correct readings (Fig. 3). For example, one tree is counted as "i-ppo-n," 2 trees as "ni ho-n", and 3 trees as "sa-n bo-n."

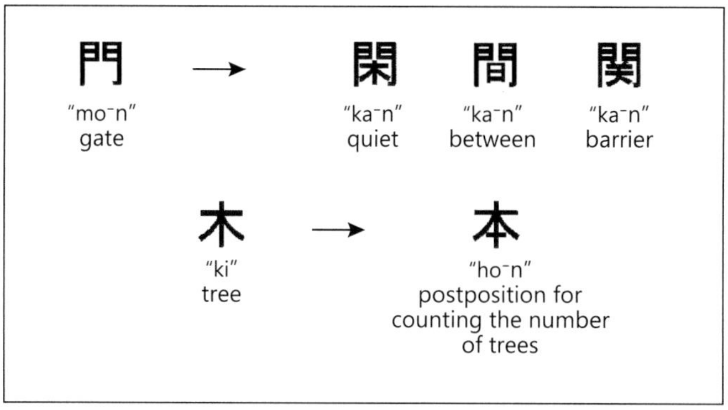

Fig. 2. Reading performance of Imura's case E. Confusion of kanji forms. The patient misread the first kanji "mo-n" in Figure 1 as "ka-n" which is like in form with such characters meaning quiet, between, or barrier. Also he misread the third kanji "ki" in Figure 1 as "ho-n," which is similar in form.

外 soto, *hoka, hazu, gai, ge*
本 bon, *hon, pon, moto*

Fig. 3. Reading performance of Imura's case E. Selection errors of pronunciation. The upper kanji in the table has 5 ways of pronunciation. The lower kanji has four. The patient read the upper one (the second kanji in Figure 1) meaning outside as "ga-i, " which is one of 5 correct readings for the character but wrong for the text. It should be read as "soto." Similarly, he read the lower kanji (the fifth kanji in Figure 1) as "po-n" which is wrong, although the pronunciation itself for the character is correct. It should be "bo-n."

Writing

He wrote his name and address correctly. He could write a few words with kana for dictation but impossible with kanji.

Copying Characters

He showed no difficulty in copying characters either in kanji or kana.

As this illustrative case demonstrates, the most conspicuous linguistic symptom of Gogi aphasia manifests itself in the patient's verbal behavior. A typical patient would spontaneously respond to a question by picking up and repeating the substantive word in the question he does not understand. This peculiar verbal behavior was repeatedly confirmed and emphasized as a hallmark of Gogi aphasia by later researchers [7, 8]. The author's experience coincides with the opinion [9].

Thus, the patient could grasp an acoustic form of the word quite easily but could not understand what it means. His spontaneous tendency to repeat the word suggests he is trying to stabilize the sound image of the word in his mind. Imura insisted this difficulty in grasping word meaning in the face of normal capacity to grasp its sound form is an isolated difficulty because their ability to deal with syntax is intact. Later studies support this claim [8, 10].

Historical Background

When he proposed the concept of Gogi syndrome, he cited semantic aphasia proposed by Head [11], or Namenaphasie by Kleist [12] or mixed transcortical aphasia by Goldstein [13] for discussion but did not identify it with them. Of these, Imura regarded Goldstein's mixed transcortical aphasia most akin to Gogi aphasia [14]. Although Imura failed to mention, almost identical aphasic symptom complex had been reported by Arnold Pick in 1898 [15]. In this article, Pick introduced Arnaud's contribution. According to Pick, this Arnaud described a type of transcortical aphasia he termed as "surdite verbale representative." As the name suggests, this "representative verbal deafness" is characterized by good grasp of spoken word and inability to comprehend its meaning as if it were completely foreign. The patient would correctly repeat an incomprehensible word he just heard. It is not the problem of word sound reception, but the problem of understanding the sound as a symbol of concept. Pick himself described several cases of this type of aphasia. One of them (case F, 67-year-old female) grasped a word sound correctly and repeated the word consciously as if asking its meaning. For instance, she responded to a command to close her eyes, by repeating the word eyes: "What are eyes?" Likewise, to a command to bring a piece of soap, she questioned: "What is soap?"

The existence of Gogi aphasia has been repeatedly confirmed in Japan [8]. Unfortunately, this has not been the case in Europe and America. This may be due to the difference of the mode of spoken language. Indo-European languages belong to a group called reflected language, while Japanese is one of the agglutinated languages in which semanteme (substantive words) and morpheme (grammatical words) are clearly separated [4].

Neuropsychological Interpretation

Imura thought the essential trouble in Gogi aphasia is an impairment of the "dictionary" meaning of words, which is rather fixed and has relatively independent meaning even in a sentence. He asserted that impairment of sentence comprehension even if present is only secondary, compared to the primary impairment of word comprehension [16].

He further argued that word meaning should not be regarded as referent or things meant. In other words, meaning is not an entity. Rather it is a relation between a name and its concept. A name evokes a mental image, while at the same time the evoked image evokes back the name. This "close co-occurrence" of 2 psychological processes is the basis of meaning. In Gogi aphasia, this co-occurrence becomes unstable. This is reflected in the patient's difficulty not only in comprehending word meaning but also in evoking a sound image of the word [16, 17]. Imura called Gogi aphasia "semantic form of aphasia" [14] or "semantic-form aphasia" [17] contrasting it with "phonetic form of aphasia" such as Broca's and Wernicke's aphasia.

As for the fourth feature of Gogi aphasia, Imura's stance was rather vague. Although he included it as one of the core features of Gogi aphasia, he was prudent to regard the difficulty as an integral part of the syndrome. Thus, in the original paper [1], he admitted that no complete correspondence between symptoms of speech and written language could be confirmed, since every case he had encountered did not necessarily show this pattern of difficulty in written language. But in the subsequent papers, he seemed to have gained confidence to claim that this particular pattern of kanji-kana dissociation is an essential part of the syndrome [14, 16, 17]. Imura also argued that the selective difficulty in kanji handling in Gogi aphasia is caused by its logographic nature, in which a single kanji character stands for multiple sounds and concepts simultaneously [16]. This complexity necessarily burdens a reader with the decision making to choose a correct pronunciation from possible candidates every time he has to read a sentence aloud.

Later studies either included the fourth feature of Imura's Gogi aphasia as one of the core symptoms [5, 9] or excluded it as coincidental [18, 19].

Responsible Lesions

Imura speculated that responsible lesions for Gogi aphasia are rather diffuse, involving the second and third temporal gyri and adjacent parietal lobe on the left side [16].

One of his cases (the above quoted case E) had been slowly deteriorating, leading Imura to presume a possibility of presenile dementia for its etiology [6]. The autopsy finding described by Pick of the case with "surdite verbale representative" (case F) which had also been slowly progressive showed the presence of diffuse cerebral atrophy, mainly affecting the left temporal lobe [15].

In 1991, Kurachi and Matsubara reported their experience on 11 cases of clinically diagnosed Pick's disease, of them three had been autopsy confirmed [20]. Of the three, one had been reported as a typical case of Gogi aphasia 7 years earlier [21]. The case showed prominent bilateral atrophy of the middle and inferior temporal gyrus and the fusiform gyrus, but the extent of atrophy was much stronger on the left side.

In the following year, Tanabe et al. [7] reported their experience on 7 cases of Gogi aphasia, of which 6 were diagnosed as suffering from Pick's disease of temporal lobe type. All the diagnosis was based on the findings of CT or MRI studies, which showed bilateral atrophy of the anterior and middle temporal lobes, the left being more affected. The present author also encountered 2 cases of typical Gogi aphasia caused by temporal lobe degeneration [9, 22].

But it has to be emphasized that Pick's disease is not the only cause of Gogi aphasia. Imura's 2 other cases suffered from non-progressive brain pathology, that is, hemorrhage and infarction. The patient of Sasanuma and Monoi [5] suffered from a head trauma. A surgical operation confirmed the presence of brain contusion as well as hematoma in the left second and third temporal gyri and the parietal lobe. Tanabe's experience includes a case of herpes simplex encephalitis [7]. Such non-progressive etiology continues to be reported. For instance, Matsuda et al. [10] described 2 cases of stroke and one case of head trauma with MRI confirmation. Funayama described a case of cerebral infarction caused by sinus thrombosis [23].

Thus, it seems there are 2 types of Gogi aphasia. One is progressive, and wider mental deterioration eventually ensues. This type is closely associated with Pick's disease of temporal lobe type [20]. The lesion involves bilateral temporal lobes even though the atrophy of the left side is much more prominent. The other is caused by various etiologies such as stroke, trauma, and encephalitis involving the lower temporal lobe. Symptoms of this type either remain stable or improve. The herpes simplex case and traumatic cases almost certainly must have suffered from bilateral damage of the temporal lobes. Even with stroke cases, bilateral lesions were demonstrated by MRI studies [10]. Thus, bilateral lesions of the temporal lobes seem to be a necessary condition for the emergence of Gogi aphasia. But the possibility of a left unilateral lesion causing this unique loss of lexical meaning cannot be easily discarded [23].

Gogi Aphasia and Semantic Dementia

In 1989, Snowden et al. [24] reported three cases of "semantic dementia," characterized by progressive breakdown in language and visual perception. All three showed loss of symbolic meaning affecting both verbal and non-verbal domains. All suffered from progressive lobar degeneration limited to bilateral anterior temporal lobes (temporal lobe type of Pick's disease in older terminology). The linguistic part of the syndrome is characterized by impaired comprehension and naming, but with well articulated speech with normal syntax and preserved repetition [24]. Based on experiences of 5 cases, Hodges et al. [25] further elaborated the nature of this "semantic dementia" as characterized by fluent dysphasia with severe anomia, reduced vocabulary, and prominent impairment of single-word comprehension. Of course, the concept of "semantic dementia" implies combined deterioration of linguistic meaning such as words and non-linguistic meaning such as faces, the linguistic part of the clinical picture corresponds with Gogi aphasia [26, 27].

Preferred occurrence of single-word meaning loss by damage of the left temporal lobe at a certain stage of progressive lobar degeneration suggests that a yet to be identified region or regions in the lobe occupies a pivotal part of a distributed neural network responsible for such a complex cognitive experience as "meaning" of a word.

References

1 Imura T: Aphasie, ihre eigenartigen Ersheinungen in der Japanischen Sprache. Folia Psychiatrica et Neurologica Japonica 1943;47:196–218. (in Japanese with German title)

2 Panse F, Shimoyama T: Zur Auswirkung aphasischer Störungen im Japanischen. I. Agrammatisums und Paragrammatismus. Arch f Psychiatr u Z Neur 1955; 193:131–138.

3 Panse F, Shimoyama T: Zur Auswirkung aphasischer Störungen im Japanischen. II. Schreib und Lesestörungen. Arch f Psychiatr u Z Neur 1955;193:139–145.

4 Panse F, Shimoyama T: On the effects of aphasic disturbance in Japanese: agrammatism paragrammatism; in Goodglass H, Blumstein S (eds): Psycholinguitics and Aphasia. Baltimore, MA, The Johns Hopkins University Press, 1973, pp 171–182.

5 Sasanuma S, Monoi H: The syndrome of Gogi (word-meaning) aphasia. Selective impairment of Kanji processing. Neurology 1975;25:627–632.

6 Imura T: Apraktische Ersheinungen bei Aphasikern. Folia Psychiatrica et Neurologica Japonica 1940;44:393–426. (in Japanese with German title)

7 Tanabe H, Ikeda M, Nakagawa Y, Yamamoto H, Ikejiri Y, Kazui H, Hashikawa K, Harada K: Gogi (word meaning) aphasia and semantic memory for words. Higher Brain Funct Res 1992;12:153–167. (in Japanese with English abstract)

8 Tanabe H, Nakagawa Y, Ikeda M, Hashimoto M, Yamada N, Kazui H, Nishikawa T, Okuda J: Selective loss of semantic memory for words; in Ishikawa K, McGaugh LI, Sakata H (eds): Brain Process and Memory. Amsterdam, Elsevier Science B.V., 1996, pp 141–152.

9 Yamadori A: Aphasia in ideograph readers: the case of Japanese; in Coppens P, Lebrun Y, Basso Y (eds): Aphasia in Atypical Populations. London, Lawrence Erlbaum, 1998, pp 143–174.
10 Matsuda M, Mizuta H, Hara K, Kumakura I: Three cases with transcortical sensory aphasia presenting disturbance of word comprehension as a cardinal feature. Higher Brain Funct Res 1993;13:279–287. (in Japanese with English abstract)
11 Head H: Aphasia and Kindred Disorders of Speech, vol. II. New York, NY, Hafner Publishing Company, 1963, pp xix–xxiv. (originally published in 1928 by Cambridge University)
12 Kleist K: Gehirn Pathologie Vornehmlich auf Grund der Kriegserfahrungen. Verlag von Johann Ambrosiuas Barth, 1934, pp 748–780.
13 Goldstein K: Language and Language Disturbances. New York, NY, Grune and Stratton, 1948, pp 301–303. (Original idea on mixed transcortical aphasia published in 1915.)
14 Imura T, Nogami Y, Asakawa K: Gogi aphasia – a semantic form of aphasia; in Imura T (ed): Studies on Psychiatry Volume 2. Tokyo, Misuzu Shobo Publishers, 1967, pp 292–303 (in Japanese).
15 Pick A: Studien zur Lehre vom Sprachverständnis. Beitrage zur Pathologie und pathologischen Anatomie des Centralnervensystems mit Bemerkungen zur normalen Anatomie desselben. S. Karger, Berlin, 1898 (translated into Japanese by Kurachi M, Enokido H; in Akimoto H, Ohashi H, Sugishita M, Torii H (eds): The Origins of Neuropsychology. Aphasia Part 2. Tokyo, Souzou Shuppan Publishers, 1984, pp 71–113. (in Japanese)
16 Imura T: Aphasia; in Imura T (ed): Studies on Psychiatry, vol 2. Tokyo, Misuzu Shobo Publishers, 1967, pp 142–195. (in Japanese) (The article originally published as a lecture for abnormal psychology in 1954)
17 Imura T, Nogami Y, Asakawa K: Aphasia in Japanese Language. Nihon Univ J Med 1971;13:69–90.
18 Jibiki I, Yamaguchi N: The Gogi (word-meaning) syndrome with impaired Kanji processing: alexia with agraphia. Brain Lang 1993;45:61–69. (in Japanese with English abstract)
19 Nakagawa Y, Okuda J, Tanabe H: Gogi Aphasia. Japanese Society of Biological Psychiatry: Neuropsychology and Psychiatry. Gakkai Shuppan Center, 1995, pp 46–58. (in Japanese)
20 Kurachi M, Matubara S: Clinicopatholgy and brain imaging of Pick's disease. Jpn J Neuropsychol 1991;7:10–18. (in Japanese with English abstract)
21 Matsubara S, Enokido H, Torii H, Hiraguchi M, Ainoda N: A case of presenile dementia with Gogi (word-meaning) aphasia. Higher Brain Funct Res 1984;4:59–69. (in Japanese with English abstract)
22 Miura R, Tabuchi M, Endo K, Fujii T, Yamadori A: Word meaning disorder in a case with word meaning (Gogi) aphasia. Higher Brain Funct Res 2000;20:157–164. (in Japanese with English abstract)
23 Funayama M: Semantic memory and Gogi-aphasia. Jpn J Neuropsychol 2012;28:116–123 (in Japanese with English abstract).
24 Snowden JS, Goulding PJ, Neary D: Semantic dementia: a form of circumscribed atrophy. Behav Neurol 1989;2:167–182.
25 Hodges JR, Patterson K, Oxbury S, et al: Semantic dementia: progressive fluent aphasia with temporal lobe atrophy. Brain 1992;115:1783–1806.
26 Ralph MA, Howard D: Gogi aphasia or semantic dementia? Simulating and assessing poor verbal comprehension in a case of progressive fluent aphasia. Cogn Neuropsychol 2000;17:437–465.
27 Komori K, Ikeda M, Nakagawa Y, Tanabe H: The role of the right temporal lobe in semantic memory: evidence from semantic dementia. Higher Brain Funct Res 2003;23:107–118. (English abstract)

Atsushi Yamadori
Tohoku University Graduate School of Medicine
1-23 Iwazono-cho
Ashiya 659-0013 (Japan)
E-Mail dfckf900@kcc.zaq.ne.jp

Bogousslavsky J, Boller F, Iwata M (eds): A History of Neuropsychology.
Front Neurol Neurosci. Basel, Karger, 2019, vol 44, pp 39–52 (DOI: 10.1159/000494951)

Alexia and Agraphia from 1861 to 1965

Victor W. Henderson

Departments of Health Research and Policy (Epidemiology) and of Neurology and Neurological Sciences, Stanford University, Stanford, CA, USA

Abstract

Studies of alexia and agraphia have played historically important roles in efforts to understand the relation between brain and behavior. In the second half of the 19th century, works by Paul Broca and Carl Wernicke led to the concept of delimited cortical centers in the left cerebral hemisphere concerned with discrete aspects of spoken and written language. These specialized centers were linked by white matter pathways. Charlton Bastian, Jean-Martin Charcot, Sigmund Exner, and Jules Dejerine championed center–pathway models of reading and writing. Dejerine played a dominant role, rejecting the idea of a left frontal lobe center that mediated writing and proposing a unique, specialized role for the left angular gyrus in both reading and writing. In 1891 and 1892, he detailed the symptoms of alexia and agraphia that resulted from injury to the left angular gyrus and from the isolation of the left angular gyrus from visual input required for reading. During the early 20th century, his work and that of other so-called diagram makers was confronted and largely discredited by Pierre Marie, joined later by Henry Head and Kurt Goldstein. In the 1960s, the center–pathway model was resurrected and refined by Norman Geschwind. He drew upon foundational works of Dejerine, Hugo Liepmann, and others to describe syndromes resulting from cortical disconnections and, in doing so, helped to establish a framework for the modern discipline of behavioral neurology.

Introduction

Aphasia is an acquired disorder of language defined principally by deficits in speech and speech understanding. Reading and writing are the visual counterparts of spoken language. Disorders of reading and writing, viz., alexia and agraphia, are often considered in relation to the language impairments of aphasia. Studies of aphasia, alexia, and agraphia play a historically important role in understanding the relation between brain function and complex behaviors.

1861 is a useful starting point for the history of alexia and agraphia. This is the year in which the French surgeon and anatomist Paul Broca (1824–1880) described his first case of aphemia (Broca's aphasia) [1]. A convenient place to conclude is 1965, when Boston neurologist Norman Geschwind (1926–1984) ushered in the modern era of brain-behavior studies with his publication on cerebral disconnection syndromes [2]. Aspects of this topic have been reviewed [3, 4].

Broca proposed an anatomical center within the cerebral cortex that mediated articulate language. This model, expanded by others to accommodate reading and writing, came to include several cortical centers with discrete functional roles, interconnected by subcortical white matter pathways. As in Broca's original case, the role of a center was inferred from symptoms after tissue destruction within a delimited cortical area. The role of a pathway was often inferred from the function of centers that it connected. Early proponents of the center–pathway model included Wernicke, Bastian, Charcot, and particularly Dejerine, who provided a key theoretical framework for alexia with and without agraphia. Opposing views were espoused by Hughlings Jackson and later by Marie, Head, and Goldstein. Geschwind's work represented a rediscovery and elaboration of earlier models in the mode of Broca and his successors.

Setting the Stage

Franz Gall (1758–1828), an accomplished neuroanatomist linked to the pseudoscience of phrenology, observed physical features of the head and related these to mental faculties. While still a student, he famously associated protruding eyes with an excellent memory for words. During the early 19th century, Gall described regional anatomical variations in the human brain, which he associated with mental abilities and behaviors observed during life [5]. He proposed cerebral organs as the morphological substrates for an intellectual faculty, psychological trait, or moral tendency. Thus, Gall reasoned that brain tissue behind the orbits represented organs for word memory and language sense, and their enlargement led to protruding eyes [5]. Gall did not identify organs for writing or reading. His controversial doctrines were popular throughout the 19th century but were opposed by the Catholic Church and by the scientific establishment.

Beginning in 1825, the French physician Jean-Baptiste Bouillaud (1796–1881) reported series of patients who had lost the ability to speak but understood what was said to them. At autopsy, he described areas of injury within the anterior (frontal) lobes, and Bouillaud proposed that a "special cerebral center…distinct and independent" (p 42) was responsible for speech [6]. This interpretation accorded with Gall's organ for language sense, which Gall had located within a more delimited portion of the anterior lobes [5].

Building on Bouillaud's work, Louis Victor Marcé (1828–1864) in 1856 described patients whose speech or writing was impaired; 2 patients wrote well despite speaking poorly [7]. By way of explanation, Marcé proposed that the agent responsible for speech coordination, but not the agent for writing coordination, had been damaged. These cases implied that a brain faculty coordinated the graphic representation of ideas, the formation of letters, and the assembly of letters into syllables and words. The role of this writing faculty was analogous to the speech center described by Bouillaud [6]. Marcé recognized, as had Bouillaud, that speech and writing were usually impaired together after brain injury. He reasoned that the speech and writing faculties were separate but intimately connected, but Marcé did not propose anatomically distinct centers.

1861: Broca's Aphemia

Bouillaud's notion of a speech center in the anterior lobes was refined by Broca. In 1861, members of the Anthropological Society of Paris, co-founded by Broca the year before, debated the relation between intelligence and brain size. Noting that the brain is a complex organ, a debate participant – Bouillaud's son-in-law Ernest Auburtin (1825–1893) – asked whether different parts of the brain should be considered separately. He mentioned a patient who had lost speech but who retained the ability to understand and, further, he predicted that an autopsy would eventually confirm a softening (stroke) within the anterior lobes in accordance with Bouillaud's ideas [8].

By remarkable coincidence, a man with similar symptoms was admitted to Broca's surgical service at the Bicêtre hospital 8 days later. Years before, he had lost his ability to speak, and he was paralyzed on his right side. He died of infection shortly thereafter, and Broca reported clinical and autopsy findings to the Anthropological Society [1]. His patient "understood almost all that one said to him" (p 236), and Broca interpreted this finding as evidence that intelligence was spared. The autopsy showed that "the frontal lobe of the left hemisphere was softened in most of its extent," particularly affecting "the middle part of the frontal lobe of the left hemisphere" (p 237) [1]. This localization, according to Broca, supported Bouillaud's view that anterior lobes were affected when speech was lost.

Broca used the term aphemia (*aphemie*) to describe the disorder of articulate language shown by his patient [9]. As more cases of aphemia were reported by Broca and others, he suggested that brain injury causing aphemia consistently affected one region of the anterior lobes (the posterior portion of the third frontal convolution [gyrus]) on one side of the brain (the left side) [10]. Broca noted that the left cerebral hemisphere also controlled movements responsible for right handedness and suggested, by way of analogy, that "we speak with the left hemisphere" (p 384) [11]. It was only several years later that Broca mentioned reading and writing disturbances in relation to aphemia [12].

Alexia and Agraphia in the Wake of Broca's Discovery

Armand Trousseau (1801–1867) in Paris proposed the term aphasia (*aphasie*) for Broca's aphemia [13]. He recognized that deficits in articulate language were almost always accompanied by disturbances in other aspects of intelligence, including the inability to read and write [13, 14]. During the several years after Broca's formulation of a left hemisphere cortical center for articulate language, other physicians reported cases intended to confirm, refute, or extend Broca's observations. Key issues were the relation between language and intelligence, whether spoken language could be disturbed without impairing written language or the converse, and whether there were separate cortical centers for writing or reading [10].

Four years after Broca's first report, Moritz Benedikt (1835–1920) in Vienna used the terms alexia (*Alexie*) and agraphia (*Agraphie*) in his review of controversies surrounding aphasia as described by Broca, Trousseau, and others [15]. Two years later in England, William Ogle (1824–1905) published cases of patients with impairments in speech, most with autopsy findings. He emphasized defects in "expression of ideas in written symbols or writing" (p 99), and he provided a classification scheme [16]. Ogle, like Marcé, viewed speech and writing as parallel activities. Brain injury might disrupt articulate speech (aphasia), written communication (agraphia) or, commonly, both. He described 2 varieties of agraphia (amnemonic and atactic agraphia) [16]. Amnemonic agraphia was due to impaired memory for words. A patient with amnemonic agraphia could "form letters and words with sufficient distinctness, but he either substitutes one word for another or … writes a confused series of letters which have apparently no connection to the words intended" (p 99). Atactic agraphia occurred when the patient no longer knew how to write words, and "the power of writing even separate letters is lost" (p 99).

Ogle described a patient who wrote well after a stroke but whose speech production was sharply limited. The autopsy revealed a small area of softening in the posterior part of the left inferior frontal convolution. This location, according to Ogle, strongly supported Broca's view of the brain area affected in atactic aphasia (Broca's aphasia). However, because writing was unaffected, Ogle concluded "that the faculty of speech and the faculty of writing are not subserved by one and the same portion of the cerebral substance" (p 106). Still, the hypothesized speech and writing centers must be "closely contiguous" (p 100), since aphasia and agraphia so frequently occurred together [16].

By 1874, it was clear that aphasia was not a homogenous syndrome. This was the year in which Carl Wernicke (1848–1904) in Breslau prepared his famous monograph on the symptom complex of aphasia [17]. Wernicke was the first to offer a plausible anatomical and conceptual framework to accommodate different types of aphasia [18]. He recognized a motor center in the left frontal lobe (Broca's area) that mediated speech production, and he proposed a cortical sensory center (subsequently referred to as Wernicke's area) in the left, first temporal convolution (superior temporal gyrus) that encoded images of word sounds. The cortical centers were joined by pathways, and Wernicke described specific symptoms from damage to centers and pathways [17]. Reading and writing required the visual memory of letters, and damage to visual regions of the brain would lead to alexia and agraphia. Because writing is guided by word sound images, damage to the sensory speech area (Wernicke's area) caused agraphia as well as aphasia. Left frontal lobe injury affecting images of speech movement (Broca's aphasia) could also cause agraphia either because writing sometimes involves subliminal speech movements or because injury affecting Broca's area might encroach on a nearby center that mediated writing movements.

At this time, influential voices from the National Hospital at Queen Square, London were those of John Hughlings Jackson (1835–1911) and Charlton Bastian (1837–1915). Their perspectives on the relation between brain and behavior could not have differed more [19]. Hughlings Jackson was unwilling to localize speech to Broca's area or any other small part of the brain, recognizing, "To locate the damage which destroys speech and to locate speech are two different things" (p 19) [20]. To Hughlings Jackson, speech was "a general term for all shades of intellectual expression, from the most general to the most particular" (p 32) and included "all grades and varieties of expression of ideas, chiefly by words" (p 30) [21]. For the person with aphasia, "Written or printed words cease to be symbols of words used in speech for the simple reason that those words no longer exist to be symbolized" (p 322) [22]. "The speechless patient does not write because he has no propositions to write" (p 318) [22]. Impaired reading was simply "the same defect in another form" (p 275) [23].

Bastian proposed discrete, interconnected cortical centers. There were auditory and visual perceptive centers for the comprehension of spoken and written language [24]. To write, according to Bastian, one first revives the sound impressions of words, then revives the visual impressions of letters, and then produces muscle contractions used in the physical act of writing. Writing and speech could be impaired separately or in concert, depending on which cortical center or which set of connecting fibers was injured [24]. To read, "visual symbols of words call up or revive automatically (by means of connecting fibres between the [visual perceptive centre and the auditory perceptive centre]) the words as sound perceptions" (p 488). These combined impressions were then associated with the memory of objects [24]. Reading comprehension was impaired when "communications between the visual and auditory perceptive centres were injured" (p 484) [24].

Alexia was recognized as an isolated symptom of brain disease by Adolf Kussmaul (1822–1902) in Germany. In his 1877 monograph on disturbances of speech, he pointed out that alexia usually accompanied impairments in writing and speech, and he described different types of alexia. Some patients could read words but not letters, and some could read letters but not words. Even more striking, "a complete text-blindness may exist, although the power of sight, the intellect and the power of speech are intact" (p 775) [25]. Kussmaul devised a complex diagram that included centers for visual images of words, sound images of words, motor coordination of spoken words, and motor coordination of written words (Fig. 1). Kussmaul thought it was premature to assign discrete anatomical locations to these functional centers [25].

Born in Russia in 1852 and working in Paris, Nadine Skwortzoff wrote a medical thesis on word blindness (alexia) and word deafness in 1881 [26]. Word blindness represented

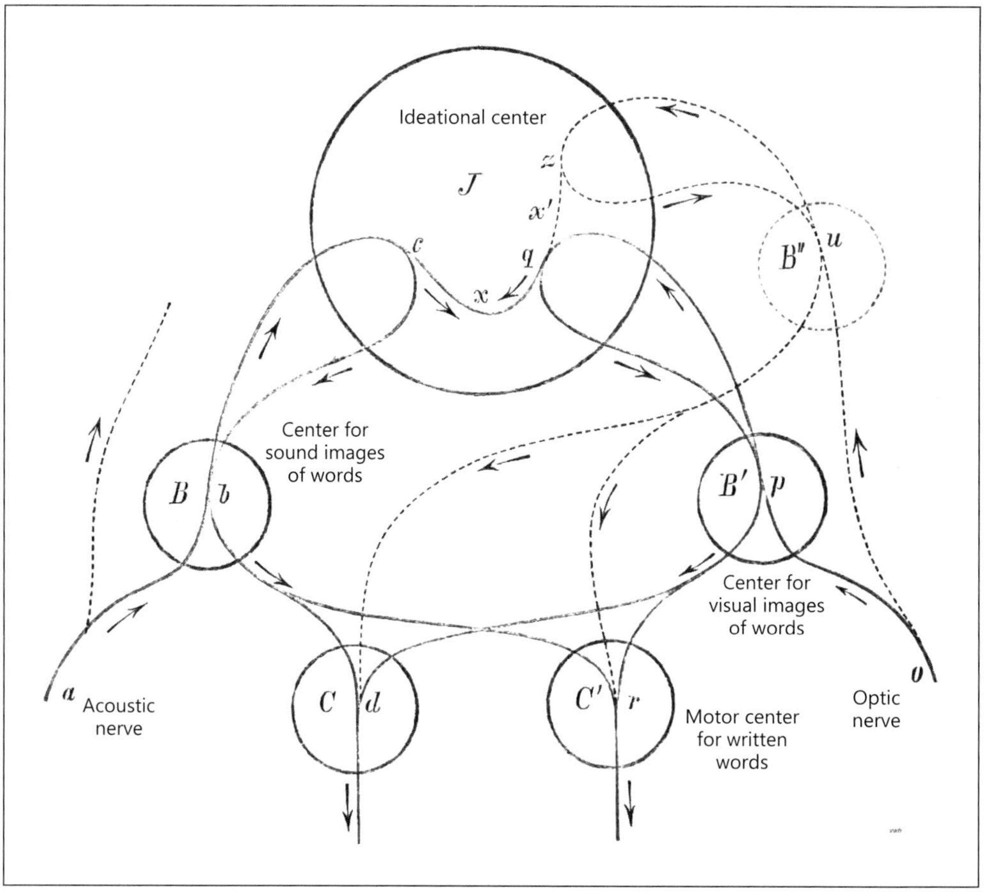

Fig. 1. Kussmaul's 1877 diagram [25] of centers and tracks involved in spoken and written language (labeling added). *J*, ideational (concept) center. *B*, center for the sound images of words. *B'*, center for the visual, or text, images of words. *C*, motor center for spoken words. *C'*, motor center for written words. *a*, acoustic (auditory) nerve. *o*, optic nerve. *o–p–q–p–r*, pathway for copy of written text. *o–p–r*, pathway for copying words that are not understood. *q–p–r*, pathway for writing spontaneously. *c–x–q*, pathway for writing to dictation by associating sound images with text images within the concept center. Pathway *p–q–p* is obstructed in word blindness (alexia) with agraphia. Pathway *p–q* is obstructed in word blindness without agraphia. Original image modified by V.W. Henderson.

the "failure to comprehend signs of thoughts represented by writing" (p 33). Her thesis included 14 cases with prominent reading impairments. She was influenced by the Scottish neurologist and physiologist David Ferrier (1843–1924). Working in England, Ferrier had mistakenly identified the angular gyrus of the parietal lobe as the primate visual center [27], and Skwortzoff suggested that the angular gyrus in the inferior left parietal lobe was damaged in cases of word blindness.

Also in 1881, Sigmund Exner (1846–1926) in Vienna reviewed literature cases where clinical and autopsy findings permitted inferences on cortical localization [28]. In his chapter on cortical fields for speech, 4 cases mentioned writing disturbances; lesions in these cases included the posterior part of the left middle frontal gyrus. This region is immediately in front of the part of the motor cortex involved with hand movement and immediately above Broca's area in the inferior frontal gyrus. In one patient, only this area was involved. Exner suggested that this region, later referred to as Exner's area, played a role in written expression similar to that played by Broca's area in spoken expression.

The identification of specific centers for reading and writing were a logical extension of ideas advanced by Broca and Wernicke. Bastian, in 1887, produced a new brain diagram that now included "word centres" for auditory impressions, visual impressions, "glosso-kineasthetic" impressions (based on speech movements; Broca's area), and "cheiro-kinaesthetic" impressions (based on writing movements; Exner's area) [29]. Damage of the visual word center led to word blindness, and damage of the cheiro-kinaesthetic center led to isolated agraphia. Word blindness and agraphia occurred together when the visual word center and the white matter pathway connecting it to the cheiro-kinaesthetic center were affected all together. Agraphia resulted when this pathway was damaged in isolation.

Jean-Martin Charcot (1825–1893), first recipient of the chair in Clinical Diseases of the Nervous System at the Salpêtrière hospital in Paris, was intensely interested in problems of aphasia [19]. His center-pathway model was based on component memories. Word memories consisted of an auditory image, a visual image, a motor image for articulatory movements, and a motor image for movements required for writing (Fig. 2) [30]. Charcot was interested in partial forms of memory loss, which he believed provided convincing evidence for the existence of independent cerebral centers. Charcot used word blindness (alexia) and agraphia to illustrate 2 of the partial forms of aphasia [31].

Charcot's student Albert Pitres (1848–1928) in Bordeaux provided the first detailed description of isolated agraphia [32]. Like Charcot, he accepted that the posterior part of the left second frontal convolution (Exner's area) played a role in graphic memory similar to the role of the posterior part of the third frontal convolution (Broca's area) in phonetic memory. Pitres described a patient with "pure motor agraphia" affecting the right hand. He had developed aphasia 18 months before, but speech, speech understanding, reading, and spelling aloud were normal when Pitres examined him. He wrote legibly with his left hand. With his right hand, he wrote neither words nor letters, but he easily drew geometric figures. He could copy printed text with his right hand, albeit, as if copying a design; he could not copy cursive text. Pitres interpreted the problem as the written counterpart of motor aphasia (Broca's aphasia); that is, the loss of memory for movements needed to guide the right hand in writing.

Alexia with and without Agraphia

Jules Dejerine (1849–1917) is linked to syndromes of alexia with agraphia and alexia without agraphia. His seminal work occurred at the Bicêtre hospital in Paris, and later he became the third person to hold the chair in Clinical Diseases of the Nervous System at the Salpêtrière hospital.

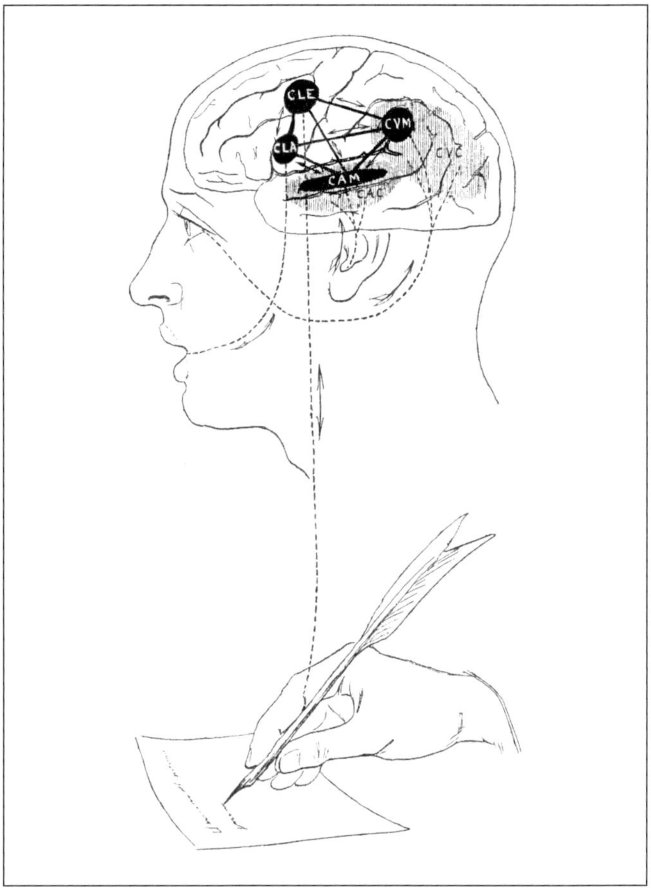

Fig. 2. Charcot's diagram of cortical centers for oral and written language, prepared by Marie in 1888 [30]. CAM, auditory word center. CLA, motor center for articulate language; CLE, motor center for written language; CVM, visual word center; CVC, common visual center; CAC, common auditory center. Original image modified by V.W. Henderson.

Dejerine, like Charcot and others, recognized alexia and agraphia as distinct and dissociable manifestations of aphasia. However, he rejected the existence of a separate specialized writing center near Broca's area. Agraphia was a feature of damage that caused motor (Broca's) or sensory (Wernicke's) aphasia. In addition, reading and writing were selectively impaired by injury to the left angular gyrus [33].

In 1891 and 1892, Dejerine published 2 highly influential case reports in which he provided the anatomical and theoretical basis for word blindness (alexia) with agraphia and word blindness without agraphia [34, 35]. Dejerine's first case was a 63-year-old man who suddenly discovered that he could not read his morning newspaper [34]. In contrast to relatively preserved spoken language, he could not read or write (p 198; translation from [3]):

> When one gives him a newspaper or a written phrase, he looks at the newspaper or the paper for a moment, then faces the examiner, stating, "I do not understand." The same for letters of the alphabet, which he could scarcely name.... When one tells the patient to write, he holds the pen or pencil quite awkwardly ... and if sometimes he wishes to write spontaneously, to dictation or copy, he always writes [only] his name. [34].

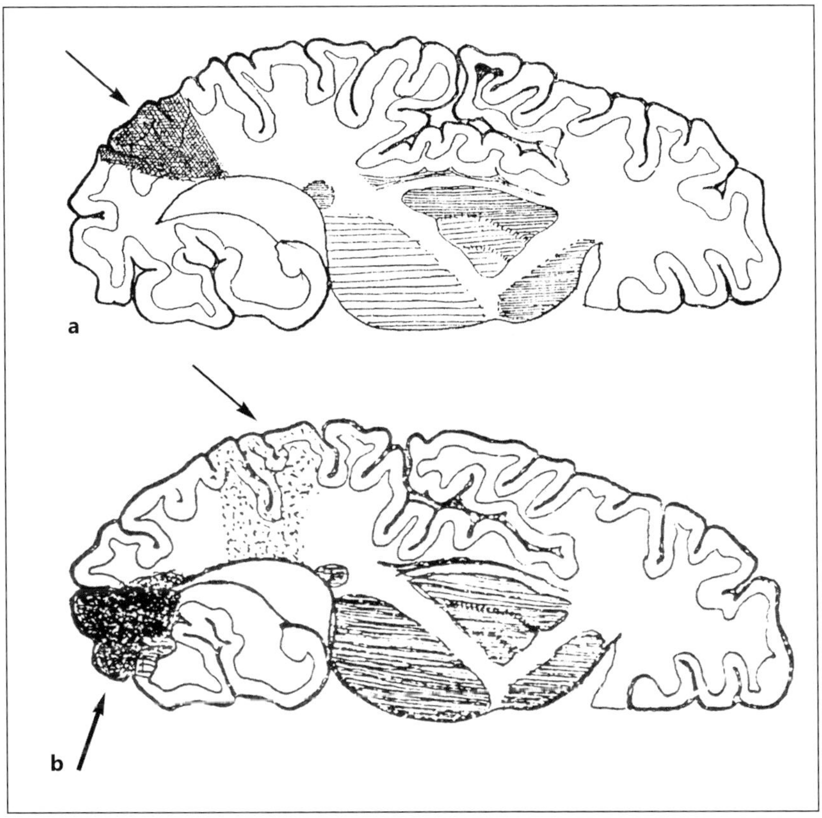

Fig. 3. Horizontal sections through the left cerebral hemisphere, which depict softenings caused by stroke affecting angular gyrus cortex and subcortical white matter (thin arrows) in Dejerine's patient with word blindness (alexia) with agraphia [34] (**a**, top) and with word blindness without agraphia followed by word blindness with agraphia [35] (**b**, bottom). The thick arrow in **b** indicates the occipital lobe site of the first stroke. Original images modified by V.W. Henderson.

Autopsy 10 months later revealed a small area of cortical softening that involved the left angular gyrus, extending inward from the surface [34] (Fig. 3a). Dejerine inferred that alexia and agraphia were caused by the angular gyrus softening, which resulted in the "loss of optical images of letters" (p 200) [34].

The following year, Dejerine established the theoretical basis for pure word blindness. He described the remarkable case of a 68-year-old man who had 2 strokes. The first caused pure word blindness and the second caused word blindness with agraphia [35]. According to Dejerine, the critical lesion of pure word blindness isolated the left angular gyrus from visual input, required for letters and words to be perceived as linguistic symbols. After the first stroke, Dejerine's examination revealed no weakness or sensory loss. Speech was normal and writing nearly so, except that the patient wrote as if he were copying a drawing. He could not read (Fig. 4a–c; pp 67–69; translation from [3]):

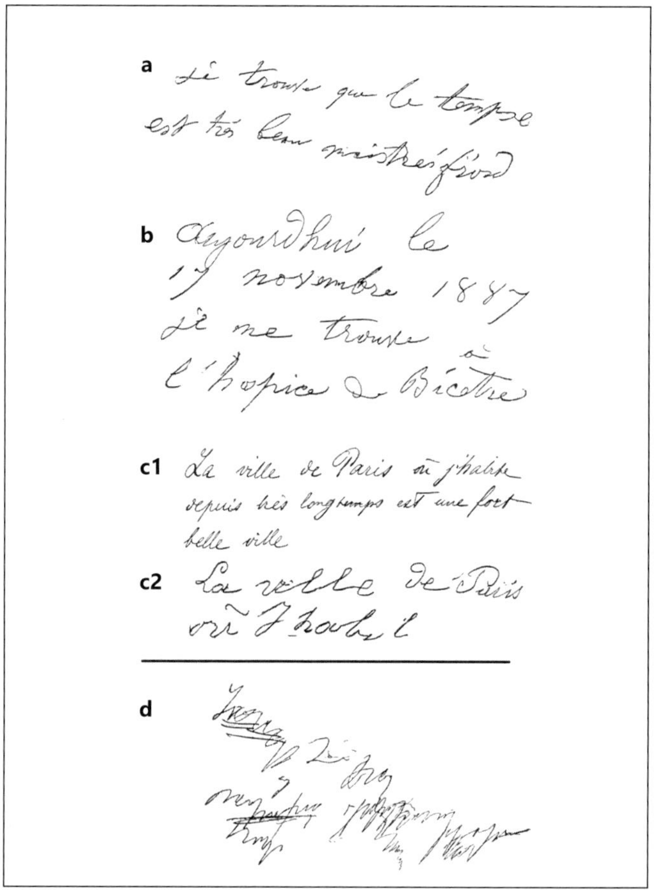

Fig. 4. Writing samples from Dejerine's 1892 patient after his first (**a–c**) and second (**d**) stroke [35]. **a** Spontaneous writing. **b** Writing to dictation. **c1** and **c2** Model text (**c1**) and patient's copy (**c2**). **d** Illegible writing after second stroke. Original image modified by V.W. Henderson.

His spoken language is very correct, even carefully selected; he always uses appropriate terms and shows no trace of paraphasia. ... The patient understands perfectly all that one says to him. ... Writing spontaneously and to dictation is perfectly preserved. ... *Spontaneously*, the patient writes as well as he speaks. In comparing the many writing specimens that I had him write, one notices no mistakes, no spelling error, no transposition of letters. ... Writing *to dictation* is executed equally easily and fluently, but reading what the patient has written is absolutely impossible. Here it is indeed a question of a case of absolutely pure word blindness. The patient recognizes not a letter, not a word except, however, his name." [35].

The second stroke caused slurred speech and right-sided weakness. Although he soon regained his strength, his speech contained naming errors, and he could not write (Fig. 4d). He died soon after the second stroke, and the autopsy showed 2 lesions (Fig. 3b). Dejerine summarized the case as follows (pp 83–84; translation from [3]):

During the first phase, which lasted 4 years, the patient presented the purest clinical picture that one can imagine of ... *pure word blindness without any alteration in spontaneous writing or [writing] to dictation.* During the second phase, which lasted only 10 days, complete agraphia with paraphasia came to complicate word blindness. In this second phase, the clinical picture then corresponded to ... *word blindness with marked alteration of writing.* To these two clinical phases correspond, as the autopsy shows, two anatomically distinct lesions in the left hemisphere: one old, occupying the occipital lobe and more particularly the convolutions at the occipital point, the base of the cuneus, as well as those of the lingual and fusiform lobules.... The other lesion of a recent date occupies the angular gyrus and inferior parietal lobule, that is to say the region that we are accustomed to see lesioned in the case of word blindness with writing difficulties. It perfectly explains symptoms observed during the last days of this patient's life. [35].

The key consequence of the first stroke was to interrupt tracts coursing from visual cortex in the occipital lobes to the left angular gyrus. For Dejerine, the left angular gyrus was a center interposed between visual cortex and the auditory center for words (Wernicke's area) in the temporal lobe, wherein "the visual image of letters simultaneously arouses the auditory image and the articulatory image" (p 87) [35]. The auditory word center was linked to the frontal lobe center for motor articulation (Broca's area). Angular gyrus destruction led to both alexia and agraphia. Dejerine suggested that letters of a specific word evoked meaning through connections between the left angular gyrus and other parts of a left hemisphere "language zone."

Deconstruction

In 1906, the dominant Broca-Wernicke-Dejerine paradigm was unexpectedly and doggedly assailed by Pierre Marie (1853–1940) [36, 37]. Marie had trained with both Broca and Charcot, and later he succeeded Dejerine to Charcot's neurology chair at the Salpêtrière. Marie did not accept the dogma of cerebral centers specialized for language. He pointed out that during the long course of human evolution and culture, reading and writing were relatively recent developments. It was illogical to presume that specialized centers had evolved for these purposes [38]. Marie acknowledged but one variety of aphasia. This was Wernicke's aphasia, which occurred after lesions within a broadly defined left hemisphere Wernicke's "zone" that included cortex and white matter tracts of the angular and supramarginal gyri and the posterior superior and middle temporal gyri [36]. Broca's aphasia was simply mild Wernicke's aphasia from a Wernicke zone lesion, coupled with dysarthria when the lesion extended beneath Broca's area to the lenticular nucleus (caudate and putamen). Because it lay within the same vascular territory, the left third frontal convolution was often affected by a stroke that caused symptoms of Broca's aphasia. However, injury to Broca's area was incidental and irrelevant.

Wernicke zone lesions affected not just language but all aspects of intelligence dependent on didactic learning [37]. Alexia and agraphia did not exist apart from aphasia. Like Broca's area, the angular gyrus had no special role: "*One cannot recognize in the [angular gyrus] the role of the center for visual images of words*" (p 500) [37].

Marie's iconoclasm resonated with English neurologist Henry Head (1861–1940), who in 1926 published his monumental *Aphasia and Kindred Disorders* [39]. Studying patients with brain trauma suffered during World War I, Head conceived all aphasia as impairment in "symbolic formulation and expression" (vol 1, p 218) in which speech, reading, and writing were affected in concert. He denounced "diagram makers" like Bastian and Wernicke for "serene dogmatism" (vol 1, p 57) [39] and championed Hughlings Jackson's writings.

Along similar lines, Kurt Goldstein (1878–1965), a pupil of Wernicke who worked in Germany and the United States, proposed that the fundamental impairment in brain-injured patients was in "abstract attitude." Like Hughlings Jackson, Goldstein denied "a simple relation between a symptom and a lesion in a circumscribed area" (p 50) [40]. Symptoms were influenced by the "condition of the rest of the brain, and even of the whole organism" (p 256) [41].

Apraxia and Agraphia

Hugo Liepmann (1863–1925) in Berlin offered a theoretical framework for apraxia, disorders characterized by the failure to carry out motor tasks despite the ability to do so [42]. In 1907, Liepmann and Otto Maas (1874–1965) reported the case of a man with unilateral agraphia [43]. He had right-sided weakness. Despite normal speech and speech understanding, he was unable to follow commands requiring the use of his left arm. He could not write, copy text, or use anagram letters to spell his name. An autopsy showed damage from a large stroke in the distribution of the anterior cerebral artery. Involvement of the rostral corpus callosum and white matter tracts disrupted connections between anterior regions of the 2 cerebral hemispheres. Liepmann and Maas [43] attributed agraphia to apraxia of the left hand due to the disruption between motor cortex of the right hemisphere, which controlled left hand movements, and left hemisphere areas responsible for goal-oriented movements.

1965: Rediscovery and New Directions

There were exceptions, such as Solomon Henschen (1877–1930) in Sweden and Johannes Nielsen (1890–1969) in Los Angeles, but the center–pathway model fell out of vogue during the early and middle decades of the 20th century. Ascendant views of Marie, Head, and Goldstein were reinforced by the works of Swiss pathologist Constantin von Monakow (1853–1930) on diaschisis (focal brain lesions exerted distant effects) and the American psychologist Karl Lashley (1890–1958) on equipotentiality (one part of the cortex could take over when another part was damaged).

In Boston, Geschwind revived earlier formulations of alexia and agraphia based on Dejerine's center-pathway model. He was inspired by unexpected findings described by Roger Sperry (1913–1994) in split-brain patients, who had undergone corpus collosotomy, the surgical separation of the 2 cerebral hemispheres, to control intractable epilepsy [44]. With neuropsychologist Edith Kaplan (1924–2009), Geschwind reported a patient with agraphia of the left hand, which they interpreted as a functional disconnection of the

2 cerebral hemispheres [45]. Delving into the older neurological literature, Geschwind was "troubled by the fact that people who had left their mark so indelibly in many areas of neurology, such as Wernicke, Bastian, Dejerine, Charcot, and many others, could apparently have shown what was asserted to be the sheerest naiveté and incompetence in the area of higher functions" (p 215) [46]. In his landmark article of 1965, "Disconnexion syndromes in animal and man," [2] Geschwind discussed Dejerine's case of alexia without agraphia [35] and Liepmann and Maas's case of unilateral agraphia [43]. These cases and others were adduced in support of a critical role for pathway lesions in disconnecting functionally discrete cortical regions [2]. Geschwind reinterpreted the left angular gyrus as a center for visual-auditory associations required for memories of the "'rules of translation' from written to spoken language" (p 279) [2]. For alexia without agraphia, the disconnection was between visual cortex and the left angular gyrus. For apraxic agraphia, the disconnection lay between right hemisphere motor cortex and left hemisphere language areas.

Geschwind's disconnection theory – in conjunction with research of colleagues Harold Goodglass (1920–2002), Frank Benson (1928–1996) and others at the Boston University Aphasia Research Center – rekindled interests in what has become known as behavioral neurology [47] and led to new approaches to the study of aphasia, alexia, and agraphia, and of brain-behavior relations more generally. More than half a century after their rediscovery, the classic formulations of Dejerine and Liepmann retain their heuristic value.

References

1 Broca P: Perte de la parole, ramollissement chronique et destruction partielle du lobe antérieur gauche du cerveau. Bull Soc Anthropol (Paris) 1861;2:235–238.

2 Geschwind N: Disconnexion syndromes in animals and man. Brain 1965;88:237–294, 585–644.

3 Henderson VW: Alexia and agraphia. Handb Clin Neurol 2010;95:583–601.

4 Henderson VW: History of disorders of writing and reading; in Barr WB, Bieliauskas LA (eds): The Oxford Handbook of History of Clinical Neuropsychology. Oxford, Oxford University Press, 2018.

5 Gall FJ: Sur les Fontions du Cerveau, vol 5. Organologie ou Exposition des Instincts, des Penchans, des Sentimens et des Talens, ou des Qualités Morales et des Facultés Intellectuelles Fondamentales de l'Homme et des Animaux, et du Siége de leurs Organes. Paris, J-B Ballière, 1825.

6 Bouillaud J: Recherches cliniques propres à démontrer que la perte de la parole correspond à la lésion des lobules antérieurs du cerveau, et à confirmer l'opinion de M. Gall, sur le siège de l'organe du langage articulé. Arch Gen Med 1825;8:25–45.

7 Marcé LV: Mémoire sur quelques observations de physiologie pathologique tendant a démontrer l'existence d'un principe coordinateur de l'écriture et ses rapports avec le principe coordinateur de la parole. C R Mem Séances Soc Bio (Paris) 1856;3:93–115.

8 Aubertin E: Reprise de la discussion sur la forme et le volume du cerveau. Bull Soc Anthropol (Paris) 1861;2: 209–220.

9 Broca P: Remarques sur le siège de la faculté du langage articulé, suivies d'une observation d'aphémie (perte de la parole). Bull Soc Anatom (Paris) 1861;6 (2nd series): 330–357.

10 Henderson VW: Alalia, aphemia, and aphasia. Arch Neurol 1990;47:85–88.

11 Broca P: Sur le siége de la faculté du langage articulé. Bull Soc Anthropol (Paris) 1865;6:377–393.

12 Henderson VW: Paul Broca's less heralded contributions to aphasia research. Historical perspective and contemporary relevance. Arch Neurol 1986;43:609–612.

13 Trousseau A: De l'aphasie, maladie décrite récemment sous le nom impropre d'aphémie. Gaz Hop Civ Milit 1864;37:13–14, 25–26, 37–39, 49–50.

14 Trousseau A: Clinique Médicale de l'Hôtel-Dieu de Paris, ed 2, vol 2. Paris, J.-B. Ballière et Fils, 1865.

15 Benedikt M: Über Aphasie, Agraphie und verwandte pathologische Zustände. Wiener Med Presse 1865;6: 897–899, 923–926, 945–948, 997–999, 1020–1022, 1067–1070, 1094–1097, 1139–1142, 1167–1169, 1189–1190, 1264–1265.

16 Ogle W: Aphasia and agraphia. St George Hosp Rep 1867;2:83–122.

17 Wernicke C: Der Aphasische Symptomencomplex. Eine Psychologische Studie auf Anatomischer Basis. Breslau, Max Cohn & Weigert, 1874.
18 Henderson VW: Sigmund Freud and the diagram-maker school of aphasiology. Brain Lang 1992;43:19–41.
19 Henderson VW: Alexia and agraphia: contrasting perspectives of J.-M. Charcot and J. Hughlings Jackson. Neurology 2008;70:391–400.
20 Hughlings Jackson J: On the nature of the duality of the brain. Med Press Circ 1874;17 (new series):19–21, 41–44, 63–65.
21 Hughlings Jackson J: Loss of speech: its association with valvular disease of the heart and with hemiplegia on the right side. – Defects of smell. – Defects of speech in chorea. – Arterial lesions in epilepsy. Clin Lect Rep Med Surg Staff London Hosp 1864;1:388–471.
22 Hughlings Jackson J: On affections of speech from disease of the brain. Brain 1878;1,2:304–330, 203–222, 323–356.
23 Hughlings Jackson J: On the physiology of language. Med Times Gaz 1868;54:275–276.
24 Bastian HC: On the various forms of loss of speech in cerebral disease. Brit Foreign Med Chirurg Rev 1869;43: 209–236, 470–492.
25 Kussmaul A: Disturbances of speech. An attempt in the pathology of speech; in von Ziemssen H (ed): Cyclopedia of the Practice of Medicine, vol 14. Diseases of the Nervous System, and Disturbances of Speech. New York, William Wood and Company, 1877, pp 581–893.
26 Skwortzoff N: De la Cécité et de la Surdité des Mots dans l'Aphasie. Paris, Delahaye et Lecrosnier, 1881.
27 Ferrier D: The Croonian lecture. Experiments on the brain of monkeys. Philosophical transactions of the royal society of London series B. Biol Sci 1875;165:433–488.
28 Exner S: Untersuchungen über die Localisation der Functionen in der Grosshirnrinde des Menschen. Vienna, W. Braumuller, 1881.
29 Bastian HC: On different kinds of aphasia, with special reference to their classification and ultimate pathology. Brit Med J 1887;2:931–936, 985–990.
30 Marie P: De l'aphasie en général et de l'agraphie en particulier, d'après l'enseignement de M le professeur Charcot. Prog Med 1888;7(2nd series):81–84.
31 Charcot JM: Des différentes formes de l'aphasie [collated by C Féré]. Prog Med 1883;11:441–444, 469–471, 487–488, 521–523, 859–861.
32 Pitres A: Considérations sur l'agraphie. Rev Med 1884;4: 855–873.
33 Dejerine J: Contribution à l'étude des troubles de l'écriture chez les aphasiques. Mem Soc Biol 1891;43: 97–113.
34 Dejerine J: Sur un cas de cécité verbale avec agraphie, suivi d'autopsie. C R Séances Soc Biol 1891;43:197–201.
35 Dejerine J: Contribution à l'étude anatomo-pathologique et clinique des différentes variétés de cécité verbale. C R Séances Mem Soc Biol 1892;44:61–90.
36 Marie P: Revision de la question de l'aphasie: la troisième circonvolution frontale gauche ne joue aucun rôle spécial dans la fonction du langage. Semaine Med 1906;26:241–247.
37 Marie P: Revision de la question de l'aphasie: que faut-il penser des aphasies sous-corticales (aphasies pures)? Semaine Med 1906;26:493–500.
38 Marie P: L'évolution du langage considérée au point de vue de l'étude de l'aphasie. Presse Med 1897;5:397–399.
39 Head H: Aphasia and Kindred Disorders of Speech. Cambridge, Cambridge University Press, 1926.
40 Goldstein K: Language and Language Disturbances. New York, Grune and Stratton, 1948.
41 Goldstein K: The Organism: A Holostic Approach to Biology Derived from Pathological Data in Man. New York, American Book Company, 1938.
42 Liepmann H: Drei Aufsätze aus dem Apraxiegebiet. Berlin, Karger, 1908.
43 Liepmann H, Maas O: Fall von linksseitiger Agraphie und Apraxie bei rechtseitiger Lämung. J Psychol Neurol 1907;10:214–227.
44 Gazzaniga MS, Bogen JE, Sperry RW: Some functional effects of sectioning the cerebral commissures in man. Proc Natl Acad Sci U S A 1962;48:1765–1769.
45 Geschwind N, Kaplan E: A human cerebral deconnection syndrome. A preliminary report. Neurology 1962; 12:675–685.
46 Geschwind N: The paradoxical position of Kurt Goldstein in the history of aphasia. Cortex 1964;1:214–224.
47 Benson DF: The history of behavioral neurology. Neurol Clin 1993;11:1–8.

Victor W. Henderson, MD, MS
Departments of Health Research and Policy (Epidemiology) and of Neurology and Neurological Sciences
Stanford University
259 Campus Drive, HRP Redwood Building
Stanford, CA 94305-5405 (USA)
E-Mail vhenderson@stanford.edu

Bogousslavsky J, Boller F, Iwata M (eds): A History of Neuropsychology.
Front Neurol Neurosci. Basel, Karger, 2019, vol 44, pp 53–63 (DOI: 10.1159/000494952)

Kanji (Morphogram) and Kana (Phonogram) Problem in Japanese Alexia and Agraphia

Yasuhisa Sakurai

Department of Neurology, Mitsui Memorial Hospital, Tokyo, Japan

Abstract

The kanji and kana (or kanji vs. kana) problem in the Japanese language denotes the dissociation between kanji (morphograms) and kana (phonograms) in reading/comprehension and writing. Since paragraphia of kana in a patient with amyotrophic lateral sclerosis was first reported in 1893, kanji-kana dissociation has been the central topic in Japanese aphasiology. Recent advancements in lesion-to-symptom analyses and functional imaging studies have identified some areas whose damage causes dissociative disturbances of reading or writing between kanji and kana. That is, (1) angular alexia with agraphia causes kanji agraphia; alexia of kana with an angular gyrus lesion is the result of a damage to the middle occipital gyrus; (2) alexia with agraphia for kanji is caused by a posterior inferior temporal cortex (mid-fusiform/inferior temporal gyri; visual word form area) lesion, whereas pure agraphia for kanji is caused by a posterior middle temporal gyrus lesion; and (3) pure alexia, particularly for kanji, results from a mid-fusiform gyrus lesion (Brodmann's Area [BA] 37), whereas pure alexia for kana results from a posterior fusiform/inferior occipital gyri lesion (BA 18/19).

Two Writing Systems in the Japanese Language

The Japanese language has 2 writing systems: kanji (morphograms) and kana (phonograms). Originally, kanji borrowed their form from Chinese characters. Kanji can be read in 2 ways: *on*-reading and *kun*-reading. *On*-reading derives from Chinese pronunciation and conveys the phonetic value, whereas *kun*-reading is a Japanese way of reading that is associated with the meaning. Many kanji characters have multiple *on*-readings, depending on the era when a kanji pronunciation was transported from China. In contrast, a kanji character has usually only one *kun*-reading.

A single character kanji is itself a word with inherent meaning. The combination of 2 or more kanji characters can produce a new word associated with the meaning of each kanji. In fact, there are far more 2-character kanji words than 3- or more-character kanji words. A kanji word can be transcribed to kana character sequences. Kana make up Japanese phonetic writing, comparable to the Roman alphabet, consisting of 46 letters/characters with consistent consonant-vowel combinations. Kana are further divided into 2 types: hiragana (cursive type of kana that are normally used for grammatical morphemes) and katakana (square type of kana that are used primarily for representing loan words). The relationship between hiragana and katakana orthographically resembles that between capitals and small letters in English in the sense that both hiragana and katakana have the same phonetic value and 10 out of 46 kana are orthographically similar (e.g., hiragana う [u] and katakana ウ [u]). Therefore, they can be regarded as allographs [1].

Because of the above-mentioned unique writing systems, Japanese patients with aphasia, alexia, and agraphia have been reported to show better performance in kanji than in kana processing (reading aloud, reading comprehension, or writing), and vice versa. The kanji and kana (or kanji vs. kana) problem refers to dissociative disturbance in reading or writing between kanji and kana. In the next sessions, we will see how Japanese patients with aphasia, alexia, and agraphia show these dissociations as well as other characteristic symptoms.

Table 1 illustrates the correspondence between English and Japanese words. This table may serve to understand how Japanese kanji and kana are related to English words.

Kanji and Kana Problem before World War II

As early as in 1893, Watanabe [2] reported a patient with progressive bulbar palsy and muscular atrophy who showed motor aphasia. The patient wrote some kanji words, but could not write their kana transcription, leading to phonemic paragraphia. This may be the first case report on kanji-kana dissociation in Japan. From a modern perspective, the patient had frontotemporal dementia with motor neuron disease (pathologically, frontotemporal lobar degeneration with TDP43) or progressive bulbar palsy type amyotrophic lateral sclerosis. Kana phonemic paragraphia is characteristic of frontal pure agraphia in Japan [3].

Miura [4], professor of Tokyo Imperial University, presented a patient with Broca's aphasia whose writing was paragraphic in kana, and claimed that kana reading and writing were sometimes poor in aphasics because kana were only a phonetic sign whereas kanji had shape and meaning, in addition to a phonetic sign. Subsequently, a similar case of Broca's aphasia with alexia and agraphia, particularly for katakana, was reported [5]. The author explained this dissociation based on the fact that kana are phonographic, like the Roman alphabet, whereas kanji are visual or ideographic.

Table 1. The correspondence between English and Japanese words (Revised from Sakurai [36])

English Example	Letter strings fgtp	Regular nonword (pseudoword) beed	Regular word lunch	Irregular word yacht
Kana Example		Kana nonword うよひ /uyohi/	Kana word あした /ashita/ (tomorrow)	
Kanji Example		Kanji nonword 味想 /misou/	Kanji word (typical) 石油 /sekiyu/ (oil)	Kanji word (exceptional) 煙草 /tabako/ (tobacco)
Pronunciation Word form	LBL* None	Regular None	Regular Present	Irregular Present

* LBL is letter by letter, that is, pronouncing letter by letter.

Asayama [6] published a German paper on selective kana alexia and agraphia in a patient with motor and sensory aphasia, being the first to introduce kana-kanji dissociation throughout the world. Imura [7] reviewed his 51 cases of Japanese aphasia patients (the paper was later translated into German). In this paper, he described a type of transcortical sensory aphasia called Gogi (word-meaning) aphasia. The typical example was caused by a cortical degenerative disease, and is now thought to be equivalent to semantic dementia in Western countries. In contrast to previous reports, patients with Gogi aphasia showed selective impairment of kanji reading and writing with preserved kana reading and writing (for details of Gogi aphasia, see Yamadori of this volume).

Paradis et al. [8] reviewed 69 cases of Japanese alexia and agraphia published from 1901 to 1983, and found that 20 were able to read aloud and comprehend kanji but not kana characters, whereas 16 were able to read aloud and comprehend kana but not kanji characters. A problem is whether there is a neural substrate underlying kanji processing or kana processing.

Kanji and Kana Problem after the War

Since the introduction of brain CT in the 1970s and magnetic resonance imaging (MRI) in the 1980s, lesion-to-symptom studies have markedly accumulated, and many new findings have been reported. Sasanuma and Fujimura [9], a pioneering speech pathologist in Japan, successively published works focusing on the kanji vs. kana problem in aphasia and pure alexia. She retrospectively analyzed 378 patients who were admitted to a large rehabilitation center and administered a kanji and kana reading and writing battery, constituting a total of 17 subtests [10]. The main finding was that predominant impairment of kana processing was observed in Broca's aphasia, Wernicke's aphasia, and conduction aphasia whereas predominant impairment of kanji processing was observed in the mixed-form of

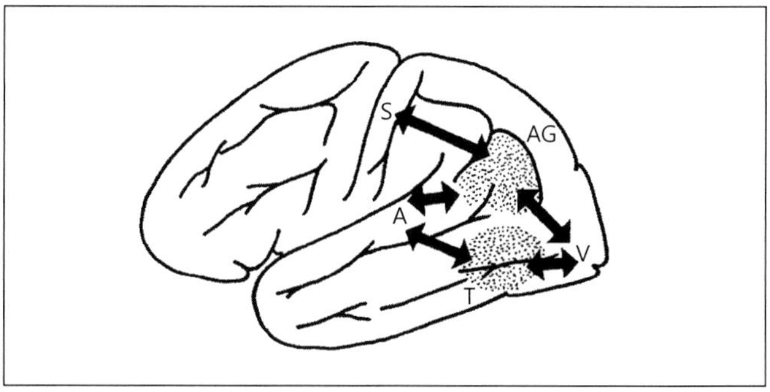

Fig. 1. Iwata's dual-route hypothesis of reading and writing (reproduced with permission from Iwata [13]). A, Wernicke's area; AG, angular gyrus; S, somatosensory area; T, posterior inferior temporal area; V, visual area.

transcortical aphasia. Her series of works has drawn attention of kanji versus kana problem in the Japanese language from the Western investigators. Later, she adopted cognitive neuropsychological models to explain the kanji-kana dissociation.

Yamadori [11] reported an interesting case of alexia with agraphia caused by damage to the angular artery region. The patient had difficulty reading kana words but read kanji words with ease. Writing was markedly impaired for both kanji and kana. He hypothesized that the alexia was caused by the disconnection between the visual cortex and auditory-oral system. This was a case of parietal (angular) alexia with agraphia. Yamadori later reviewed additional cases of alexia with agraphia, and argued that data were still insufficient to conclude that kana reading is specifically impaired in angular alexia with agraphia.

Another notable case was reported by Iwata [12, 13]. In contrast to Yamadori's case, the patient could not read or write kanji but could read and write kana characters. This was the first reported case of alexia with agraphia for kanji due to a posterior inferior temporal cortex (PITC; Brodmann's Area [BA] 37) lesion. Based on these dissociations, Iwata proposed a dual-route hypothesis of reading and writing in the Japanese language (Fig. 1). In this model, visual information on graphemes is conveyed from the visual cortex to Wernicke's area through 2 different pathways: a dorsal route via the angular gyrus, and a ventral route via the PITC. The dorsal route is mainly used for phonological processes in kana reading, whereas the ventral route is indispensable for semantic processes in kanji reading. Later, the model was modified so that the angular gyrus was replaced by the lateral occipital gyri.

Since Iwata's paper, a number of similar cases have been reported, and several problems have been raised. For example, Soma et al. [14] observed that alexia with agraphia due to a PITC lesion resolved to pure agraphia for kanji in 3 patients, and claimed that it is equivalent to lexical agraphia in Western countries. According to Sakurai et al. [15], whether alexia with agraphia or pure agraphia occurs with nearly the same PITC lesion depends on differences in lesion localization (described later). Another important finding was that alexia with agraphia due to a PITC lesion accompanies anomia, and the severity of anomia parallels that of kanji reading [16]. It was not until 20 years later that alexia with agraphia for irregular words accompanied by anomia, which is equivalent to Japanese alexia with agraphia for kanji in the strict sense, became known in Western countries [17].

Kawamura [18] compared the symptoms among parietal pure agraphia (6 patients), angular alexia with agraphia (2 patients), and alexia with agraphia due to a PITC lesion (4 patients). He found that selective kanji writing impairment occurred in parietal pure agraphia, and that angular alexia with agraphia was characterized by kana alexia and kanji agraphia. Later, Sakurai et al. [1] claimed that the alexic symptom in angular alexia with agraphia was not caused by damage to the angular gyrus but to the middle occipital gyrus adjacent to the angular gyrus.

Sugishita et al. [19] criticized previous reports for the paucity of reliable data, and examined a total of 50 patients with Broca's aphasia, Wernicke's aphasia, alexia with agraphia, and pure alexia using a 46 single-character kanji and kana reading test. They found that kanji reading and kana reading were unselectively impaired in most patients, irrespective of the type of alexia. However, the problem cannot be resolved unless we subdivide each type of alexia further into a kanji-impairment group and a kana-impairment group.

Isolated agraphia also occurs due to damage to the frontal lobe. Phonemic paragraphia of kana has been frequently reported [3, 20], although kanji agraphia due to impaired character recall was also observed [3]. The lesion of frontal pure agraphia is located in the posterior middle and inferior frontal gyrus, near the so-called Exner's area.

Based on lesion-to-symptom analyses, Sakurai et al. [3, 15, 21] proposed a dual-route hypothesis for writing (Fig. 2b). In this model, the phonological route coveys phonemic sequences along the arcuate fasciculus, whereas the orthographic route coveys orthographic information of grapheme sequences. According to this model, disruption of the phonological route results in phonemic paragraphia. As kana words are composed of consonant-vowel phonemic sequences, kana word spelling is more affected. In contrast, disruption of the orthographic route results in the impairment of character recall. As kanji abound in orthographic features, recall of kanji characters is more affected. This is why there is dissociation between kanji writing and kana writing.

The Role of the Right Hemisphere in the Recognition of Kanji

The ideographic features of kanji have led to European investigators erroneously concluding that kanji were processed in the right hemisphere whereas kana were processed in the left hemisphere. This was ruled out by the fact that patients with transection of the splenium of the corpus callosum could not read kanji or kana presented with a short duration in the left visual field, but could do so when presented in the right visual field [22]. However, there are some findings that suggest the involvement of the right hemisphere in reading. First, the patients with transection of the splenium described above recovered the ability to read kanji but not kana. Second, a patient with a lesion in the posterior part of the splenium showed reading and writing (with either hand) impairment of kana in the left visual field with relatively preserved reading and writing of kanji [23]. These findings suggest that the right BA 37 and 19 store some orthographic information on characters and compensate for the dysfunction of the left hemisphere.

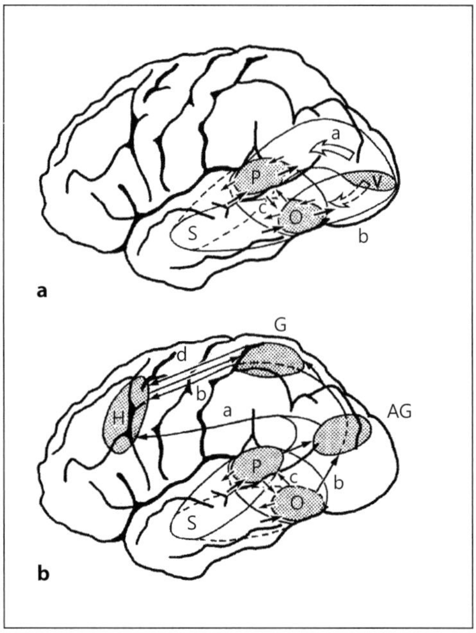

Fig. 2. Weighted dual-route hypothesis for reading (**a**) and dual-route hypothesis for writing (**b**; Reproduced with permission from Sakurai [37]). **a** The phonological (dorsal) route (a) proceeds from the primary visual cortex (V) to the posterior superior temporal gyrus (P; Wernicke's area) via the lateral occipital gyri (middle and inferior occipital gyri) and deep perisylvian temporoparietal cortex. This route is used for the sequential visual recognition of character sequences. The phonological lexical information (P) is stored around the end of this route. The orthographic (ventral) route (b) proceeds from the primary visual cortex (V) to the inferior temporal gyrus via the fusiform gyrus. This route is used for the holistic visual recognition of words, and plays a dominant role in reading. The orthographic lexical information (O) is stored around the end of this route. a, dorsal (phonological) route; b, ventral (orthographic) route; c, interaction between P and O; O, orthographic lexicon (visual word form area); P, phonological lexicon; S, semantic storage; V, visual cortex. **b** The phonological route (a) proceeds from the primary auditory cortex (Heschl's gyri) and the posterior superior temporal gyrus (P; Wernicke's area) to the angular (AG) and supramarginal gyri and joins the arcuate fasciculus to travel to the frontal motor and premotor hand area (H). This route is used for the transmission of phonological information via the arcuate fasciculus or phoneme-to-grapheme conversion at the angular/lateral occipital gyri. The orthographic route (b) goes from the posterior inferior temporal cortex and proceeds upward under the angular gyrus and superior parietal lobule to travel to the frontal motor and premotor hand area (H). The orthographic route is divided into direct and indirect pathways in the parietal lobe. The direct pathway conveys holistic visual information on words and letters to the frontal motor and premotor hand area (H), whereas the indirect pathway enters the graphemic area (G) where visuokinesthetic and sequential motor engrams for words and letters are stored, and goes further to the hand area. a, phonological route; b, orthographic route; c, interaction between P and O; d, interaction between G and H; AG, angular/lateral occipital gyri; G, graphemic area; H, hand area; O, orthographic lexicon; P, phonological lexicon; S, semantic storage.

Table 2. A classification of alexia and agraphia (Revised from Sakurai et al. [1])

I	Aphasic alexia/agraphia: Broca's, Wernicke's, Conduction, Transcortical, and Global aphasias		
II	Primary non-aphasic alexia/agraphia		
	1	Pure alexia	
		A	Splenium type: medial occipital gyri (or optic radiation, lateral geniculate body) + splenium (or callosal radiation, forceps major)
		B	Non-splenium type
			Fusiform type: mid-fusiform gyrus (Area 37)[a]
			Posterior occipital type: posterior fusiform/inferior occipital gyri (Area 18/19)[b]
	2	Alexia with agraphia	
			Angular type: angular/lateral occipital gyri (Area 39/19)[b, c]
			Posterior inferior temporal type: mid-fusiform/inferior temporal gyri (Area 37)[a, c]
	3	Pure agraphia	
			Posterior middle temporal gyrus (Area 21/37)[c]
			Angular gyrus (Area 39)[c]
			Supramarginal gyrus (Area 40)[d]
			Superior parietal lobule (intraparietal sulcus, Area 7)[c]
			Posterior middle frontal gyrus (Area 6)[c, d]
III	Secondary non-aphasic alexia/agraphia		
	1	Alexia	
			Hemianopic alexia
			Neglect dyslexia
			Callosal alexia
			Thalamic alexia
	2	Agraphia	
			Neglect dysgraphia (spatial agraphia)
			Callosal agraphia
			Constructional agraphia
			Thalamic agraphia

[a] Kanji > Kana (Kanji reading is more impaired than kana reading).
[b] Kana > Kanji (Kana reading is more impaired than kanji reading).
[c] Kanji > Kana (Kanji writing is more impaired than kana writing).
[d] Kana > Kanji (Kana writing is more impaired than kanji writing).

Recent Advancement in Understanding of Kanji and Kana Problem

Lesion-to-symptom analyses with precise lesion localization and functional imaging studies have clarified the detailed anatomical subdivision of alexia and agraphia. Table 2 is an example of such classification.

Positron Emission Tomography and Functional MRI Studies

Sakurai et al. [24–26] conducted positron emission tomography studies on reading kanji words, kana words, and kana nonwords each to a different group with region of interest-based analysis, and later with statistical parametric mapping (Sakurai et al. [27–29]). Their results were summarized as follows: (1) kanji words specifically activated the mid-fusiform/posterior inferior temporal gyri (BA 37), whereas kana words specifically activated posterior fusiform/middle and inferior occipital gyri (BA 18/19); (2) kana nonwords activated more extensive areas of the occipital and occipito-temporal cortices bilaterally than kana words; (3) conjunction of kana words and kana nonwords activated the middle occipital gyrus and temporo-parietal cortex (BA 40/22) deep to the Sylvian fissure; and (4) subtraction of kanji words from kana words revealed activation of the middle occipital gyrus, whereas subtraction of kana words from kanji words revealed no activation.

Based on these results, Sakurai et al. [28] modified Iwata's model for Japanese [12, 13] and proposed a weighted dual-route hypothesis for reading that is applicable to language in general (Fig. 2a). According to this model, the inferior occipital, fusiform/posterior inferior temporal gyri (O) constitute a ventral route for reading (b) and process orthography (whole-word recognition) for words, whereas the middle occipital gyrus, deep perisylvian temporo-parietal area (BA 40/22), and posterior superior temporal gyrus (P; Wernicke's area) constitute a dorsal route for reading (b) and process phonology (grapheme to phoneme conversion) for words. Pseudoword (kana nonword) or unfamiliar word reading requires both routes. However, as we become familiar with the word, the whole-word image and meaning are stored around the mid-fusiform/posterior inferior temporal gyri (BA 37); thus, the ventral route gains dominance (weighted dual-route) in reading real words (kanji and kana words or irregular and regular words). Kanji are processed exclusively in the orthographic route, whereas kana are processed both in the orthographic and phonological routes.

The PITC or mid-fusiform/posterior inferior temporal area that was activated by kanji words is identical to the so-called visual word form area (VWFA). This area was also activated in kanji character writing and recall together with the intraparietal sulcus and posterior middle and inferior frontal gyri, but not in kana character writing in functional MRI studies [30]. Clinically, damage to the VWFA itself causes alexia with agraphia for kanji or more generally alexia with agraphia for irregular words [16] (orthographic alexia with agraphia; Sakurai [31]), as described earlier.

Pure Alexia for Kana or Pure Alexia for Letters

Sakurai et al. (2001) [32] reported a patient with pure alexia who showed selective impairment of kana reading with preserved reading of kanji after hemorrhage in the left posterior occipital gyri. Later, Sakurai et al. [33] analyzed symptoms of 6 patients (including 2 previously reported patients) with pure alexia for kana. The cardinal feature is a reading impairment of kana single character and nonwords; kana real word reading is relatively preserved. Comparing the lesion site common to 6 patients with the activated area during covert reading of kana words [29], they identified the responsible lesion in the posterior fusiform/inferior occipital gyri (BA 19). This area is posterior to the VWFA. As kana are comparable to the Roman alphabet, pure alexia for kana can be more generally designated as pure alexia for letters. This type of alexia may occur due to damage to the earlier stage of the orthographic or phonological route.

Pure Alexia Particularly for Kanji or Pure Alexia for Words

In contrast to pure alexia for kana, pure alexia particularly for kanji is characterized by pronounced kanji reading impairment with relatively preserved kana reading [34]. The lesion is in the left mid-fusiform gyrus, medial to the PITC or the VWFA. From a cognitive neuropsychological point of view, pure alexia particularly for kanji is thought to arise from an inability to access the VWFA or the disconnection of visual information between the visual cortex and VWFA. As a kanji character has both sound and meaning, kanji are comparable to real words in Western languages. Therefore, pure alexia particularly for kanji can be more generally designated as pure alexia for words. Although kanji-predominant alexia has been reported in pure alexia, few studies have identified the responsible lesion. Further evidence is needed to locate the lesion responsible for kanji alexia.

Kanji Agraphia due to a Posterior Middle Temporal Gyrus Lesion

Pure agraphia for kanji due to a lesion of the left posterior middle and inferior temporal gyri was reported [15]. Kanji agraphia is characterized by impaired recall of characters, and corresponds to lexical agraphia in Western languages. The lesion occurs in BA 37, and is located above and posterior to the VWFA (mid-fusiform/posterior inferior temporal gyri). It is thought that agraphia results from interrupted input from the phonological lexicon to the orthographic lexicon (VWFA) or interrupted output from the orthographic lexicon to the parietal graphemic area where visuokinesthetic information is stored (Fig. 2b). Pure agraphia for kanji due to a posterior middle temporal gyrus lesion should be anatomically differentiated from alexia with agraphia for kanji due to a PITC lesion: the lesion responsible for pure agraphia for kanji is located more dorsally and laterally in the posterior temporal lobe than that causing alexia with agraphia for kanji.

Apraxic Agraphia

Apraxic agraphia is characterized by: (i) the production of illegible graphemes in writing that cannot be accounted for by sensorimotor dysfunction, (ii) grapheme production improvement with copying, and (iii) preserved oral spelling or typing. In Japanese apraxic agraphia, both kanji and kana configurations are disturbed. What is notable is that patients make writing stroke sequence disorders [35]. Although this symptom was also observed in patients from European countries, it is more pronounced in the Japanese language, in which kanji characters require more complex sequential writing strokes.

Allographic Agraphia

Allographic agraphia refers to the inability to select appropriate letter shapes in spelling. In the English literature, the disruption of allographic conversion manifests as, for example, confusion over upper- and lower-case letters. A similar phenomenon was reported in Japanese angular alexia with agraphia [1]. The patient confused 2 allographs, hiragana and katakana, and wrote character sequences mixing hiragana and katakana, when dictated to, for example, いきる ([ikiru], live, all hiragana) was written as イキる ([ikiru], the first 2 characters were replaced by katakana).

References

1 Sakurai Y, Asami M, Mannen T: Alexia and agraphia with lesions of the angular and supramarginal gyri: evidence for the disruption of sequential processing. J Neurol Sci 2010;288:25–33.
2 Watanabe E: About a patient with cortical motor aphasia, medullary bulbar palsy and progressive muscular atrophy. Okayama Igakukai Zasshi 1893;40:138–144.
3 Sakurai Y, Matsumura K, Iwatsubo T, Momose T: Frontal pure agraphia for kanji or kana: dissociation between morphology and phonology. Neurology 1997;49:946–952.
4 Miura K: Clinical lecture. Iji Shinbun 1901;584:249–256.
5 Yamamoto S: About motor aphasia. Dai Sankai Nihon Igakukaishi 1911;1233–1234.
6 Asayama T: Über die Aphasie bei Japanern. Dtsch Arch Klin Med 1914;113:523–529.
7 Imura T: Aphasia, its characteristic manifestation in the Japanese language. Seishin Shinkeigaku Zasshi 1943;47: 196–218.
8 Paradis M, Hagiwara H, Hildebrandt N: Neurolinguistic Aspects of the Japanese Writing System. Orlando, Academic Press, 1985.
9 Sasanuma S, Fujimura O: Selective impairment of phonetic and non-phonetic transcription of words in Japanese aphasic patients: kana vs kanji in visual recognition and writing. Cortex 1971;7:1–18.
10 Sasanuma S: Kana and Kanji processing in Japanese aphasics. Brain Lang 1975;2:369–383.
11 Yamadori A: Ideogram reading in alexia. Brain 1975;98: 231–238.
12 Iwata M: Kanji versus Kana. Neuropsychological correlates of the Japanese writing system. Trends Neurosci 1984;7:290–293.
13 Iwata M: Neural mechanism of reading and writing in the Japanese language. Funct Neurol 1986;1:43–52.
14 Soma Y, Sugishita M, Kitamura K, Maruyama S, Imanaga H: Lexical agraphia in the Japanese language. Pure agraphia for Kanji due to left posteroinferior temporal lesions. Brain 1989;112:1549–1561.
15 Sakurai Y, Mimura I, Mannen T: Agraphia for kanji resulting from a left posterior middle temporal gyrus lesion. Behav Neurol 2008;19:93–106.
16 Sakurai Y, Sakai K, Sakuta M, Iwata M: Naming difficulties in alexia with agraphia for kanji after a left posterior inferior temporal lesion. J Neurol Neurosurg Psychiatry 1994;57:609–613.
17 Rapcsak SZ, Beeson PM: The role of left posterior inferior temporal cortex in spelling. Neurology 2004;62: 2221–2229.
18 Kawamura M: Localization and symptomatology of pure alexia, pure agraphia and alexia with agraphia. Shinkeishinrigaku 1990;6:16–24.
19 Sugishita M, Otomo K, Kabe S, Yunoki K: A critical appraisal of neuropsychological correlates of Japanese ideogram (kanji) and phonogram (kana) reading. Brain 1992;115(pt 5):1563–1585.
20 Tohgi H, Saitoh K, Takahashi S, Takahashi H, Utsugisawa K, Yonezawa H, Hatano K, Sasaki T: Agraphia and acalculia after a left prefrontal (F1, F2) infarction. J Neurol Neurosurg Psychiatry 1995;58:629–632.
21 Sakurai Y, Onuma Y, Nakazawa G, Ugawa Y, Momose T, Tsuji S, Mannen T: Parietal dysgraphia: characterization of abnormal writing stroke sequences, character formation and character recall. Behav Neurol 2007;18: 99–114.
22 Sugishita M, Iwata M, Toyokura Y, Yoshioka M, Yamada R: Reading of ideograms and phonograms in Japanese patients after partial commissurotomy. Neuropsychologia 1978;16:417–426.
23 Suzuki K, Yamadori A, Endo K, Fujii T, Ezura M, Takahashi A: Dissociation of letter and picture naming resulting from callosal disconnection. Neurology 1998;51: 1390–1394.
24 Sakurai Y, Momose T, Iwata M, Watanabe T, Ishikawa T, Takeda K, Kanazawa I: Kanji word reading process analysed by positron emission tomography. Neuroreport 1992;3:445–448.
25 Sakurai Y, Momose T, Iwata M, Watanabe T, Ishikawa T, Kanazawa I: Semantic process in kana word reading: activation studies with positron emission tomography. Neuroreport 1993;4:327–330.
26 Sakurai Y, Momose T, Iwata M, Ishikawa T, Sato T, Kanazawa I: Regional cerebral blood flow in the covert reading of kana words: a comparison with the study of reading aloud tasks. Eur Neurol 1996;36:237–239.
27 Sakurai Y, Momose T, Iwata M, Sudo Y, Kumakura Y, Ohtomo K, Kanazawa I: Cortical activation in reading assessed by region of interest-based analysis and statistical parametric mapping. Brain Res Brain Res Protoc 2001;6:167–171.
28 Sakurai Y, Momose T, Iwata M, Sudo Y, Ohtomo K, Kanazawa I: Different cortical activity in reading of Kanji words, Kana words and Kana nonwords. Brain Res Cogn Brain Res 2000;9:111–115.
29 Sakurai Y, Momose T, Iwata M, Sudo Y, Ohtomo K, Kanazawa I: Cortical activity associated with vocalization and reading proper. Brain Res Cogn Brain Res 2001;12:161–165.
30 Nakamura K, Honda M, Hirano S, Oga T, Sawamoto N, Hanakawa T, Inoue H, Ito J, Matsuda T, Fukuyama H, et al.: Modulation of the visual word retrieval system in writing: a functional MRI study on the Japanese orthographies. J Cogn Neurosci 2002;14:104–115.
31 Sakurai Y: Varieties of alexia from fusiform, posterior inferior temporal and posterior occipital gyrus lesions. Behav Neurol 2004;15:35–50.
32 Sakurai Y, Ichikawa Y, Mannen T: Pure alexia from a posterior occipital lesion. Neurology 2001;56:778–781.
33 Sakurai Y, Terao Y, Ichikawa Y, Ohtsu H, Momose T, Tsuji S, Mannen T: Pure alexia for kana. Characterization of alexia with lesions of the inferior occipital cortex. J Neurol Sci 2008;268:48–59.

34 Sakurai Y, Yagishita A, Goto Y, Ohtsu H, Mannen T: Fusiform type alexia: pure alexia for words in contrast to posterior occipital type pure alexia for letters. J Neurol Sci 2006;247:81–92.
35 Otsuki M, Soma Y, Arai T, Otsuka A, Tsuji S: Pure apraxic agraphia with abnormal writing stroke sequences: report of a Japanese patient with a left superior parietal haemorrhage. J Neurol Neurosurg Psychiatry 1999;66:233–237.
36 Sakurai Y: Neural substrates of reading and writing. Shinkei Naika 2008;68:248–255.
37 Sakurai Y: Reading and writing impairments: basic and clinical. High Brain Funct Res 2010;30:25–32.

Yasuhisa Sakurai, MD, PhD
Department of Neurology, Mitsui Memorial Hospital
1 Kanda-Izumi-cho, Chiyoda-ku
Tokyo 101-8643 (Japan)
E-Mail ysakurai-tky@umin.ac.jp

Bogousslavsky J, Boller F, Iwata M (eds): A History of Neuropsychology.
Front Neurol Neurosci. Basel, Karger, 2019, vol 44, pp 64–74 (DOI: 10.1159/000494953)

Early History of Amnesia

Karen G. Langer
Rusk Rehabilitation, NYU Langone Medical Center, New York, NY, USA

Abstract

Memory and forgetfulness have been viewed since antiquity from perspectives of physical, emotional, and spiritual states of well-being, and conceptualized philosophically. Numerous discussions of memory loss, or case reports, existed, but a fundamental advance in conceptualization of memory loss as a pathological clinical phenomenon originated when Sauvages classified "amnesia" as a medical disorder, in 1763. Originally, amnesia was recognized as a weakening or dissolution of memory, according to a taxonomy that ascribed known causes to the disorder. Etiologic factors included neurological disorders of stroke, hemorrhage, and head injury, metabolic dysregulation, alcohol and substance abuse, toxicity, anoxia, and other acute or chronic (sometimes progressive) brain disorders. Clinical descriptions of amnesia appeared internationally in medical dictionaries and scientific encyclopedias in the early 19th century. The possibility that amnesia could be either idiopathic, or symptomatic of another illness, was proposed based on the wide range of recognized etiologies and associations. Debate ensued regarding the status of amnesia as an illness or a symptom, but regardless, amnesia was soon recognized as an independent disorder of memory, distinguishable from disorders of global intellect, or of consciousness, or of language. Distinctions of amnesia considered its temporal gradient, duration and natural course, nature of onset, severity or depth of memory loss, course, and prognosis. Concepts of retrograde (forgetting knowledge preceding onset) and anterograde (difficulty learning, recalling new information) further specified the nature of amnestic memory difficulty. Alcoholic amnesia in Korsakoff's syndrome generated much attention. Amnesia as a clinical feature was critical to the development of notions of dissociation of conscious from subconscious recall in hysteria, and differentiation of neurogenically-based from psychogenically-based amnesia became central to understanding post-traumatic states. Amnesia studied as a disorder of memory remains an avenue to enrich clinical understanding of a condition that continues to be powerfully challenging to this day.

Introduction

Memory has been viewed since antiquity through the lens of physical, emotional, and spiritual states of well-being. Biblical references to forgetting and memory abound. Concepts of memory and remembrance are recognized in the works of Hippocrates, Plato, Aristotle, Cicero, Avicenna, Averroes, and Maimonides, among others.

The term amnesia derives from the Greek ἀμνησία, meaning loss of memory [1]. The river of oblivion or forgetting in classical Greek mythology, Lethe (λήθη, forgetting), was thus named. A very early appearance of the term ἀμνησία has it as a synonym for 'amnesty' (etymologically related, as a noun: "Forgetfulness, oblivion; an intentional overlooking" [1].

The physician Galen used the term "lethe" (translated as amnesia) [2] to describe symptoms with "destruction of function;" Thucydides' description of the Plague of Athens and Hippocrates' mention of the term were noted, but there is question of whether the term is "too strong for" amnesia, and a milder "forgetfulness" is more accurate [2]. Galen credited his predecessors for the designation of "such conditions by different names, lack of memory (ἐπιλησμοσύνη), forgetfulness (λήθη), or the loss of memory (μνήμηςἀπώλεία), but also qualified them indistinctly as damage (βλάβη), affect or illness (πάθος), illness (νόσος), or even symptom (σύμπτωμα) or infirmity (ἀρρώστημα)" [3]. It appears that cases of forgetfulness or memory loss were well-recognized, but as can be seen, the term "amnesia" as a pathologic clinical medical entity with substantive semiological classifications did not develop until the late 18th century.

Classic conceptions of memory may have paved the way for the clinical use of amnesia, seeding notions of forgetting contents of the past, inability to recollect ideas or experiences, or inability to imagine or conceptualize new ideas through learning, imagination or deliberation. These concepts took form in the definitions of disordered memory or its pathology, and although this review is not intended to be exhaustive, and other early sources for memory loss exist, it traces the early history of amnesia from the time it began to be classified as a medical disorder.

Historically, descriptions of what is now recognized as amnesia occurred largely in case reports or first-person descriptions of memory disturbances. A fascinating exposition sketching the literary portrayal of amnesia over time contrasts concepts in scientific literature with the depiction of amnesic memory disorders and repressed memories in various genres [4]. Scholars Montaigne and Rousseau vividly portrayed their own post-traumatic amnesia in concussion and head injury [5]. Reports of forgetfulness or memory loss included anecdotal cases of memory loss [6, 7] or descriptions of large-scale events or epidemics found in classical works (e.g., Thucydides' description of memory loss in Athens, soldiers with typhus in Vilna and in Mayence), used as testimony of adverse effects of pandemics [8, 9].

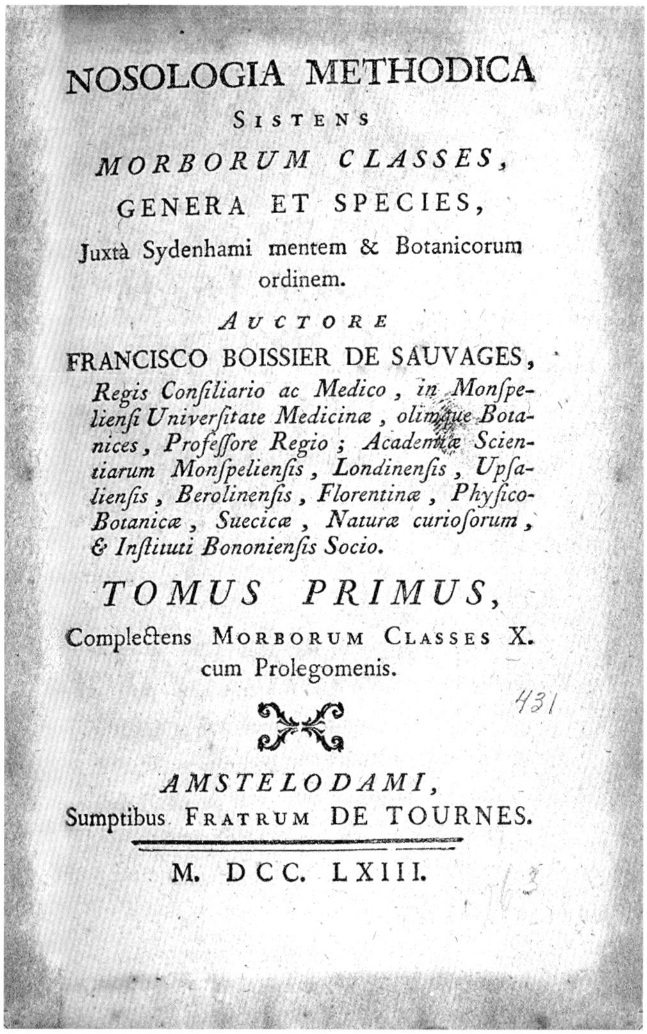

NOSOLOGIA METHODICA
SISTENS
MORBORUM CLASSES,
GENERA ET SPECIES,
Juxtà Sydenhami mentem & Botanicorum ordinem.
AUCTORE
FRANCISCO BOISSIER DE SAUVAGES,
Regis Consiliario ac Medico, in Monspeliensi Universitate Medicinæ, olimque Botanices, Professore Regio; Academiæ Scientiarum Monspeliensis, Londinensis, Upsaliensis, Berolinensis, Florentinæ, Physico-Botanicæ, Suecicæ, Naturæ curiosorum, & Instituti Bononiensis Socio.
TOMUS PRIMUS,
Complectens MORBORUM CLASSES X. cum Prolegomenis.
431
AMSTELODAMI,
Sumptibus FRATRUM DE TOURNES.
M. DCC. LXIII.

Fig. 1. Title page from the "Nosologia Methodica" of de Sauvages, 1763. Courtesy of the US National Library of Medicine.

Amnesia: The Term

The original application of "amnesia" to a medical condition, in the 18th century, is credited to Boissier de Sauvages [10, 11], whose methodical nosology classifies illnesses (Fig. 1). The French translation [11] describes "Oubli" (Forgetting), an abolition or diminution of memory. The classification system listed memory loss whose types included:

(1) Venereal, (2) Senile, (3) Traumatic, (e.g., contusion, head injury), (4) Plethoric (i.e., an excess of blood, or fullness of blood vessels due to suppressed blood flow), (5) Pathematic (from emotional suffering or afflictions of the spirit, following strong emotions such as fear, terror or chagrin), (6) Cephalalgic (following headache), (7) Intoxication (i.e., abuse of substances, such as alcohol and opium; ingestion of poison), and (8) Febrile (i.e., following acute fever) (Table 1). Of note, the eighth category, febrile, though not in the original edi-

Table 1. Classification of amnesia

Sauvages 1763/1768		Sauvages (trans. Nicolas) 1771		Sagar 1776	
amnesia a venere	amnesia from venery (i.e., pursuit of sexual pleasure)	oubli vénérien/ amnesia a venere	venereal oblivion [French]/ amnesia from venery [Latin]	a venere	from venery
a. senilis	senile a.	o. des vieillards/ a. senilis	o. of the elderly/ senile a.	senilis	senile
a. traumatica	traumatic a. (i.e., from [head] wounds)	o. traumatique/ a. traumatica	traumatic o./ traumatic a.	traumatica	traumatic
a. plethorica (a suppressis haemorrhoidibus)	plethoric a. (from suppressed blood flow) (i.e., excessive fullness of blood vessels)	o. pléthorique/ a. a suppressis haemorrhoidibus	plethoric o./ a. from suppressed blood flow [Latin lacks *plethorica*]	plethorica	plethoric
–		–		ab inedia*	from lack of food
a. a pathemate	pathematic a. (i.e., from emotional suffering)	o. ensuite d'une affection de l'âme/ a. a pathemate	o. after an ailment of the soul/ pathematic a.	–	
a. cephalalgica	cephalalgic a. (i.e., from a headache)	o. céphalalgique	cephalalgic o./ [no Latin]	cephalalgica	cephalalgic
a. a temulentia	a. from intoxication	o. d'ivresse/ a. a t[e]mulentia	drunken o./ a. from intoxication	crapulosa	drunken
–		–		apoplectica	apoplectic
a. febrisequa	a. following fever	o. qui suit la fièvre	o. following fever/ [no Latin]	febrisequa	following fever

* Under *amnesia plethorica*, the preceding category of amnesia, Sauvages cites Jacob Horstius (1537–1600), who noted similar symptoms when someone ate heavily after a long fast. Following this cue, Sagar creates a new category, *amnesia ab inedia*, but he omits Sauvages's next category, *amnesia a pathemate*. Color Key: Green: Original in Sauvages 1763 and constant through Sagar. Orange: New in Sauvages 1768 (rev. ed.). Red: New in Sagar.

tion [10], appeared in the revised 1768 edition, published posthumously, then in the first French translation [11], and in subsequent translation (e.g., that of Gouvion; Lyon, J.-M. Bruyset, 1772), and sources that followed. Various etiology- and age-specific treatments were proposed. Sauvages stated that among "authorities," the preferred term was "oblivio morbosa," indicating that the reference to weakened memory had been used previously, though he used the term amnesia. About 14 inaugural dissertations were written between 1622 and 1760 on memory and forgetfulness (oblivione) and hurt or damaged memory (Memoriae laesione), plus other published work on memory and its loss (e.g., Vogel's *Mnemosynologia,* 1676), as cited [12]. Numerous individual cases or discussions of memory loss existed, but the fundamental advance and analysis of memory loss as a clinical phenomenon originated when Sauvages used amnesia in the medical sense, categorized taxonomically.

Sagar [13] largely adopted Sauvages' classification, adding categories "apopleptica," amnesia after stroke, and "ab inedia," related to famine (Table 1). One may speculate that Sagar's addition of famine-related amnesia is based on the notation within Sauvages' category "plethoric" that forgetting can be observed in persons who resume eating after long abstinence, thus possibly related to the lack of food. Sagar omitted "pathemate" (due to strong emotions) for unknown reasons, possibly unintentionally.

Another Latin medical text by a German bibliographer [14] defines amnesia as: "memoriae debilitas, defectus" (weakness, defect of memory), provides a bibliography of earlier texts that discuss memory loss (likely oblivion in his sources), and lists causes and therapies. There is also an entry for partial amnesia ("Amnesia Partialis") [14], though references largely refer to language disorders, reflecting a probable confounding of "verbal amnesia" and aphasia, as later proposed [15]. By the early 19th century, descriptions of "amnesia" began to appear internationally. A Spanish medical dictionary defined amnesia as "the complete loss of memory," adding: "Amnesia is a weakness of the mind relating to memory, such that patients do not recall the relations of objects ... when the lack of memory increases, it always leads to amentia" [16]. Etiologic classifications were based on Sauvages' 8 subtypes.

Shortly thereafter, an Italian entry depicts amnesia as "the temporary suspension, the diminution, or the complete loss of memory" [17]. This may be an early implication of transience, the "temporary suspension" of memory, likely sowing seeds of later notions of transitory states of amnesia, possibly as transient global amnesia ("les ictus amnésiques" as noted in review, the original term used [18]). An Italian philologist [19] elegantly traced the word's etymology:

"Amnesia oblivio [Latin, = 'amnesia,' 'forgetfulness'], amnésie, oubli [French, = 'amnesia', 'forgetting'], Gedächtnisschwäche [German, = 'weakness of memory'] (Medicine). [From privative α-[alpha] and from μνάομαι (mnaomai), 'to remember,' and from φρὴν (phren), 'mind.' A type of disease that takes away the ability to recognize and reproduce ideas in the mind, that is, the abolition or diminution of memory, whose symptom is the utterance of words disconnected from their meaning." Sauvages], thereby linking the term to illness, disability, and symptom.

Clinical usage of amnesia in English medical literature appears late in the 18th century, defined as "loss of memory" [20]. The London Encyclopedia [21] elaborated: "Amnesia, in medicine, loss of memory; sometimes the consequence of febrile diseases, when it generally recedes as the patient gains strength. As the consequence of old age it can hardly be expected to be cured." This definition effectively distinguished reversible from irreversible causes and transitory states from permanence. The description of "amnésie" (amnesia) as a clinical entity began to flourish in French specialized medical dictionaries and scientific encyclopedias in the early 19th century [8, 12, 22–24], and theses on amnesia appeared in French throughout the century [9, 15, 25]. Primary features of amnesia began to include distinctions of general or complete (total) and partial, durable or lasting only for a specific time [8].

Descriptive and Diagnostic Considerations

Debate soon ensued as to whether amnesia was more correctly an illness or a symptom. Those favoring the illness designation attempted to demonstrate its independent status. Questions arose related to whether amnesia could be found to exist independently of other cognitive difficulties, as an isolated defect of memory, or whether it was part of a more global intellectual decline. One perspective suggested that not only is amnesia a symptom, and not an illness [9], but that other distinctions (e.g., partial or complete) are not valid, as they represent only differing points on the continuum of amount of memory loss (e.g., dysmnesia and amnesia), and differ only in degree [24]. Another interesting possibility proposed that amnesia could be considered idiopathic and essential when existing independently, and symptomatic when due to primary maladies or an accessory component of certain illnesses, acute or chronic, often cerebral in origin (e.g., apoplexy, epilepsy, etc.) [8].

Prognosis for recovery in amnesia was believed to be more favorable for traumatic onset [15], with the cure of an associated illness, or for hemorrhagic origin (once the clot had resorbed) [22]. Amnesia of generally slow onset with more progressive nature was considered prognostically ominous [15]. Prognosis was also considered pessimistic for static and long-lasting variants, or complete amnesia, such that chronicity and intensity were key considerations for prognosis and expectation.

Distinctions of complete or incomplete amnesia were enhanced with classifications for acquired (rather than congenital) types. Acquired amnesia could be traumatic or illness-based, the latter remarkably detailed, including inflammation, epilepsy, mania, ossification of the dura or arachnoid membrane, circulatory effusion, tuberculosis, cancerous tumor), appetitive or corporeal excesses, and toxicologic [22]. Further etiologic precision detailing causes beyond those categories already proposed by Sauvages and followers included: cerebral illnesses involving dural or arachnoid fungus, brain softening, meningoencephalitis, cysts, abscesses, syphilitic tumors, metabolic effects, illnesses such as typhoid or tuberculosis, hypoxia/anoxia, temperament (e.g., melancholy) and occupational health, and environmental issues (e.g., smoking in closed spaces, solar-induced inflammation, mining and other subterranean work). Drawing from prior sources and compiling a rather comprehensive list of causes known at the time (i.e., in addition to unknown sources) individual origins of amnesia were specified [12]: hereditary, head injury, concussion/contusion, weaknesses of aging and senility, climate (e.g., cold, wind, heat), substance ingestion, such as alcoholism, narcotic use, or poisons; fatigue, sedentary lifestyle, states of anger, fear or terror; cholera, bleeding excesses; fevers, especially pestilent-induced; headaches; illnesses, and conditions such as encephalitis, hydrocephalus, apoplexy/stroke, mania, and epilepsy. Many of these, though drawn from earlier sources, can be classified within the nosological system(s) outlined by Sauvages and followers.

Memory-specificity was recognized in amnesia; different memories, or types of memories (i.e., skills or modalities) might be lost, and progression and duration could vary. Remarkably, even then cases of transient amnesia were described that persisted just hours, days, or weeks. Transient amnesia that lasted only seconds [24], or that was otherwise momentary [22], was recognized, alongside the more common variants, which were more lasting, or persisted indefinitely. Amnesia was further characterized by defining features [15]: nature of onset (sudden or progressive), duration (temporary or lasting and stable), and periodicity (periodic or continuous). Progressive forms, typically reflecting brain diseases, are characterized by slow and continuous dissolution of memory, often presenting as partial amnesia in earliest phases [26].

By the late 19th century, Korsakoff had sparked much interest in amnesia [27], owing to the vivid clinical descriptions of the alcoholic syndrome named after him, characterized by a severe defect of retention related to the onset of the illness and a few weeks before, without a corresponding disorder of consciousness [27]. Korsakoff expressed much theoretical interest regarding the peculiarities of memory loss in this alcoholic amnesia.

Amnesia could be classified as pure and simple (no other faculty affected) or complicated [23]. Delirium and confusional states, importantly, were distinguished from amnesia. Differentiation of amnesia for words from that of events and facts, or amnesia from aphasia, assumed clinical significance [28, 29], as it was suggested that the 2 conditions had been enmeshed or confounded, and that much of what was called amnesia from antiquity until the first half of the 19th century was really aphasia [15].

Amnesia was noted to conform to Ribot's law, such that older memories were better preserved than more recent ones, certainly in temporal proximity to the brain injury or psychic trauma. Memory restitution also progressed in reverse order of loss [15, 25]. Temporal order of loss and resolution of memory was considered important, both for the course of recovery and for remediation [25]. Order of dissolution of content in amnesia is first for recent events, then ideas, then sentiments and affections (i.e., emotions), and then actions (i.e., habits and routines) [26]; applying the law of regression, progression of dissolution or loss is from the unstable to the stable, from most recent (least organized, least fixed) to more permanent, sensorial, and instinctive memory.

Various designations were introduced that went beyond complete or partial in their depiction of the temporal nature of amnesic memory difficulties. The term retro-anterograde amnesia was introduced in France by Charcot [30] in his lectures, in a case of probable hysteria. Anterograde amnesia was defined [31] as a difficulty in registering or learning new facts (though "amnésie antérograde de conservation" was used by Ribot [26]), and retrograde amnesia (attributed to Azam [32]) as a forgetting of facts occurring prior to trauma or accident. (As noted above, much earlier case examples also documented the phenomenon.)

Amnesia was additionally distinguished [33] based on processes of conservation or reproduction. Methodical clinical assessment introduced by Sollier [33] included consideration of consequences of amnesia, interval for disappearance of impressions, and ways to fix and conserve or restore and revivify impressions. Sollier's innovative approach to amnesia rehabilitation included intensification of impressions by fixing attention and by association with preserved sensory images, stabilization via repetition, multi-modal associations, recording, repetition, and emotional emphasis. The extent to which memories could be fixed or revivified was further considered. Retroactive amnesia was considered as loss of memory extending only a short period before the onset of the cause, with shock or other factors interfering with the process of fixation, and was thus distinguished from dissociative amnesia (where memories can be revivified by "psychological methods"), and from retrograde amnesia, where memory is eliminated for a longer period [34].

In the latter part of the 19th century, French alienists turned their attention to amnesia. Amnesia as a clinical feature was critical to the development of notions of subconscious, and of dissociation of memories and conscious from subconscious recall [35] in hysteria. These notions were fueled by the practice of hypnosis popular in case demonstrations of the period, in works by Charcot and followers, in vivid descriptions of multiple personality by Azam (e.g., Félida) and Janet, among others, and other psychogenic forms of amnesia, which presupposes a need to forget fueled by psychological trauma. The implications of psychogenic amnesia, fugue, or dissociation for legal cases, involving crimes or other forensic issues, including sanity, culpability, and social justice, began to be broadly considered in psycho-legal texts. Differentiation of neurogenically-based from psychogenically-based amnesia was for some practitioners a key to understanding patients' clinical manifestations. Psychological or emotional imbalances, with states of depression and melancholy, jealousy, fear or horror [25], later became essential to distinguishing between amnesias of psychogenic versus neurogenic origin. However, it began to be well recognized that there is a dynamic interplay between emotional factors and recollection even in cases of neurogenic amnesia.

In amnesia, clinicians noted that recollection of trauma may seem real and current, due to disturbance of judgement of time perception, such that the patient experiences the past as present [27], the traumatic past as currently real, with deleterious effects on psychological integrity. On the other hand, it was recognized that psychological factors might affect development of amnesia, and sources of intense emotional reaction could be identified with its origins and progression or resolution.

Early writings on amnesia had identified potential psychological factors. Psychological imbalances were considered amenable to distraction, passage of time, and restoration of vitality [25]. Later, psychological methods, including hypnosis or psychotherapy, were used in treatment. The psychological or secondary benefit of amnesia and forgetting is thought to be linked to the quality of contents of recollection, or lack thereof. Concurring with prior philosophical and psychological perspectives, it was poignantly noted [25] that loss of memory may sometimes be a blessing, as after psychological trauma, and recollection of more pleasant times or experience may be the basis of wisdom or serenity.

By early in the 20th century, commonly recognized characteristics of amnesia retained from earlier classifications were attributes of complete or partial, stable and continuous or temporary, and anterograde or retrograde forms [36], in addition to nosology used by Sauvages and followers. Precise delineation categorized amnesia based on pathogenesis (i.e., dynamic or organic), duration (transient or persistent), degree (partial or general), onset and natural course (i.e., sudden, progressive, or periodic, intermittent), and chronology (i.e., retrograde, anterograde, or retro-anterograde) [37].

Lastly, amnesia was understood to be due to disruption in any of 3 memory processes: reception or registration, conservation, and reproduction of the mental impressions [36, 37]. It has remained, apparently throughout history, important to understand and distinguish causes of memory loss to more properly approach, respond to, or treat cases.

Discussion and Summary

Memory loss has been described since antiquity. Memory loss was noted in individual cases, associated with environmental extremes and epidemics, primary illnesses, and head injuries. As amnesia began to be classified as a medical disorder, first attributed to Sauvages in 1763, its nosology and etiological origins were delineated, with further clinical distinctions. Principal among specific causes identified were organic neurological conditions associated with memory loss; apoplexy or stroke, hemorrhage, head injury, syphilitic conditions, bodily or metabolic dysregulation, excesses and abuse of consumption (including alcohol or opium), ingestion of toxic substances, other diseases and illnesses (e.g., cholera, typhus), following febrile episodes, and other acute or chronic (sometimes progressive) brain disorders.

Recognition of memory loss or weakening presupposes that one knows the normal state of memory and its different types [23]. Attention has been drawn to the range between normal forgetfulness and the pathological aspects of memory loss in amnesia.

Scholars of the period noted that amnesia could also be differentiated from the more global losses of intellectual function that characterized dementia; amnesia thus took its place alongside other neurological disorders depicted by semiological descriptions. Amnesia and amnestic states were clearly established via detailed clinical observations and reports of pathological findings as independent disorders of memory.

Disease classification systems of the period have been considered [38]. The amnesic syndromes and their historical roots remain a focus of interest and inquiry [39–43], supported by increasingly sophisticated psychological and neurological investigations.

Acknowledgments

Deepest gratitude is expressed for the kindness and inspiration of Andre Langer.

At NYU Libraries, Michael Agnew, Librarian for Romance Languages, Bobst Library, provided invaluable assistance in the preparation of Table 1 and instrumental guidance. Mr. Agnew thoughtfully provided all translations from Latin, Spanish, German, and Italian appearing in this work.

David DeSimone provided invaluable reference support and consistent encouragement. W. Gerald Heverly, Librarian for Classics, Hellenic Studies, and Philosophy, Bobst Library, provided translation of Greek and guidance on Classic sources. At the New York Academy of Medicine, Ms. Arlene Shaner, Historical Collections Librarian is thanked for support and guidance.

References

1 amnesia, n.: OED Online. Oxford University Press, December 2018. Web http://www.oed.com (accessed May 2017; February 2019).

2 Johnston I (trans): Galen: On Diseases and Symptoms. New York, NY, Cambridge University Press, 2006, pp 263–264.

3 Boudon-Millot V: What is a mental illness, and how can it be treated? Galen's reply as a doctor and philosopher; in Harris WV (ed): Columbia Studies in the Classical Tradition vol 38. Boston, Leiden, Brill, 2013, pp 129–146.

4 Dieguez S, Annoni JM: Stranger than fiction: literary and clinical amnesia; in Dieguez S, Bogousslavsky J (eds): Literary Medicine: Brain Disease and Doctors in Novels, Theater, and Film, vol 31. Basel, Karger, 2013, pp 137–168.

5 Feinsod M, Langer KG: The philosopher's swoon – The concussion of Michel de Montaigne: a historic vignette. World Neurosurg 2102;78:371–374.

6 Académie Royale des Sciences: Diverses Observations Anatomiques [Various Anatomical Observations]. Histoire de l'Académie Royale des Sciences, 1705, pp 49–58.

7 Segerus G [Seger G]: Observation CXCVIII: Sur une perte de mémoire, sans cause apparente, que le malade recouvra dans la suite par l'usage des remédes appropriés à son état [Observation 198: Regarding a loss of memory, without apparent cause, which the patient later recovered by taking remedies suited to his age]. In [Jean] Nadault, Trans., Collection académique, composée des mémoires, actes, ou journaux des plus célèbres académies & sociétés littéraires étrangères [...]: Tome III. Contenant les Ephémérides des Curieux de la Nature d'Allemagne, depuis l'année 1670 jusqu'en 1686. Dijon, François Desventes. Auxerre, François Fournier, 1755, pp 165–166.

8 Louyer-Villermay JB: Essai sur les maladies de la mémoire. Mém de Soc de méd de Par 1817;68–96.

9 Tavernier A: Quelques Considérations sur l'Amnésie. Paris, Didot le Jeune, 1825.

10 Boissier de Sauvages F: Nosologia methodica sistens morborum classes, genera et species, juxta Sydenhami mentem & botanicorum ordinem [...] Tomi tertii pars prima, complectens genera et species morborum ad classes VII and VIII pertinentium, nempe dolores et vesaniae. [Methodical nosology, with the classes, genera, and species of diseases, according to the Sydenham's reasoning and the botanists' order...First part of the third volume, including the genera and species of diseases belonging to classes VII and VIII, namely, pains and mental illnesses] (vol 3.1). Amsterdam, Sumptibus fratrum de Tournes, 1763, pp 408–410. (Revised and enlarged edition, Nosologia methodica sistens morborum classes, juxta Sydenhami mentem and botanicorum ordinem [...] Editio ultima, auctior, and emendatior, Tomus secundus. [Methodical nosology, with the classes of diseases according to Sydenham's reasoning and the botanists' order...Last edition, enlarged and revised] (2 vols.), vol 2. Amsterdam, Sumptibus fratrum de Tournes, 1768, pp 269–271).

11 Boissier de Sauvages F: Nosologie Methodique, dans laquelle les Maladies sont Rangées par Classes, Suivant le Systême de Sydenham, and L'ordre des Botanistes [Methodical nosology, in which diseases are arranged by classes, according to Sydenham's system and the botanists' order]. (Nicolas, Trans., vols. 1–3), vol 2. Paris, Hérissant le Fils, 1771, pp 752–755.

12 Frank J: De l'amnésie; in Bayle (ed): Encyclopédie des Sciences Médicales. Paris, Bureau de l'Encyclopédie, 1838, pp 123–131.

13 Sagar JBM: Systema morborum symptomaticum secundum classes, ordines, genera et species, cum characteribus, differentiis et therapeiis: filum ariadnaeum ad lectulos aegrorum [Symptomatic system of diseases according to classes, orders, genera, and species, with characteristics, differences, and therapies: an Ariadne's thread for sickbeds]. Vienna, Impensis Joannis Pauli Kraus, 1776, pp 735–755.

14 Ploucquet WG: Initia bibliothecae medico-practicae et chirurgicae realis, sive, Repertorii medicinae practicae et chirurgiae [Beginnings of a royal library on the practice of medicine and surgery, or, Repertoire of practical medicine and surgery], vol 1. Tübingen, Apud Joannem Georgium Cottam, 1793, pp 124–130.

15 Rouillard AMP: Essai sur les Amnésies: étiologie des troubles de la mémoire. Paris, Jules Le Clere, 1885.

16 Ballano A: Diccionario de Medicina y Cirugía, o, Biblioteca Manual Médico-Quirúrgica [Dictionary of medicine and surgery, or, Manual library of medicine and surgery] (vols. 1–7). Madrid, Imprenta Real, 1805–1807, vol 1, p 171; vol 7, pp 422–423.

17 Aquilino B, Marchi MA: Dizionario Etimologico di Tutti i Vocabuli Usati delle Scienze, Arti e Mestieri Che Traggono Origine dal Greco [Etymological dictionary of all the words used in the sciences, arts, and trades that have their origin in Greek], vol 1. Milan, Tipografia di Giacomo Pirol, 1819–1821, pp 158–159.

18 Pearce J, Bogousslavsky J: 'Les ictus amnésiques' and transient global amnesia. Eur Neurol 2009;62:188–192.

19 Marchi MA: Dizionario Technico-Etimologico-Filologico [Technical etymological philological dictionary], vol 1. Milan, Tipografia di Giacomo Pirola, 1828–1829, p 41.

20 Rush B: An oration, delivered before the American Philosophical Society, held in Philadelphia on the 27th of February, 1786; An Enquiry into the Influence of Physical Causes upon the Moral Faculty. Philadelphia, Charles Cist, 1786.

21 The London Encyclopedia. Universal Dictionary of Science, Art, Literature, and Practical Mechanics. London, Thomas Tegg, 1829.

22 Calmeil L: Amnésie; in Adelon et al. (eds): Dictionnaire de Médecine ou Répertoire Général des Sciences Médicales, vol 2. Paris, Béchet, 1833, pp 401–410.

23 Voisin A: Amnésie; in Jaccoud (ed): Nouveau Dictionnaire de Médecine et de Chirurgie Practiques, vol 2. Paris, J. B. Baillière et Fils, 1865, pp 52–56.

24 Falret J: Amnésie; in Dechambre (ed): Dictionnaire Encyclopédique des Sciences Médicales, vol 3. Paris, P Asselin, Sr. de Labé; Victor Masson et Fils, 1865, pp 725–742.
25 Ribault J: Dissertation sur l'Amnésie. Montpellier, Jean Martel, 1827.
26 Ribot T: Diseases of Memory. London, Kegan Paul, Trench & Co., 1882. (Translation of 1st French ed., les Maladies de la Mémoire, 1881.)
27 Korsakoff S: Étude médico-psychologique sur une forme des maladies de la mémoire. Rev Phil France L'et 1889; 28:501–530. (Korsakoff SS. Medico-Psychological Study of a Memory Disorder (WP Banks, SJ Karam, translators), Conscious Cogn 1996;5:2–21.)
28 Bouillaud J: Amnésie; in Andral et al. (eds): Dictionnaire de Médicine et de Chirurgie Pratique, vol 2. Paris, Gabon, Méquignon-Marvis, J.-B. Baillière, 1829, pp 166–169.
29 Bastian HC: The Brain as an Organ of the Mind. London, C. Keegan Paul & Co., 1880, pp 613–672.
30 Charcot JM: Sur un cas d'amnésie rétro-antérograde probablement d'origine hystérique. Rev Méd 1892;12: 81–96.
31 Souques AA: Essai sur l'amnésie rétro-antérograde dans l'hystérie, les traumatismes cérébraux et l'alcoolisme chronique. Rev Méd 1892;12:367–401 and 867–881.
32 Azam E: Les troubles intellectuels provoqués par les traumatismes cérébraux. Arch Gén de Méd 1881;7:291–315.
33 Sollier P: Les Troubles de la Mémoire. Paris, J. Rueff et Cie., 2nd ed., 1901 (First published 1892).
34 Burnham WH: Retroactive amnesia: Illustrative cases and a tentative explanation. Am J Psychol 1903;14:118–132.
35 Janet P: Étude sur quelques cas d'amnésie antérograde dans la maladie de la désagrégation psychologique. International Congress of Experimental Psychology. London, Williams & Norgate, 1892, pp 26–30.
36 Holbrook CS: Amnesia; in Piersol GM, Bortz EL (eds): The Cyclopedia of Medicine, vol 1. Philadelphia, F.A. Davis & Co., 1931, pp 379–381.
37 Dromard G, Levassort J: L'amnésie. Paris, Felix Alcan, 1907.
38 Munsche H, Whitaker HA: Eighteenth century classification of mental illness: Linnaeus, de Sauvages, Vogel, and Cullen. Cogn Behav Neurol 2012:25:224–239.
39 Berrios GE: Historical aspects of memory and its disorders; in Berrios GE, Hodges JR (eds): Memory Disorders in Psychiatric Practice. Cambridge, Cambridge University Press, 2000, pp 3–33.
40 Levin HS, Peters BH, Hulkonen DA: Early concepts of anterograde and retrograde amnesia. Cortex 1983;19: 427–440.
41 Whitty CWM, Zangwill OL (eds): Amnesia. London, Butterworths, 1966.
42 Markowitsch HJ: Intellectual Functions and the Brain. An Historical Perspective. Seattle, Hogrefe & Huber Publishers, 1992.
43 Finger S: Origins of Neuroscience: A History of Explorations into Brain Function. New York, Oxford, 1994.

Karen G. Langer, PhD
Rusk Rehabilitation, NYU Langone Medical Center
301 East 17th Street
New York, NY 10003 (USA)
E-Mail karen.langer@nyumc.org

Bogousslavsky J, Boller F, Iwata M (eds): A History of Neuropsychology.
Front Neurol Neurosci. Basel, Karger, 2019, vol 44, pp 75–82 (DOI: 10.1159/000494954)

History of Anosognosia

Guido Gainotti[a, b]

[a]Institute of Neurology, Catholic University of the Sacred Heart, Rome, Italy;
[b]Department of Clinical and Behavioral Neurology, IRCCS Fondazione Santa Lucia, Rome, Italy

Abstract

Even if Babinski (1914) is usually considered as the discoverer of anosognosia, other authors before him contributed to the development of this construct. Von Monakow (1885) and Dejerine and Vialet (1893) gave the first descriptions of patients with cortical blindness who were unaware of their disability, but did not distinguish this unawareness from the rest of the clinical description. Anton (1999) described patients with cortical deafness and cortical blindness, considering these defects of awareness as a symptom independent from the neurological dysfunction. He conceptualized them as a phenomenon in its own right and tried to link this unawareness of a disability with specific neuro-anatomical changes. Finally, Babinski (1914) coined the term "anosognosia" to designate the clinical entity conceptualized by Anton (1899) and extended this concept from the unawareness of cortical deafness and blindness to the unawareness of hemiplegia. The choice of the term "anosognosia" to denote the observed phenomenon was important, because referring to "lack of knowledge of the disease" (anosognosia), he not only emphasized the separation between "lack of knowledge" and "disease, " but also suggested a general use of this term, because disease can refer to many other disabilities besides hemiplegia. Further investigations have shown that: (a) brain-damaged patients may be unaware of different kinds of disabilities; (b) anosognosia can be selective, in that an affected person with multiple impairments may be unaware of only one handicap, while appearing fully aware of any others; and (c) lack of acknowledgment of a disease may not necessarily be due to a defective awareness, but must sometimes be considered as an extreme but understable pattern of adaptation to stress. For this condition, the term "Denial of Illness" seems preferable to that of anosognosia. Anosognosia must perhaps be viewed as a multifaceted phenomenon, resulting from both cognitive and motivational factors.

Introduction

It is reasonable to assume that our current knowledge about the origins of "anosognosia" may be only in part correct, just as our current knowledge about the origins of any other complex construct. For this reason it can be useful to start from the French neurologist Joseph Babinski [1], who coined in 1914 the term "anosognosia" and who is usually considered as the discoverer of this condition, in which a person with a severe disability seems to be unaware of the existence of this defect. In reality, Babinski's original description concerned 2 patients with right hemispheric stroke and left-sided hemiplegia, who were unaware of their paralysis, but other forms of unawareness of important disabilities had been reported by previous authors. In particular, the German neuropsychiatrist Gabriel Anton had described in 1899 [2] two patients with cortical deafness and one with cortical blindness (see references [3] and [4] for detailed descriptions) and, for this reason, visual anosognosia is often reported as Anton-Babinski syndrome. The description of this phenomenon, however, dates back to a much more ancient time, because, according to Bisiach and Geminiani [5] more than 2,000 years ago the stoic philosopher Seneca (c. 4 BC – AD 65) gave a clear description of a case of unawareness of blindness in a letter to Lucilius, in which he wrote: "This foolish woman suddenly lost her sight…Incredible as it may appear…she does not know she is blind."

The Main Three Steps Identified in the Construction of the Concept of Anosognosia

In recent years, and in a context of quickly growing knowledge of the brain organization and of its pathology, other authors [6, 7] reported before Anton [2] the clinical description of patients who were unaware of their cortical blindness. However, as rightly noted by Marková and Berrios [4], both these authors, although highlighting the fact that these patients were unaware of their blindness, considered this fact as part of the pathology related to blindness and did not view this unawareness as a separate phenomenon.

Starting from the difference between this attitude and that embraced by Anton [2] and by following authors, Marková and Berrios [4] distinguish 3 steps in the construction of the concept of anosognosia. The first step was purely descriptive and corresponded to the position adopted by von Monakow [6] and Dejerine and Vialet [7]. It consisted of a detailed description of the curious behavior shown by some patients unaware of their disability, without considering their unawareness as an independent phenomenon and rather focusing attention on the lesion causing the clinical impairment as a whole. The second step was taken by Anton [2], who considered the unawareness of a neurological disability as a symptom independent from the neurological dysfunction and conceptualized it as a phenomenon in its own right. To be sure, Anton [2] conceptualized the observed clinical phenomenon as a lack of self-awareness (*Selbstwahrnehmung*) of the neurological dysfunction and observed that this lack of self-awareness encompassed more than the visual or hearing loss. For example, the patients seemed to have missed the memory of the lost functions, as if they had never seen or heard in their life. Anton [2] sought to understand this phenomenon clinically (by exploring in great detail the patients' verbal and non-verbal behaviors) as well as pathologically (by trying to link this unawareness of a disability with specific neuro-anatomical changes). The third and last step was taken by Babinski [1] and consisted of coining the term "anosognosia" (from the ancient greek – *a*-, "without," *nosos*, "disease" and *gnōsis*, "knowledge") which corresponded to the clinical entity conceptualized by Anton [2], but extended this concept from the unawareness of cortical deafness and blindness to the unawareness of hemiplegia of cerebral origin. Therefore, even if the coining of the term "anosognosia" contributed little to the original conceptualization developed by Anton [2], it certainly served to generalize, consolidate and stabilize it as a phenomenon present in various kinds of disabilities resulting from brain damage and requiring a specific interpretation. It is worth noting from this point of view that, while the eponym "Anton's syndrome" is generally used to refer to cortical blindness [8], the general term "anosognosia" has come to signify a state of unawareness of different kinds of neurological impairments. These specific deficits can include motor defects (hemiplegia), sensory disorders (cortical deafness and blindness), spatial deficits (unilateral neglect), language disorders (Wernicke's aphasia), memory disturbances, dementia, and personality changes and are due to impairment of anatomo-functionally discrete monitoring systems [8].

How Prior History and Personal Research Perspectives Influenced Anton's and Babinski's Contribution to the Development of the "Anosognosia" Construct

To better understand the role played by Anton and Babinski in the development of the construct of anosognosia, it is necessary to consider the influence of eminent neurologists who contributed to form their scientific personality and addressed their general research perspectives. According to Kumbier et al. [3], Anton (1858–1933) developed, while he was working as Pick's assistant in Prague, an early interest in the anatomical study of brain lesions, interest that was consolidated during his work in Vienna in the psychiatric clinic of Theodor Meynert. Marková and Berrios [4] suggest that Anton's conceptualization of unawareness of neurological impairments as an independent phenomenon may have been influenced by Pick's early ideas on awareness and insight into madness [9] because Pick had explicitly studied awareness of illness in relation to mental diseases during the period in which Anton was working with him in Prague. Furthermore, Anton's interest for the anatomo-clinical correlations suggested that "unawareness of dysfunction" as a phenomenon in itself should be localized in the nervous system. However, being "unawareness" linked to processes different from those provoking the disability, the corresponding lesion should not be searched in the disability related cortical structures (e.g., in the visual cortex), but in association fibers connecting these structures with other cortical areas. This view of Anton, which considered unawareness of a disability as being due to the interruption of fibers connecting the destroyed cortical areas with other cortical centers, anticipated the disconnection account of anosognosia that was proposed by Geschwind [10] several decades later. On the contrary, Babinski (1857–1932) though being of Polish descent, worked all his life in Paris, where he became in 1885 chief resident to Charcot at the Salpetrière. Babinski was undoubtedly the favorite pupil of Charcot, of whom he wrote: "To take away from neurology all the discoveries made by Charcot would be to render it unrecognizable" [11]. After Charcot's death in 1893, Babinski pursued his research on hysteria, orienting his interest only towards "semiology," with the purpose of finding clinical means of distinguishing organic brain pathology from hysteria. Working along this line of research, Babinski [12] had already discovered the important difference between the dorsiflexion of the foot and toes (Babinski's sign) and the normal (flexor) response observed when the sole of the foot is firmly stroked. The identification of objective signs allowing to distinguish hysterical from organic paralysis became particularly important during World War I, when many young people tried to avoid getting involved in the war, which was one of the deadliest conflicts in history. Babinski's focus was, therefore, on the identification of features or signs that were associated with organic brain pathology, rather than on localization of brain functions. Related to this semiological perspective was the choice of "anosognosia" as the name denoting the observed phenomenon, because referring to "lack of knowledge of the disease" (anosognosia), he not only emphasized the difference between "lack of knowledge" and "disease," but also suggested a general use of this term, since disease can refer to many other disabilities besides hemiplegia.

The Selective Nature of Anosognosia

We have previously said that brain-damaged patients may be unaware of different kinds of disabilities: of sensory defects such as cortical blindness or hemianopia; of (usually left-sided) hemiplegia; of language comprehension and expression; of neglect for the left half of space; of memory disorders, of Alzheimer's disease (AD), and of personality change. It must also be underlined that anosognosia can be selective in that an affected person with multiple impairments may be unaware of only one handicap, while appearing fully aware of any others [13]. This phenomenon of double dissociation between disorders of which the patient is aware and unaware can be an indicator of domain-specific disorders of awareness mechanisms, meaning that in anosognosia, brain damage can selectively impact the self-monitoring process of one specific physical or cognitive function rather than affecting a general control function, probably located in the frontal lobes. A problem which has often been discussed while investigating the mechanisms underlying anosognosia for lateralized disorders, such as hemiplegia, hemianopia or unilateral neglect concerns the fact that these forms more commonly follows injury to the right hemisphere. Geschwind [10] viewed anosognosia for left-sided hemiplegia as a consequence of an interhemispheric disconnection. He proposed that patients might fail to verbally report hemiparesis when injury to the non-dominant hemisphere isolates this hemisphere's motor system from the dominant hemisphere's language centers. According to this model, "...many of the patient's responses can only be described as confabulating – that is, they are attempts to fill gaps in the information available to the speech area." This interpretation could explain confabulations reported by von Monakow [6], Dejerine and Vialet [7], and Anton [2] in the early descriptions of unawareness of cortical blindness and by Feinberg et al. [14] in more recent interpretations of anosognosia. However, the disconnection hypothesis was not confirmed by results obtained by Adair et al. [15], using right carotid barbiturate injection as a model for anosognosia for hemiplegia and providing the left hemisphere with explicit information regarding the left upper extremity function.

Motivational Factors Can Influence Unawareness of Illness

In a further discussion of patients with left-sided hemiplegia who ignored or seemed to ignore their severe motor defect, Babinski [16] made the paradoxical observation that some of these patients had been for many years very afraid of the condition that they now apparently ignored. This mismatch between previous anxious expectancies and present lack of concern could suggest that, at least in some patients, the subject's apparent unawareness of illness might be influenced by motivational factors. This interpretation, assuming that defense mechanisms may lead some patients to deny a condition that they are unable to accept, was formally advanced after the development by Freud (1856–1939) of the psychoanalytical theory. At that time, some authors suggested that the lack of awareness of a disease could be a form of organic suppression of unacceptable defects or disabilities. These theories had their ancient roots in Charcot's demonstration of unawareness in patients with hysterical disabilities in the absence of organic lesions [17] and were not inconsistent with the view proposed by Anton that unawareness may be a phenomenon independent of the neurological dysfunction. The idea that lack of acknowledgment of a disease may not necessarily be due to a defective awareness, but must sometimes be considered as an extreme but understable pattern of adaptation to stress was first expressed by Schilder [18], who spoke of an "organic repression" whereby the patient excluded from consciousness the unacceptable facts of hemiplegia or blindness. Some years later Weinstein and Kahn [19] coined, in a book which represented the culmination of several years of intensive investigation of the behavioral changes in patients with severe brain disease, the term "Denial of Illness," to define the "form of social behavior in which the patient by an altered mode of interaction in the environment adapts to the stress of his disability." In more recent times, it has been generally acknowledged that denial serves a useful purpose in helping people to cope with sudden intolerable changes, but is harmless as long as it is not maintained too long, as it is fortunately observed in most cases. Several observations suggest that in the acute stage of left-sided hemiplegia, lack of awareness and denial of hemiplegia may co-exist. For instance, Marcel et al. [20] noticed that patients who show no awareness of their deficits in response to a direct verbal question often demonstrate reluctance or verbal circumlocution when asked to perform an online task. Thus, they may find excuses for not performing a bimanual task, even though they may not admit that it is because of their paralyzed arms. An objection that has been raised to the construct of anosognosia as a denial of illness consists of the fact that many common forms of anosognosia concern the left side of the body or of extrapersonal space and that there are studies [21] showing that vestibular stimulation can temporarily improve both the syndrome of spatial unilateral neglect and of anosognosia for left-sided hemiplegia. Several reasons suggest, however, that neither of these objections is decisive. As a matter of fact, in the study by Cappa et al. [21], neglect phenomena improved in all patients after vestibular stimulation, while an effect on anosognosia was found only in some cases. Furthermore, Ramachandran [22], replicating the Cappa et al. [21] observation, showed that anosognosic patients who admitted their paralysis during the vestibular stimulation, a few hours later when the effects of the caloric stimulation wore off relapsed into anosognosia, in spite of recalling in great detail the caloric episode. Finally, the prevalence of right-sided lesions in patients with anosognosia is not necessarily at variance with the motivated suppression hypothesis, because Gainotti has shown that the right hemisphere plays a critical role in emotional behavior [23] and has suggested [24] that the right hemisphere dominance may concern not only the "preverbal implicit memories," considered by Freud [25] as a form of "non-removed" unconscious, but also dynamic unconscious phenomena, such as anosognosia/denial of hemiplegia. It is, therefore, possible that the right hemisphere may play a critical role in unconscious emotional phenomena, resulting from an active process of repression [26].

Anosognosia of Patients with Impaired Cognition

Even though most early studies of anosognosia have focused on hemiplegia and other symptoms resulting from focal brain lesions, in more recent times the weight that AD and other forms of dementia have assumed in today's neuropsychology has led to pay much more attention to anosognosia of patients with impaired cognition. The neuroanatomical correlates of anosognosia in AD have often been investigated with functional imaging studies which have shown, in agreement with the hypothesis of a link between right hemisphere, emotions [23] and anosognosia, that disease unawareness in AD is associated with right-sided abnormalities in the frontal region (e.g., [27, 28]), while the medial temporal lobe, which is usually damaged in mild AD, is not associated with anosognosia [29]. These anatomo-clinical data are consistent with neuropsychological investigations which have shown that the severity of memory disorders alone does not account for anosognosia in AD (e.g., [27, 29]), whereas frontal lobe involvement [30] and the presence of intrusions on memory tasks [31] may be important determining factors of disease unawareness.

Concluding Remarks

We have repeatedly claimed in the previous sections of this chapter that, if we draw on the distinction proposed by Marková and Berrios [4] between the 3 main steps that have contributed to build the construct of "anosognosia," different responses can be given to the question: "How was anosognosia discovered?" As a matter of fact, if we use the term "discovered" to indicate the first description of a strange and unexpected phenomenon, we can say that this discovery was probably made by the stoic philosopher Seneca in a letter to Lucilius, but was inserted in a context of scientific investigations concerning the brain and its pathology by von Monakow [6] and Dejerine and Vialet [7], who gave detailed descriptions of clinical cases and searched for correlations between behavioral findings and anatomical lesions. If, on the contrary, we use this term to indicate a conceptual entity ("disease unawareness") independent from the disease itself and that should be studied by its own, we must certainly attribute this discovery to Anton [2], who singled out the "unawareness of disability" as a phenomenon by itself, that can be present or absent in a given disability and should be subsumed by a specific neural dysfunction. Finally, if we use the term discovery in a still more general acceptation, that is, the unification under the same verbal label of behavioral patterns observed in different disabilities and having in common the fact of pointing to an unawareness of these disabilities, this discovery must be attributed to Babinski [1], who coined a term "anosognosia" that can be applied to every kind of disease unawareness. This unification has facilitated the assumption that "awareness" may be conceptualized and investigated as an independent function in neuropsychology [32] and legitimized the development of accounts, such as that of "denial of illness," that have strongly changed the traditional meaning of "anosognosia." This motivational account has, indeed, proposed that, besides cognitive and sensorimotor factors, emotional factors also play a role in the pathophysiology of disease unawareness, because the suppression of intolerable conscious information can allow the patient to take the time necessary to approach the problem more rationally and to cope effectively with a challenging situation. Many different accounts have been given on anosognosia, usually focusing on hemiplegia for left-sided hemiplegia. Thus Heilman et al. [33] explained it as a specific deficit of feed-forward motor mechanisms, whereas Berti et al. [34] proposed that anosognosia may result from the combination of sensory deficits and higher-order cognitive disorders such as confusion, confabulation, and memory impairments. The problem with all these models is that they can only account for one specific aspect of anosognosia (namely for anosognosia for hemiplegia) neglecting the fact that after Babinski (1914) the general term "anosognosia" has come to signify a state of unawareness of different kinds of neurological impairments. It is, therefore, possible, that anosognosia must be viewed as a multifaceted phenomenon, in which both the disruption of sensorimotor mechanisms and the emergence of neuromotivational factors need to be taken into account [20, 22, 35]. From this point of view, anosognosia should be considered as a work in progress, whose discovery concerns only the foundations of the whole building, whereas the details concerning the mechanisms underlying the different forms of anosognosia and its motivational aspects remain the object of a lively discussion.

References

1 Babinski J: Contribution à l'étude des troubles mentaux dans l'hémiplégie organique cérébrale (Anosognosie). Rev Neurol (Paris) 1914;27:845–848.
2 Anton G: Ueber die Selbstwahrnehmung der Herderkrankungen des Gehirns durch den Kranken bei Rindenblindheit und Rindentaubheit. Arch Psychiatr Nervenkr 1899;32:86–127.
3 Kumbier E, Haack K, Herpertz S: [Considerations on the work of the neuropsychiatrist Gabriel Anton (1858–1933)]. Nervenarzt 2005;76:1132–1136, 1138–1140.
4 Marková IS, Berrios GE: The construction of anosognosia: history and implications. Cortex 2014;61:9–17.
5 Bisiach E, Geminiani G: Anosognosia related to hemiplegia and hemianopia; in Prigatano GP, Schacter DL (eds): Awareness of Deficit after Brain Injury. New York, Oxford University Press, 1991, pp 17–52.
6 von Monakow C: Experimentelle und pathologisch-anatomische Untersuchungen über die Beziehungen der sogennanten Sehsphare zu den infracorticalen Opticuscentren und zum N. opticus. Arch Psychiatr Nervenkr 1885;16:151–199, 317–352.
7 Dejerine JJ, Vialet N: Sur un cas de cecité corticale diagnostiquée pendant la vie et confirmée par l'autopsie. Comptes Rendus de la Societé de Biologie 1893;45:983–987.
8 Prigatano GP, Schacter DL: Awareness of Deficit after Brain Injury: Clinical and Theoretical Issues. Oxford [Oxfordshire], Oxford University Press, 1991.
9 Pick A: Ueber Krankheitsbewusstsein in psychischen Krankheiten. Arch Psychiatr Nervenkr 1882;13:518–581.
10 Geschwind N: Disconnexion syndromes in animals and man. Brain 1965;88:237–294.
11 Tan SY, Shigaki D: Jean-Martin Charcot (1825–1893): pathologist who shaped modern neurology. Singapore Med J 2007;48:383–384.
12 Babinski J: Sur le réflexe cutané plantaire dans certaines affections organiques du système nerveux central. Comptes rendus de la Societè de Biologie 1896;48:207–208.
13 Alajouanine T, Lhermitte F: Des anosognosies electives. Encephale 1957;46:505–519.
14 Feinberg TE, Roane DM, Kwan PC, Schindler RJ, Haber LD: Anosognosia and visuoverbal confabulation. Arch Neurol 1994;51:468–473.
15 Adair JC, Schwartz RL, Na DL, Fennell E, Gilmore RL, Heilman KM: Anosognosia: examining the disconnection hypothesis. J Neurol Neurosurg Psychiatry 1997;63: 798–800.
16 Babinski J: Sur l'anosognosie. Rev Neurol 1923;36:731–732.
17 Charcot JM: L'hystérie. Textes choisis et présentés par E. Trillat, Toulouse, Privat, 1971.
18 Schilder P: Localization of the body image (postural model of the body). Assoc Research Nerv Mental Disorders 1932;13:466–484.
19 Weinstein EA, Kahn RL: Denial of Illness. Sprinfield, IL, Charles C. Thomas, 1955.
20 Marcel AJ, Tegnér R, Nimmo-Smith I: Anosognosia for plegia: specificity, extension, partiality and disunity of bodily unawareness. Cortex 2004;40:19–40.
21 Cappa S, Sterzi R, Vallar G, Bisiach E: Remission of hemineglect and anosognosia during vestibular stimulation. Neuropsychologia 1987;25:775–782.
22 Ramachandran VS: Phantom limbs, neglect syndromes, repressed memories and Freudian psychology. Intern Rev Neurobiol 1994;37:291–333.
23 Gainotti G: Emotional behavior and hemispheric side of lesion. Cortex 1972;8:41–55.
24 Gainotti G: Unconscious processing of emotions and the right hemisphere. Neuropsychologia 2012;50:205–218.
25 Freud S: Group Psychology and the Analysis of the Ego. London, The International Psychoanalytical Press, 1922.
26 Turnbull OH, Solms M: Awareness, desire, and false beliefs: Freud in the light of modern neuropsychology. Cortex 2007;43:1083–1090.
27 Reed BR, Jagust WJ, Coulter L: Anosognosia in Alzheimer's disease: relationships to depression, cognitive function, and cerebral perfusion. J Clin Exp Neuropsychol 1993;15:231–244.
28 Sedaghat F, Dedousi E, Baloyannis I, Tegos T, Costa V, Dimitriadis AS, Baloyannis SJ: Brain SPECT findings of anosognosia in Alzheimer's disease. J Alzheimers Dis 2010;21:641–647.
29 Fujimoto H, Matsuoka T, Kato Y, Shibata K, Nakamura K, Yamada K, Narumoto J: Brain regions associated with anosognosia for memory disturbance in Alzheimer's disease: a magnetic resonance imaging study. Neuropsychiatr Dis Treat 2017;13:1753–1759.
30 Michon A, Deweer B, Pillon B, Agid Y, Dubois B: Relation of anosognosia to frontal lobe dysfunction in Alzheimer's disease. J Neurol Neurosurg Psychiatry 1994; 57:805–809.
31 Dalla Barba G, Parlato V, Iavarone A, Boller F: Anosognosia, intrusions and 'frontal' functions in Alzheimer's disease and depression. Neuropsychologia 1995;33:247–259.
32 McGlynn SM, Schacter DL: Unawareness of deficits in neuropsychological syndromes. J Clin Exp Neuropsychol 1989;11:143–205.
33 Heilman KM, Barrett AM, Adair JC: Possible mechanisms of anosognosia: a defect in self-awareness. Philos Trans R Soc Lond B Biol Sci 1998;353:1903–1909.
34 Berti A, Ladavas E, Della Corte M: Anosognosia for hemiplegia, neglect dyslexia and drawing neglect: clinical findings and theoretical considerations. J Int Neuropsychol Soc 1996;2:426–440.
35 Fotopoulou A, Pernigo S, Maeda R, Rudd A, Kopelman MA: Implicit awareness in anosognosia for hemiplegia: unconscious interference without conscious re-representation. Brain 2010;133:3564–3577.

Guido Gainotti
Institute of Neurology, Policlinico Gemelli
Largo A. Gemelli, 8
IT–00168 Rome (Italy)
E-Mail guido.gainotti@unicatt.it

Bogousslavsky J, Boller F, Iwata M (eds): A History of Neuropsychology.
Front Neurol Neurosci. Basel, Karger, 2019, vol 44, pp 83–88 (DOI: 10.1159/000494955)

History of Amusia

Mitsuru Kawamura[a] Michael W. Miller[b]

[a]Okusawa Hospital and Clinics, Tokyo, Japan; [b]Medical Research Communications Program, The University of Tokyo Postgraduate School of Medicine, Tokyo, Japan

Abstract

We live in a world surrounded by sound. Throughout life, we are exposed to music: from lullabies and songs taught at school to instrumental music both heard and played for pleasure. Every nation, along with its own language, has unique forms of music and dance. "Music knows no boundaries," as the saying goes. Just as language impairment is known as "aphasia," impairment of the perception of music is called "amusia." In this article, we will first classify the types of amusia. This will be followed by an introduction to the classical research of Salomon Eberhard Henschen (1847–1930), and to a discussion of higher auditory functions in which we highlight cases of amusia encountered in a person and through the literature.

Types of Amusia (Table 1)

Amusia is often classified in association with aphasia. Expressive amusia is the impairment of the ability to sing, whistle, and hum, and corresponds to Broca's aphasia. Receptive amusia, the impairment of the ability to distinguish between different melodies, is the musical counterpart to Wernicke's aphasia. Impairment of the ability to recognize familiar tunes is amnesic amusia. Furthermore, musical alexia with agraphia, musical agraphia, can be differentiated into separate conditions, variously affecting musical score literacy. In addition, instrumental amusia affects people trained in playing musical instruments.

This paper is translated from the Japanese article "The pathogenesis of amusia" [Clin Neurosci 2011;29(12):1422–1424].

Table 1. Types of amusia

Expressive amusia	
	Impairment of singing, whistling, and humming ability, due to lesions in the right frontal and temporal lobes
Receptive amusia	
	Impairment of the ability to distinguish between different melodies, due to bilateral or unilateral (left or right) lesions in the temporal and parietal lobes
Amnesic amusia	
	Impairment of the ability to recognize familiar melodies
	The existence of this condition is still debated
Musical alexia	
	Impairment of the ability to write musical scores, due to lesions in the left occipital and temporal lobes
Musical alexia with agraphia	
	Impairment of the ability to read and write musical scores, pure cases are due to lesions in the left angular gyrus
Musical agraphia	
	Impairment of the ability to write musical scores, pure cases are due to lesions in the vicinity of the left intraparietal sulcus
Instrumental amusia	
	Impairment of the ability to play instruments in people with musical training, due to lesions in various regions

Brain Lesions and Amusia

The study of lesions responsible for amusia has a long history. The phrenologist, Franz Joseph Gall (1758–1828), claimed the existence of brain regions governing musical skills. And in 1861, Broca proposed localization of language functions. Thereafter, there was a host of studies in the West on aphasia and amusia.

Henschen's research is of particular importance [1, 2]. He systematized cases of amusia reported in the literature, and published them together with his own cases in German in 1920 and in English in 1926 (Fig. 1). He compared linguistic impairment and musical impairment, and defined the relationship between symptoms and lesions as seen on autopsy. Henschen described musical and linguistic impairments in the following way: "The musical faculty is analogous to that of language and has analogous pathological forms. We have acoustic forms of amusia, that is inability to comprehend music as music, inability to sing, read and write music, and also to execute music, a form of musical apraxia ... and each of these forms has its peculiar localisation in the cortex." Thus, his research suggests that amusia, like aphasia, occurs in various forms, and demonstrates that cases involving musicians and people without a musical background need different approaches. However, Henschen's greatest interest was in the localization of musical functions. According to him, injury to the left temporal pole resulted in sensory amusia. The note-reading center was in the vicinity of the angular gyrus, while injury responsible for impairment of the ability to play musical instruments varied according to the type of instrument. However, singing ability was localized in the anterior part of Broca's area (the left inferior frontal gyrus). He reached the overall conclusion that musical perception and expression probably involved both hemispheres. Henschen's view provoked intense debate and is still considered relevant [3].

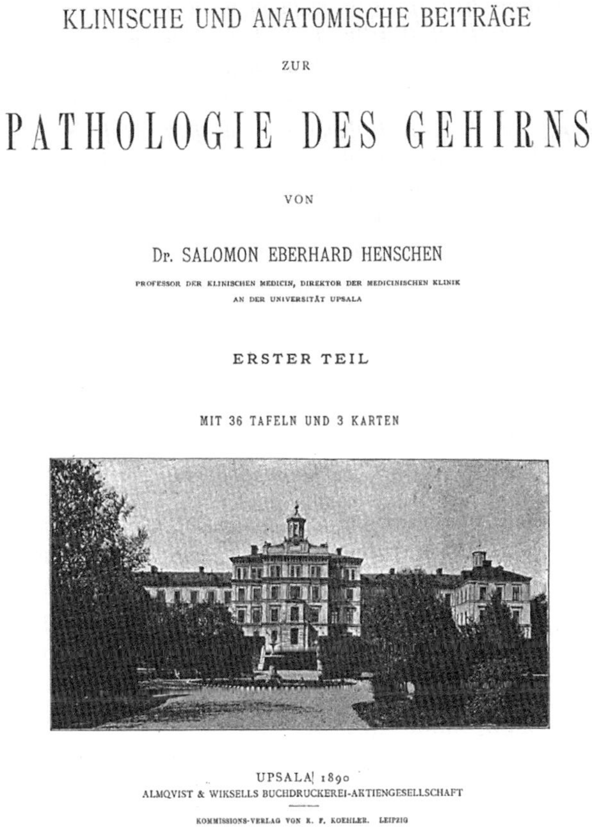

KLINISCHE UND ANATOMISCHE BEITRÄGE

ZUR

PATHOLOGIE DES GEHIRNS

VON

Dr. SALOMON EBERHARD HENSCHEN

PROFESSOR DER KLINISCHEN MEDICIN, DIREKTOR DER MEDICINISCHEN KLINIK AN DER UNIVERSITÄT UPSALA

ERSTER TEIL

MIT 36 TAFELN UND 3 KARTEN

UPSALA 1890
ALMQVIST & WIKSELLS BUCHDRUCKEREI-AKTIENGESELLSCHAFT

KOMMISSIONS-VERLAG VON K. F. KOEHLER. LEIPZIG

Fig. 1. The cover of Henschen's Klinische und anatomische Beiträge zur Pathologie des Gehirns, Teil 1 (Part 1). Part 1 was published in 1890 and Part 8, the last of the series, was published in 1930. Part 5, published in 1920, discusses amusia and acalculia. Parts 6 and 7 deal with sensory and motor aphasia, respectively. Each volume collates and tabulates detailed symptoms and lesions in cases subjected to conventional autopsy.

In fact, many of the problems raised by Henschen remain unsolved: whether brain mechanisms differ between music and language; whether brain organization for music processing differs between musicians and people without musical expertise; and whether a music center, as such, exists. The last question is the focus of recent intensive functional imaging studies. However, these reveal widespread activation.

Expressive Amusia

With regard to expressive musical function, the ability to sing was localized around Broca's area by Henschen. However, a number of reports including those by Yamadori et al. [4] and by one of the present writers, Kawamura [5], reveal that patients with Broca's aphasia and complete loss of spontaneous speech, can still sing songs correctly. Our review of cases in the literature further revealed predominance of frontal and temporal lesions in the right hemisphere in reported cases of expressive amusia [5]. In such cases, the ability to sing was impaired in melody and pitch, but rarely in rhythm.

Receptive Amusia

This results from lesions in the temporal and parietal lobes, and is often accompanied by auditory agnosia and word deafness. The lesions are usually bilateral, but can be unilateral, left or right.

One of the authors (M. Kawamura) treated a 63-year-old right-handed man [5] in whom T2-weighted magnetic resonance imaging revealed high-signal intensity suggestive of cerebral infarction, bilaterally, of temporal and parietal lobes and in the left caudate nucleus. He had relatively good, pure-tone perception but poor speech discrimination, with obvious impairment of ambient sound and music perception. His premorbid history was significant for his better-than-normal ability to sing: his hobby had been singing and he once performed in a song contest. A premorbid tape recording of his songs was available, but he could not recognize them when asked to listen. He then learned the titles and was asked to sing them, but was unable to do so or to reproduce the correct melody and pitch. Nevertheless, without accompaniment, he did sing with relatively correct rhythm and join in with traditional Japanese folk songs.

Just as patients with Wernicke's aphasia are not always capable of correct speech, so people with receptive amusia usually show concomitant impairment of musical expression in singing.

Amnesic Amusia

Although amnesic aphasia is a common type of aphasia, amnesic amusia, that is, impairment of the ability to recognize familiar tunes, has rarely been reported, and opinions differ as to whether it is a separate condition [6].

Musical Alexia: Impairment of the Ability to Read Musical Scores

This condition often accompanies aphasia.

A patient, known widely as Monsieur C, whose condition was diagnosed as alexia without agraphia (pure alexia) by Joseph Jules Déjerine (1849–1917) in 1892, had been trained as a musician [7]. This patient, with damage to the left occipital and temporal lobes, had difficulties reading not only individual words but also musical scores. Nevertheless, he could sing melodies, both familiar and new, play the piano, and write musical scores. Symptoms seen in this patient reveal the existence of aspects common to linguistic and musical expressions in people with musical background. It is interesting that the first reported case of pure alexia should be accompanied by musical alexia.

Beversdorf and Heilman [8] reported a case of posterior cortical atrophy. The patient was a 65-year-old female musician who gradually lost the ability to read new scores. At the same time she lost her ability to read, while retaining the ability to write. Positron-emission tomography revealed bilateral lesions predominantly in the occipital lobes. This is generally consistent with the case of Dejerine's Monsieur C.

Musical Alexia with Agraphia: Impairment of the Ability to Read and Write Musical Scores

In 1891, a year before publishing his case of alexia without agraphia (pure alexia), Dejerine reported impairment of reading and writing (alexia with agraphia) due to lesion in the left angular gyrus. However, he did not describe how musical functions were affected. Kawamura et al. [9] reported a similar case, affecting the ability to read and write musical scores, due to a hemorrhage in the left, angular gyrus. The patient was a professional trombonist.

Musical Agraphia: Impairment of the Ability to Write Musical Scores

Midorikawa and Kawamura [10] have also reported a case of pure musical agraphia without aphasia, or impairment of score reading. The female patient was a graduate of a college of music. A lesion was found proximate to the intraparietal sulcus of the left hemisphere. The location was pathologically significant in two ways: the intraparietal sulcus is associated with pure linguistic agraphia in the left hemisphere. Therefore, this case suggests brain regions associated with both musical and linguistic literacy in those with musical training. The patient had a good sense of pitch, but a severely impaired sense of rhythm.

The findings described in sections 7–9 above suggest that a system for remembering and responding to music is formed in the brains of those with musical training. Extensive involvement of the left hemisphere is a possibility for trained musicians. Furthermore, Midorikawa et al. [11] once treated a piano teacher with an infarct in Wernicke's area who exhibited Wernicke's aphasia with impairment of score reading. The resultant musical alexia was characterized by a preserved sense of pitch but inability to read rhythm. In general, amusia varies for those with musical training.

Instrumental Amusia: Impairment of the Ability to Play Musical Instruments

Although there are reported cases of impairment of the ability to play musical instruments, such as guitar, shamisen (a traditional Japanese string instrument), accordion, and organ, they have not been definitively linked to particular locations. Such ability may be more global and requires further study.

Concluding Remarks

While writing this article, we also considered the musician Evelyn Glennie (Dame Evelyn Elizabeth Ann Glennie, DBE). Glennie is a percussionist and keyboardist from Scotland. Her father was an accordionist, and she studied at the Royal Academy of Music. She started losing her hearing at the age of 8, and lost nearly all of it by the age of 12. Despite this, she perceives sound waves somatically and is a leading, virtuoso percussionist.

In the introduction, we stated our intention to discuss music perception in terms of higher auditory functions. However, the example of Glennie suggests that musical perception is not limited to auditory perception, and may involve, for example, somatosensory perception. Her case offers an important clue towards better understanding of music in the brain.

Acknowledgements

The research was supported by Grants-in-Aid for Scientific Research (also known as KAKENHI) for Innovative Areas (JP 25119006; JP 18H05525).

References

1 Henschen SE: Klinische und Anatomische Beiträge zur Pathologie des Gehirns, Teil 5: Über Aphasie, Amusie und Akalkulie. Stockholm, Nordiska Bokhandeln, 1920.
2 Henshen SE: On the function of the right hemisphere of the brain in relation to the left in speech, music and calculation. Brain 1926;49:110–126.
3 Basso A: Amusia; in Boller F, Grafman J (eds): Handbook of Neuropsychology. New York, Elsevier Science Publishers, 1993, vol 8, pp 391–409.
4 Yamadori A, Osumi Y, Masuhara S, et al: Preservation of singing in Broca's aphasia. J Neurol Neurosurg Psychiatry 1977;40:221–224.
5 Kawamura M: Expressive Aspects of Amusia. JPN J Logoped Phoniatr 1996;37:468–473.
6 Midorikawa A: Amusia. Brain and Nerve 2007;59:865–870.
7 Hanley JR, Kay J: Monsieur C, Dejerine's case of alexia without agraphia; in Code C, Wallesch CW, Joanette Y, Lecours AR (eds): Classic Cases in Neuropsychology. Hove, Psychology Press, 2003, vol 2, pp 57–74.
8 Beversdorf DQ, Heilman KM: Progressive ventral posterior cortical degeneration presenting as alexia for music and words. Neurology 1998;50:657–659.
9 Kawamura M, Midorikawa A, Kezuka M: Cerebral localization of the center for reading and writing music. Neuroreport 2000;11:3299–3303.
10 Midorikawa A, Kawamura M: A case of musical agraphia. Neuroreport 2000;11:3053–3057.
11 Midorikawa A, Kawamura M, Kezuka M: Musical alexia for rhythm notation: a discrepancy between pitch and rhythm. Neurocase 2003;9:232–238.

Mitsuru Kawamura, MD
Okusawa Hospital and Clinics
2-Chome-11-1
Setagaya
Tokyo 158-0083 (Japan)
E-Mail river7941@gmail.com

Bogousslavsky J, Boller F, Iwata M (eds): A History of Neuropsychology.
Front Neurol Neurosci. Basel, Karger, 2019, vol 44, pp 89–99 (DOI: 10.1159/000494956)

Hemineglect and Attentional Dysfunction

Karen G. Langer[a] Bartlomiej Piechowski-Jozwiak[b]
Julien Bogousslavsky[c]

[a]Rusk Rehabilitation, NYU Langone Medical Center, New York, NY, USA; [b]Neurological Institute, Cleveland Clinic, Abu Dhabi, United Arab Emirates; [c]Neurocenter, Swiss Medical Network, Clinique Valmont, Montreux, Switzerland

Abstract

Tracing the history of neglect is intriguing, as diverse terminologies have been used to characterize a multi-factorial disorder with rather startling manifestations. In part, heterogeneous terms may have hinted at distinct subtypes. Thus, different variants of hemi-inattention and neglect relate conceptually, but may be functionally dissociable. Patients with neglect, acting as if the world-space they perceive is full, do not phenomenally experience the omissions or absences so patently obvious to an observer. From the late 19th century, hemi-inattention was described according to its prominent manifestations, visual, bodily or spatial. Since then, diverse terms including imperception, inattention, unilateral visual inattention, unilateral spatial agnosia, and neglect, among others, reflected proposed underlying mechanisms. Major theories presented to account for this curious, even astonishing, neurological disorder, included disruption of body-scheme, perceptual rivalry and extinction, forgetting or amnesia for half the body, and highly nuanced models of distribution of directed spatial attention, and of disrupted perceptual processes. Unlike neurological counterparts, already designated as hemi-syndromes by the first part of the 20th century, not until about 1970 did neglect become so broadly recognized as a syndrome. Earlier, commonalities were identified, features conceptually clustered, and then subtypes were distinguished. Neglect was designated as an overarching term for a class of disorder with distinct subtypes, including visual, motor, extrapersonal, bodily or personal, other somatosensory, and representational. Specificity for modality, chronology, material, and symptom severity was noted. Remarkable clinical, neuropsychological, and behavioral manifestations of hemi-inattention and neglect may involve varying proposed mechanisms of higher cognitive functions, all within a spectrum of clinical disorder. Concepts of connectivity and interaction, neural networks, and functional integration enhance understanding of dysfunction, recovery, and compensation in neglect and inattention. Focus on distinct manifestations clustered under the umbrella of neglect offers a vantage point for examining historical trends in approach to the phenomenon.

Introduction

The literature on the history of the term hemi-neglect reveals heterogeneous terminology, characterizing a multi-faceted disorder that encompasses differing manifestations. The fact that these may be co-occurring or dissociable, under an umbrella term of neglect, likely also led to heterogeneity of prior classification. Even from a linguistic perspective, "neglect" in the English lexicon has multiple designations, and is used either as a verb, "Neglect, v.t., ... To omit by carelessness or design; to forbear to do, use, ... or attend to ...", or a noun, "n. Omission; forbearance to do anything that can be done or that requires to be done" [1].

The term neglect is used here as representative of a class of disorder, with sub-types that are conceptually related but functionally independent. The variants include categories of visual, other somatosensory, motor, representational [2], also called mental space [3], and bodily hemi-inattention or personal neglect. Patients with neglect seem particularly unaware of the side of space or the body, and act as if they were ignoring or disregarding objects, persons, self, or space, specific to the affected side [4]. The patient with neglect believes that the world-space as s/he perceives it is veridical, is real, is full, believes that the part of space, body, or object perceived is full, and does not realize that there is a part missing to them; it is not experienced as absent. Instead, the patient seems to have, or know, only one side of themselves, or of space [5]; the other side seems to no longer exist. That is, to the observer. For the patient, phenomenologically, the world appears complete and/or whole as it is, and s/he does not identify anything as missing. One account suggests the process of "perceptual completion" to explain this phenomenal experience, such that the patient perceives a complete whole with the incomplete part filled in or perceptually completed, escaping detection, which "must be discovered by a process of self observation and inference" (p 233) [6]. This explanation has served for both unawareness and neglect.

Unlike many other disorders related to cerebral dysfunction, neglect had not been very widely used to designate a syndrome until at least the middle of the 20th century, largely by 1970, when "neglect" was a featured term in neurological texts and neuropsychological literature. However, manifestations of hemi-inattention had been described a century earlier as case reports, and later as case series or studies. Still, despite definitions of various symptomatology, at the turn of the 20th century the remarkable manifestations of neglect begged further definition and elaboration. The history of discovery and definition of this startling, dramatic disorder is itself intriguing.

History of Terminology Describing Hemi-Inattention and Neglect

Imperception

In one of the earliest attempts to depict a curious phenomenon, Hughlings Jackson [7] (Fig. 1) described a patient with a large glioma of the "right temporo-sphenoidal lobe"

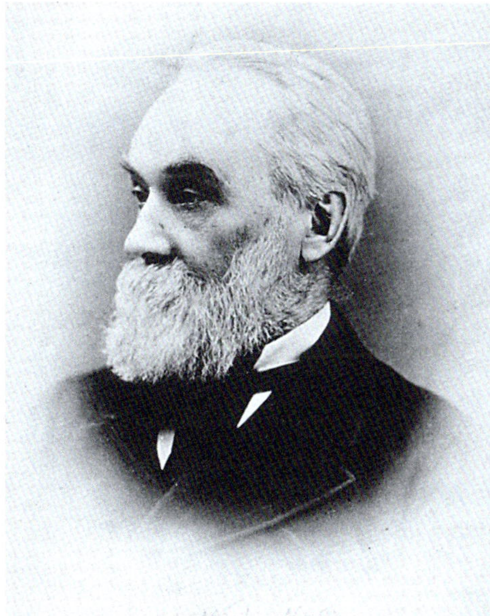

Fig. 1. John Hughlings Jackson. Courtesy of the US National Library of Medicine.

with left hemiplegia and with "imperception." Imperception involved a defect involving visual ideas, that is, a defect in knowing "objects, persons, places." The term imperception was later applied to symptoms associated with neglect. Described as "amnestic and agnostic unawareness of the impaired parts or half of the body, varying in degree from simple neglect of their presence to the experience of their nonexistence" (p 912) [8], and "imperception for one half of external space" (p 339) [5], it became a synonym for personal and hemi-spatial neglect. The patient with neglect "... may pay no attention to the paralyzed side, as though he had forgotten it; some not only neglect the defective side but even refuse to look at it or turn away to the right" (p 892) [8]. Thus conceptualized, hemi-neglect was considered a disorder of the "postural model" of the body.

Notably, imperception had at that time been associated with amaurosis. Amaurosis, defined as blindness indicating cerebral disease, without retinal or optic nerve alteration, was a unilateral visual effect difficult for the patient to lateralize, reflecting imperception [9].

Dyschiria

Dyschiria was described as a distinct defect in appreciating unilateral excitation specific to failure to appreciate sidedness, more notable with conscious volitional mental processes than automatic processes [10].

Inattention

A classic paper [11] amply described unilateral sensory manifestations of cerebral disease, with first apparent use of term "inattention" applied to the affected hand. A specific defect of attention could be lateralized to the affected side, rather than simply a defect of gen-

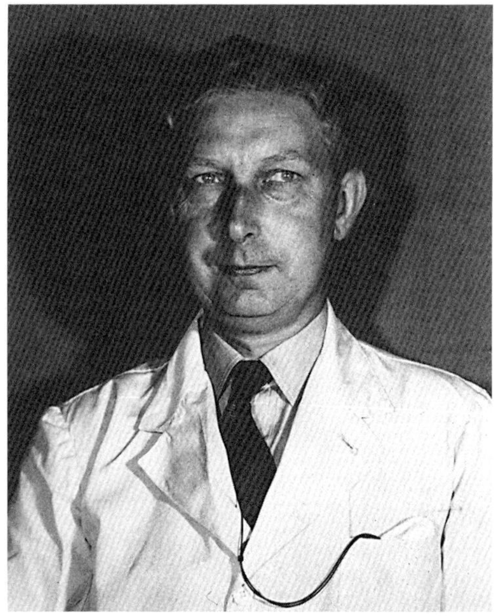

Fig. 2. Walter Russell Brain. Courtesy of the US National Library of Medicine.

eral attention [11]. The original study leading to the "postural model of the body" is attributed to Head and Holmes, though notions of topographic body schema had, under a variety of different names, been proposed earlier.

Visual Inattention

Specificity of inattention was realized shortly thereafter, with "visual inattention" [12] used in the context of disordered space perception. In 1900, a hallmark feature of visual inattention was identified, conjugate deviation of the head and eyes towards the direction of the unaffected side (i.e., ipsilesional), particularly in acute stages with hemiplegia [13]. Since then, this feature is vividly portrayed.

Unilateral visual inattention was distinguished from spatial disorientation and space perception [14]. In a series of cases, unilateral visual inattention was only variably associated with visual field defects, which is further evidence for the independent existence of visual hemi-inattention [15].

Unilateral Spatial Agnosia

Unilateral Spatial Agnosia described agnosia specific for the left half of external space, and not simply agnosia for the spatial relationships between visual objects [16]. Brain (Fig. 2) is credited with highlighting the relationship between disordered perception of the body and perception of external space. Concurring with Brain, it was noted that, "although the external space is appreciated as a unitary perception, it has been partially built up perceptually by exploring space with the limbs" (p 3660) [17], a suggestion since supported by evidence on visually guided behavior. Total unilateral spatial agnosia involves a disorder in which "The patient neglects the existence of the left half of external space…" (p 3661)

[17]. The association of spatial agnosia with inattention and neglect was widely described [18–21], and included visual spatial agnosia and neglect of the left side of the body [22], visual and personal neglect [23], and symptoms of (visual) inattention and extrapersonal hemi-spatial neglect [20].

To explain the underlying mechanism of inattention, the phenomenon of extinction was proposed [24, 25]. Bender attributed to Hippocrates the early understanding that a milder pain may be obscured or "inhibited" by a stronger pain [26], fundamentally explaining inattention and underlying extinction by means of rivalry in perception. Extinction is generally credited to Oppenheim [13], who utilized the method of double stimulation. Weaker gradations of sensory stimuli may become "imperceptible," with perceptual rivalry understood to be a mechanism of extinction [24]. Further elaboration of this hypothesis defined "visual inattention or extinction" as "the failure to notice movement of an object … in one half-field, when there is a competing stimulus in the opposite half-field" (p 51) [27].

Unilateral spatial agnosia after right hemispheric lesions was characterized by "distinctive ignorance of the opposite (left) side of the body and the ignorance of the left side of space, connected with it …" (p 165) [28]. Damage to the posterior zone of the right hemisphere leads to left-sided fixed hemianopia [28], or inattention to the left side [5, 12, 16, 18, 28], while involvement of right hemispheric middle zones leads more to inattention to the left side of the body, and sometimes of the general body schema [28].

Neglect

The term "neglect" used to depict extrapersonal spatial hemi-inattention, "an inattention to, or neglect of, the left half of external space" associated with right parietal lesions, is credited to Brain (pp 246; 257) [16]. Brain later favored concepts of "inattention, visual," and "disorders of body scheme" [27]. Parietal lesions were considered "responsible for some of the most bizarre psychophysiological disturbances. Thus, the patient may be unaware of the opposite half of his body-autotopagnosia" (p 99) [27], reflecting a general disorder of body scheme. Even as localization pointed to the involvement of parietal lobes [5] along with some other sites, there was growing awareness of varying degrees and manifestations of disturbance.

The remarkable type of neglect pertaining to the body has also been marked by different terminologies, but the symptoms associated with it have been rather uniform and classic. From the simple to the more dramatic features described in case reports [5, 29], including inattention to personal grooming (e.g., shaving, makeup, etc.) on only one side, dressing limited to one side, the striking features paint a vivid picture. These florid and unmistakable manifestations were of great neurological interest and pathognomonic of parietal disease. Critchley proposed that (motor) neglect is exhibited by a lack of spontaneous use of the arm even though it does not lack motor strength, and impoverished spontaneous movement [5] not accounted for by apraxia or sensory ataxia. Confusion may exacerbate the dramatic or bizarre presentation, such that, "To passive disregard is added active neglect" (p 227) [5]. Finally, Critchley described not just having absence of half the body image, but also "having and knowing only one side … the right" (p 229) [5].

Unilateral neglect extends outward into external space (extrapersonal), beyond the personal. Dual aspects of neglect, identified as visual and personal neglect, are reflected in case reports describing multi-faceted phenomena [23]. By the late 1960s, the term visual spatial neglect differentiated it from other types of inattention or neglect [30]. By the 1970s, however, the use of "neglect" as a syndrome proliferated, even as precise definition or interpretation of cause varied. Consideration of neglect by many distinguished clinicians flourished, from clinical, theoretical, and empirical perspectives [28, 31–33].

Other Usages of Neglect and Associated Concepts

Interestingly, evidence exists for the use of the word neglect in other languages to depict the puzzling syndrome, specifically bodily neglect. Pinéas [34] mentioned "neglect" in German, with "Vernachlässigung der linken Seite" [neglect of the left side]. This patient with dyschiria, inattention to personal hygiene, but preserved sensorium and no paresis nor hemianopia, had relatives who noticed [peculiar neglect of the left side – for example she can only turn to the right side and always forgets to get (her arm) into the left sleeve, or to put on the left shoe] (p 180) [34].

At that time, the disorder was not yet termed a syndrome nor coined "neglect" in the way that anosognosia [35] was coined to describe unawareness. However, in French, early use of "la négligence" appears to describe neglect phenomena, especially personal neglect, in patients who "act as if the limb never existed" or seem uninterested in it [36]. Patients displaying unilateral personal neglect were portrayed with "meme 'négligence' pour la jambe" [also neglect of the leg] (p 542) [29] and "il présente une amputation de son hémi-corps gauche …" (p 545) [29] [he presents (as with) an amputation of the left side of the body], dramatically depicting the phenomenon.

Additional terms were coined to capture phenomena related to neglect. Largely these reflected disturbances of body awareness, and included apractagnosia, amorphosynthesis, autotopagnosia, and somato-agnosia; these and other terms are summarized elsewhere [32].

Assessment, Recovery, and Remediation of Hemi-Inattention and Neglect

Historically, attention to features of hemi-inattention and neglect grew throughout the early part of the 20th century. Following the description of conjugate deviation of the eyes and head unilaterally [13], other behaviors associated with visual hemi-inattention (e.g., bumping into doors on the affected side) and clinical assessment techniques (e.g., rod bisection tasks, possibly a precursor of line bisection; poor performance on reading tasks) were summarized [36]. Clinical examination used double simultaneous stimulation for tactile and visual inattention, response to instruction to move one or both extremities, verbal report of side of stimulation, deviation of eyes and head, and observation of attention to details in dressing and grooming for overt signs of neglect.

Traditionally, neuropsychological assessment of visual hemi-inattention has included measures of visual scanning and lateralized attention (e.g., cancellation tasks), reading, counting scattered objects, describing pictures, and graphomotor tasks including spontaneous drawing or drawing to command, design copy and recall, clock drawing, and writing [37, 38]. Errors of omission, distortions and response biases affecting the contralesional side, deviation from midline and pull towards the ipsilesional side, perceptual distortions, spatial biases in nonverbal or visual-perceptual problem-solving, simplification, and graphic omission of material on the contralesional side, all became recognized hallmark indicators of hemi-inattention and neglect.

As neglect gained recognition as an effect of cerebral dysfunction, attempts to remediate were also developed, though largely focusing on visual inattention or visual-spatial neglect. Visual neglect was suggested to underlie some neuropsychological difficulties in complex visual perception [39]. Additional hemi-inattention problems involved telling the time on a clock or on a written schedule, making sense of a television show or movie, reading, copying designs or in arithmetic. Remediation techniques for these [38, 40] included practice with single column of text, large print, tracking and scanning to the left with moving targets, cues from verbal intelligibility and coherence, colorful highlighting and anchoring to the left in reading, and tactual-kinesthetic cues for perceptual and visual attentional deficits. Mood support has been provided for associated psychological factors. Difficulty in carry-over of attention to the left side, even when demonstrated, is an important feature [38], as patients do not realize the difficulty phenomenally, do not experience the absence of information; they must learn to discover it [6]. Systematic remedial training was suggested as beneficial for certain types of dysfunction.

Early Ideas about the Origins of Hemi-Inattention and Neglect

In the early literature describing neglect, features of attention and forgetfulness are often highlighted. A few examples illustrate this:

"The patient may pay no attention to the paralyzed side, as though he had forgotten it; some not only neglect the defective side but even refuse to look at it or turn away to the right" (p 892) [8].

"... comme si le malade avait perdu la notion de l'existence de son membre supérieur gauche. Cet oubli du membre superieur ne s'explique pas par des perturbations de sensibilité consciente." [... as if the patient has lost the notion of the existence of the upper left extremity. This forgetting of the upper limb is not explained by disturbances of conscious sensation] (p 696) [41].

"Amnesia for the limbs of one side is not a rare symptom. The patient loses these limbs from his body scheme and ignores them." (p 48) [42].

Forgetting the Limb

Ample precedence existed throughout classic French literature on anosognosia for notions of forgetting the limb or the function [36]. Indeed, Babinski observed patients' inability to pay attention to or "fix their attention" to the limb [35]. In Babinski's paper [35],

Meige described "amnésie fonctionelle motrice" (functional motor amnesia), noting that patients "neglect" to spontaneously make movements that are motorically possible, behave as if the limb no longer existed, and that memory of the function seems lost. Amnesia for half the body was a striking conceptualization of neglect.

Attentional Disorder

Roots of a current theory of neglect, involving distribution of spatial attention [33, 43, 44], were visible early in the 20th century. Difficulty in which the patient "cannot fix attention to" the limb on the impaired side, a key feature of neglect, was recognized [27]. Unlike anosognosia where patients are unaware of (or "forget") the paralysis, in neglect, it is the limb that has lost receipt of attention, and the patient is not conscious of it.

Attentional explanations of neglect abounded from the 1970s onwards. A disorder of "directed attention," or ability to direct focus of attention on "relevant" sensory events in external space, postulating an attentional-arousal disturbance [33], remains a prominent theory. Neglect was further described as a disturbance in the "spatial distribution of directed sensory attention," setting a foundation for later writers.

Psychic Amputation

Neglect has been painted powerfully. Beyond attentional disregard, neglect was described as a psychological amputation, as if there was an "amputation" of the left side of the body, with the patient remaining uninterested in the affected left side of the body, which is used either poorly or not at all [29, 45].

Body Scheme

The body scheme and concepts of the postural model of the body evolved naturally from the prototype incorporating body movement with the schemata of self [11]. Disruption of body scheme and disordered representation of limb and self were considered central to bodily neglect phenomena [5, 8, 29, 45]. Body scheme notions were popular conceptualizations of the disturbance in neglect and its related symptoms [5].

Perceptual Accounts

Perceptual accounts focus on concepts of extinction and perceptual rivalry to explain hemi-inattention. The fundamental importance of normal psychological functions [24], plus processes including perceptual rivalry, suppression and extinction, and attention mechanisms, are together explanations for unilateral visual inattention. Tachistoscopic demonstration of extinction served as further supporting evidence. Sophisticated experimentation described in split-brain studies emphasized the impact of hemispheric disconnection, though functional cognitive interpretations have been encouraged in the context of neuronal interconnection networks [46].

Another perceptual process proposed to explain the curious features of unawareness and hemi-inattention in cerebral dysfunction is perceptual completion, such that absence is not directly experienced [6]. Drawing parallel to other conditions of inaccurate bodily estimation, such as phantom limb in amputation [6], completion is suggested to account for phenomenal experience of body wholeness.

Summary and Discussion

Heterogeneous terminology proliferated throughout the century, possibly obscuring commonalities in neglect syndromes. Rightly, it is noted that the word neglect derives from the lay vocabulary and therefore, "more resistant to strict usage" [44]. Clearly, designation of the cluster of symptoms in a syndrome of neglect lagged behind earlier classification of other neurological conditions, such as heminanopsia, cortical blindness, or anosognosia.

The diversity of terms for the clinical, neuropsychological, and behavioral manifestations of hemi-inattention and neglect highlights the complexity and multi-factorial nature of the syndrome. However, the designation of neglect as a single syndrome may be theoretically problematic, as suggested, since many aspects in the spectrum of the clinical disorder are dissociable, within (temporally and symptomatically) and between patients, and may be specific to modality, spatial domain, or material [32, 47, 48].

Recent exposition of the semiology of neglect proposes distinctive anatomical and clinical subtypes, with different underlying mechanisms [49], involving spatial awareness, cognition, and attention as a higher-level disorder [50]. That different neuronal networks may be implicated is further evidence against a unitary explanation of neglect [3]. Indeed, notions of "integrative" functions of the cerebral hemispheres [3] supplant those of strictly inhibitory or rivalrous cerebral interactions, emphasizing connectivity and neural networks, compensation and recovery [3]. Recognition of distinct manifestations of the disorder clustered under the umbrella of neglect offers a vantage point for examining historical trends in approach to the phenomenon.

Acknowledgments

The first author expresses gratitude for the kindness and inspiration of Andre Langer. Also gratefully acknowledged is the thoughtful assistance of Arlene Shaner, Historical Collections Librarian at the NY Academy of Medicine, Frank Stryczek, RN, for German text translation, and Librarians Michael Agnew, NYU Bobst, and David DeSimone, NYUHSL.

References

1 Webster N: An American Dictionary of the English Language. New York, S. Converse, 1828, vol 2. (Reprinted from the original edition by Johnson Reprint Corp., New York and London, 1970).

2 Bisiach E, Luzzatti C: Unilateral neglect of representational space. Cortex 1978;14:129–133.

3 Carota A, Bogousslavsky J: Minor hemisphere major syndromes; in Bogousslavsky J (ed): Neurologic-Psychiatric Syndromes in Focus – Part I. From Neurology to Psychiatry. Front Neurol Neurosci. Basel, Karger, 2018, vol 41, pp 1–13.

4 Halligan PW, Marshall JC: The history and clinical presentation of neglect; in Robertson IH, Marshall JC (eds): Unilateral Neglect: Clinical and Experimental Studies. Hove, Lawrence Erlbaum Publishers, 1993, pp 3–25.

5 Critchley M: The Parietal Lobes. New York, NY, Hafner Press, 1953.

6 Levine DN: Unawareness of visual and sensorimotor defects: a hypothesis. Brain Cogn 1990;13:233–281.

7 Hughlings Jackson J: Case of Large Cerebral Tumour without Optic Neuritis, and with Left Hemiplegia and Imperception. Reprinted from Royal London Ophthalmic Hospital Reports, 1876, vol 8, pp 434–444.

8 Gerstmann J: Problem of imperception of disease and of impaired body territories with organic lesions. Relation to body scheme and its disorders. Arch Neurol Psychiatr 1942;48:890–913.

9 Adams JJ: A new operation for the cure of amaurosis, impaired vision and shortsightedness, in a letter addressed to John Richard Farre MD. London, John Churchill, 1841.

10 Jones E: The clinical significance of allochiria. Lancet 1907;2:830–832.

11 Head H, Holmes G: Sensory disturbances from cerebral lesions. Brain 1911;34:102–254.

12 Holmes G: Disturbances of visual space perception. Brit Med J 1919;2:230–233.

13 Oppenheim H: Diseases of the Nervous System. A Textbook for Students and Practitioners of Medicine. Translated by E.E. Mayer. (First American from the second revised and enlarged German edition.) Philadelphia, J.B. Lippincott & Co., 1900. (Originally published as Lehrbuch der Nervenkrankheiten: für Äerzte und Studirende, 1898, ed 2, Berlin, S. Karger.)

14 Riddoch G: Visual disorientation in homonymous halffields. Brain 1935;58:376–382.

15 Allen IM: Unilateral visual inattention. New Zeal Med J 1948;47:605–617.

16 Brain WR: Visual disorientation with special reference to lesions of the right cerebral hemisphere. Brain 1941; 64:244–272.

17 Duke-Elder WS: Text-Book of Ophthalmology, vol 4. The Neurology of Vision, Motor and Optical Anomalies. St. Louis, C.V. Mosby Co., 1949, pp 3619–3730.

18 McFie J, Piercy MF, Zangwill OL: Visual-spatial agnosia associated with lesions of the right cerebral hemisphere. Brain 1950;73:167–190.

19 McFie J, Zangwill OL: Visual-constructive disabilities associated with lesions of the left cerebral hemisphere. Brain 1960;83:243–260.

20 Battersby WS, Bender MB, Pollack M, Kahn RL: Unilateral "spatial agnosia" ("inattention") in patients with cerebral lesions. Brain 1956;79:68–93.

21 Hécaen H, De Ajuriaguerra J, Massonnet J: Les troubles visuo-constructifs par lésion pariéto-occipitale droite; role des perturbations vestibulaires [Visuo-motor difficulties due to parieto-occipital lesion; role of vestibular perturbations]. Encéphale 1951;40:122–179.

22 Hécaen H, Penfield W, Bertrand C, Malmo R: The syndrome of apractognosia due to lesions of the minor cerebral hemisphere. Arch Neurol Psychiatr 1956;75:400–434.

23 Ettlinger G, Warrington E, Zangwill OL: A further study of visual-spatial agnosia. Brain 1957;80:335–361.

24 Bender MB, Furlow LT: Phenomenon of visual extinction in homonymous fields and psychologic principles involved. Arch Neurol Psychiatr 1945;53:29–33.

25 Wortis SB, Bender MB, Teuber HL: The significance of the phenomenon of extinction. J Nerv Ment Dis 1948; 107:382–387.

26 Bender MB: Extinction and other patterns of sensory interaction; in Weinstein EA, Friedland RP (eds): Advances in Neurology, vol 18. New York, Raven Press, 1977, pp 107–110.

27 Brain WR: Diseases of the Nervous System, ed 6. London, Oxford University Press, 1962 (1st ed published 1933).

28 Luria AR: The Working Brain. An Introduction to Neuropsychology (Translated by Basil Haigh). New York, Basic Books, 1973.

29 Van Bogaert L: Sur la pathologie de l'image de soi. Ann Méd-Psychol 1934;ser. 14, 92:519–555; 744–759.

30 Costa LD, Vaughan HG Jr, Horwitz M, Ritter W: Patterns of behavioral deficit associated with visual spatial neglect. Cortex 1969;5:242–263.

31 Kinsbourne M: A model for the mechanism of unilateral neglect of space. T Am Neurol Assoc 1970;95:143–146.

32 Weinstein EA, Friedland RP (eds): Advances in Neurology, vol 18, Hemi-Inattention and Hemisphere Specialization. New York, Raven Press, 1977.

33 Heilman KM: Neglect and related disorders; in Heilman KM, Valenstein E (eds): Clinical Neuropsychology, ed 1. New York, Oxford University Press, 1979, pp 268–307 (5th ed published 2012).

34 Pinéas H: Ein Fall von räumlicher Orientierungsstörung mit Dyschirie. Z Gesamte Neurol Psy 1931;133:180–195.

35 Babinski J: Contribution à l'étude des troubles mentaux dans l'hémiplégie organique cérébrale (Anosognosie). Rev Neurol (Paris) 1914;27:845–848.

36 Langer KG: Babinski's Anosognosia for hemiplegia in early twentieth-century French Neurology. J Hist Neurosci 2009;18:387–405.

37 Albert ML: A simple test of visual neglect. Neurology 1973;23:658–664.

38 Diller L, Weinberg J: Hemi-inattention in rehabilitation: the evolution of a rational remediation program; in Weinstein EA, Friedland RP (eds): Advances in Neurology, vol 18, Hemi-Inattention and Hemisphere Specialization. New York, Raven Press, 1977, pp 63–82.

39 Gainotti G, Tiacci C: The relationships between disorders of visual perception and unilateral spatial neglect. Neuropsychologia 1971;9:451–458.
40 Lawson IR: Visual-spatial neglect in lesions of the right cerebral hemisphere. A study in recovery. Neurology 1962;12:23–33.
41 Alajouanine T, Thurel R, Ombredane A: Somato-agnosie et apraxie du membre supérieur gauche. Rev Neurol 1934;41:695–703.
42 Cobb S: Amnesia for the left limbs developing into anosognosia. B Los Angeles Neurol Soc 1947;12:48–52.
43 Heilman KM, Pandya DN, Geschwind N: Trimodal inattention following parietal lobe ablations. T Am Neurol Assoc 1970;95:259–261.
44 Mesulam MM: Attention, confusional states and neglect; in Mesulam MM (ed): Principles of Behavioral Neurology, Contemporary Neurology Series. Philadelphia, PA, F.A. Davis, 1985, pp 125–168.
45 Garcin R, Varay A, Hadji-Dimo (no init): Document pour servir à l 'étude des troubles du schéma corporel (sur quelques phénomènes moteurs, gnosiques et quelques troubles de l'utilisation des membres du côté gauche au cours d'un syndrôme temporo-pariétal par tumeur, envisagés dans leurs rapports avec l'anosognosie et les troubles du schéma corporel). Rev Neurol 1938;69:498–510.
46 Gazzaniga MS, Ladavas E: Disturbances in spatial attention following lesion or disconnection of the right parietal lobe; in Jeannerod M (ed): Neurophysiological and Neuropsychological Aspects of Spatial Neglect. North Holland, Elsevier Science Publishers BV, 1987, pp 203–213.
47 Bisiach E, Perani D, Vallar G, Berti A: Unilateral neglect: personal and extrapersonal. Neuropsychologia 1986;24: 759–767.
48 Marshall JC, Halligan PW, Robertson IH: Contemporary theories of unilateral neglect: a critical review; in Robertson IH, Marshall JC (eds): Unilateral Neglect: Clinical and Experimental Studies. Hove, Lawrence Erlbaum Associates, 1993, pp 311–329.
49 Rode G, Pagliari C, Huchon L, Rossetti Y, Pisella L: Semiology of neglect: an update. Ann Phys Med Rehab 2017;60:177–185.
50 Vallar G, Calzolari E: Unilateral spatial neglect after posterior parietal damage; in Vallar G, Coslett HB (eds): Handbook of Clinical Neurology, vol 151, series 3, The Parietal Lobe. North Holland, Elsevier BV, 2018, pp 287–312.

Karen G. Langer, PhD
Rusk Rehabilitation, NYU Langone Medical Center
301 East 17th Street
New York, NY 10003 (USA)
E-Mail karen.langer@nyumc.org

Bogousslavsky J, Boller F, Iwata M (eds): A History of Neuropsychology.
Front Neurol Neurosci. Basel, Karger, 2019, vol 44, pp 100–107 (DOI: 10.1159/000494957)

History of "Frontal" Syndromes and Executive Dysfunction

Jonathan DeRight
Private Practice, McLean, VA, USA

Abstract

Elements of "frontal" syndromes and executive dysfunction have been pondered by humans since ancient times, perhaps because executive dysfunction often threatens the very characteristics that make us human. This chapter provides a historical account of scientific advancements related to frontal lobe functioning and how the term has transformed over time. From ancient Greek philosophy to early neuroscientific animal studies to the default mode network, knowledge about the neural underpinnings of executive functioning has blossomed, almost so broadly that the behemoth term comprising broad neuropsychological functions may struggle to be provide specificity on its own without further clarification.

Introduction

Historically, study of the human brain primarily stemmed from experiments involving excitation and lesioning of brain structures of animal brains. From the mid-1800s onward, fruits of this experimental method led to an ever-advancing collection of findings related to the functioning of the temporal, occipital, parietal, and sensorimotor portions of the cerebral cortex. Knowledge about the frontal lobes, however, was far less established, as their complex functions exceeded the limits of simpler cause and effect models. At one point, the frontal lobes were even considered by many to be "silent zones" with no clearly defined function [1], while later research proved this area to be anything but silent.

Scientific advancements have since established the area's role in complex goal-directed behavior and many other uniquely human qualities that have been pondered for centuries dating back to the ancient Greeks. Fast forwarding to the 1970s, the term "executive functioning" was created to encompass various cognitive functions of the prefrontal area of the frontal lobes including planning, working memory, attention, inhibition, self-monitoring, self-regulation, and initiation [2]. Three clusters of symptoms, termed historically as the "frontal lobe syndromes" (now more broadly encompassed by the term "dysexecutive syndromes"), were based on the location of damage to the dorsolateral, orbitofrontal, and medial frontal areas of the frontal lobe [3, 4]. These syndromes have been of significant interest over the years, possibly because their symptoms undermine qualities that we associate most with being human [3]. This chapter will outline the historical roots of inquiry into various executive functions, how the "frontal syndromes" have transformed from a structure-function model to an associational level, and the nebulous definition of what exactly comprises executive functioning.

Ancient Inquiry about Modern Executive Functions

Table 1 depicts a timeline of select works that were important in the development of executive functioning over time. Dating back to the ancient Greeks, the neural origin of executive functions such as abstract thought [5], the soul [6], long-range planning and historical reflection [3], and "madness and delirium" [7] were deliberated. The source of human thought has been contemplated since ancient times, but much of the work by Pre-Socratic philosophers has been incomplete and second-hand, whereas the works of others, such as Aristotle, Galen, and Plato, have been well-preserved [6]. While a complete review of the ancient Greek investigations into the origin of thought is well beyond the scope of this chapter, the works of many individuals specifically addressed what we now know of as executive functioning.

In the 8th century B.C.E., Homer, in his inquiry about the functioning of the soul, discussed the "psychē" as a representation of identity that appeared only during dreams. In contrast, several "body souls" were discussed as part of the daily human experience, many of which correspond to modern-day executive functioning. For example, the "noos" was thought to be responsible for rational thought and the "menos" was thought to control aggressive impulses [6]. Around 425 B.C.E., Hippocrates set the stage for a neural basis of rational thought [7] and Socrates later questioned the source of thought in the human body as well [6]. Late in the 3rd century B.C.E., Plato considered the basis of abstract thought, which he believed to be in the brain and his student, Aristotle, believed it to be in the heart [5]. Disagreement on the location of rational thought and the soul would go on for about 2 millennia, as enlightenment philosophers such as Locke and Descartes would search for the same answer.

Executive Function in the Dawn of Human Neuroscience

In the 1870s, Fritsch and Hitzig identified the motor area of the cortex, and others began to pay attention to other areas of the cerebrum, including the frontal lobes [1]. The main methods of brain research at the time involved stimulation or extirpation of various brain

Table 1. Timeline of selected works important to executive functioning

~750 B.C.E.	Homer discusses "body souls" including the "noos" (rational thought) and the "menos" (aggressive impulses) [6]
~400 B.C.E.	Socrates questions the source of thought in the human body [6]
1573	Varolio first describes frontal lobes in the literature [24]
1848	Phineas Gage injury [8]
1861	Broca discusses the frontal lobes' role in judgment, reflection, comparison, and reflection [11]
1874	Hitzig describes the role of the frontal lobes in higher mental functions based on his experiments with dogs [11]
1876	Ferrier describes an "alteration in character" following frontal ablations of monkeys [11]
1888	Jastrowitz discusses the "so-called moria" (a childlike or foolish state) following frontal atrophy [12]
1922	Bianchi introduces "frontal lobe syndrome" [13]
1932	Jackson – loss of influence of "higher centers" on "lower centers" following frontal injury [14]
1941	Goldstein and Scheerer produce early work on the concept of abstraction [15]
1953	Broadbent publishes details of automatic and controlled processes [16]
1963	Milner discusses the role of frontal lobe dysfunction on WCST [17]
1966	Luria describes problems with everyday tasks following frontal lobe damage [1]
1971	Fuster and Alexander publish the role of prefrontal cortex in working memory [21]
1973	Luria promotes the functional mosaic, highlighting interaction rather than solitary function [22]
1973	Pribram first uses the term "executive" for frontal cortex functioning [23]
1975	Posner and Snyder discuss the concept of cognitive control [26]
1977	Schiffrin and Schneider discuss selective attention and controlled processes [27]
1986	Norman and Shallice introduce the supervisory system [19]
1993	Cummings provides neural circuitry for the three "frontal syndromes" [28]

areas. Due to what we now know as the nature of the frontal lobes' functioning, results from these studies often appeared null and confused researchers, as there was not a simple cause and effect relationship following stimulation or extirpation of the frontal lobes.

As time passed, researchers were able to learn that, although no changes in vision, hearing, sensation, or movement were noted after extirpation of the frontal lobes, animals began to change their behavior and demeanor. Following frontal damage, animals would no longer recognize their master, chewed on any object rather than just food, and were highly distractible. Researchers such as Hitzig (1874), Ferrier (1876), and Wundt (1873) were in some sort of a difficult scenario, as these symptoms did not directly correspond to neurological counterparts, as much of brain research to that point had, and instead reflected psychological terms such as "abstract intelligence," "active attention," and "apperception" [1].

Meanwhile, in the United States, a young man named Phineas Gage had a very unlucky day at work that would change the course of neuroscience. On September 13, 1848 in a remote town of Cavendish, Vermont, Phineas Gage was working as a railroad foreman when a 3 1/2 foot tamping iron was forced through his head following a premature blast [8]. The iron entered the left side of the face, immediately anterior to the angle of the lower jaw, and passed upward near the median line at the back part of the frontal bone near the coronal suture (modern investigations [9] have mapped Gage's injury to the left prefrontal cortex). Although the explosion thrust Mr. Gage onto his back and led to mild convulsions in his extremities, he was speaking within minutes and even walked up a flight of stairs an hour later. He remained conscious and was able to recite the names and residence of nearby friends (although he did not wish to see them). His physician placed his right and left index fingers into the entire length of the wound from the right to the left to search for foreign bodies [10].

Two days after the accident, however, he was noted to have "lost control of his mind, and became decidedly delirious, with occasional lucid intervals." While previously a healthy and mild-tempered 25-year-old man, his mental state began to change dramatically. He remained oriented, but "became stupid" and "did not speak unless aroused, and then only with difficulty." Fungi were found in the wound days later, and he recovered somewhat when it was excised, but continued to appear "demented." About a month after the accident, he was noted to have had normal memory for past events, but feeble intellect and childish behaviors [10].

After details of the case were published in the Boston Medical and Surgical Journal 2 months later, Dr. Harlow received a letter from Henry J. Bigelow, a Professor of Surgery at Harvard University, requesting that Mr. Gage be transported to Boston for follow-up studies, to which they agreed. Just 2 months after the accident, Mr. Gage was noted to be "quite well" (medically) and the hole in his head had entirely closed. Still, he was noted to be "a child in his intellectual capacity…[with] the animal passions of a strong man." In light of this change, his friends and acquaintances stated the now-famous description, that he was "no longer Gage" [10]. The cause of his symptomology was not agreed upon at the time, but the change in his demeanor was clear and interest in the frontal lobes remained high thereafter.

Later in the 1800s, works by researchers such as Finger [11] and Jastrowitz [12] further identified symptoms following frontal atrophy or ablation. Many of the early works examining working memory were performed with primates. In 1922, Bianchi and Macdonald [13] described impaired ability to engage in purposeful behavior, coordinate actions, and behave in a socially appropriate manner following ablation to the frontal lobes and referred to this syndrome as the "frontal lobe syndrome" [3].

Jackson's work [14] in the 1930s set up the more modern view of the frontal lobes as the aggregator and coordinator of "lower centers" of the brain. Goldstein and Scheerer [15] added to this area in the early 1940s, when they noticed difficulty with abstract thought in World War soldiers who had sustained brain injuries. In the 1950s, Broadbent [16] was one of the first to describe the nature of automatic and controlled processes, which was somewhat of a turning point in the study of frontal lobes, as information processing theory gained prominence.

Executive Function and the "Frontal Syndromes" in Modern Neuropsychology

As the field of modern neuropsychology gained traction in the 1960s with works of Milner [17] and Luria [1], tests were developed to reliably measure cognitive and emotional changes related to frontal lobe injury. Milner [17] used the Wisconsin Card Sorting Test to elucidate the various features of frontal lobe dysfunction, while Luria [1] concentrated on problems with everyday tasks, among other areas.

While the clinical symptoms of the various frontal syndromes were wide ranging, Luria [1] boiled most of the symptoms down to impairment in planning and goal-directed behavior [18]. This theory served as the basis for many later models that addressed the utility of frontal functions in the domain of control functions operating in non-routine situations [18]. Norman and Shallice [19] elaborated on Luria's approach of frontal functioning as it relates to non-routine actions by introducing the "supervisory system." This model holds that patients with frontal lobe damage will have difficulty in novel situations or inhibiting prepotent schemas. One key function of the supervisory system is planning, and in this vein Shallice [20] designed the Tower of London task [18].

Frontal lesions were shown to cause deficits in response initiation (verbal fluency) and response suppression (go/no-go and Stroop tests) in work carried out in the 1960s and 1970s by researchers like Luria [1], Drewe [18], and Perret [18]. The somewhat puzzling combination of these 2 symptoms was later examined and led to the Hayling and Brixton tests that measure response initiation, response suppression, and problem solving [18].

One of the earliest experiments that localized the short-term memory to the prefrontal cortex was completed by Fuster and Alexander [21] in 1971. In this study, the authors used single-cell recording techniques to examine what turned out to be the critical role of the prefrontal cortex in executive functioning [3]. Only 2 years later, Luria [22] promoted the "functional mosaic" and the idea that the frontal lobes served a managerial role in coordinating other functions of the brain, rather than merely having one function. That same year in 1973, Pribram [23] first used the term "executive" to describe such functions, so beginning one of the most poorly defined yet highly important domains of neuropsychology: "executive functioning."

Dozens of competing, but not mutually exclusive, models and definitions of executive functioning have arisen since the 1970s, each with similar core concepts but with varying areas of focus. Since the inception of the term "executive functioning" in 1973, over 30 constructs have been included under the umbrella term [2] and Goldstein et al. [2] outlined 33 related, but ultimately different definitions of executive functioning. Consequently, Benton [24] aptly described his attempt to tell the story of executive functioning as "necessarily sketchy and fragmentary" (p 3). Thus, the chapter could not possibly cover the extremely broad nature of all models and theories of executive functioning, but select studies and theories will be highlighted.

The executive functions, at their most basic level, consist of capacities that allow an individual to engage successfully in independent, purposive, self-directed, and self-serving behavior [25]. The idea of the frontal lobes' function in helping humans decide on what to concentrate was illuminated in the works by Posner and Snyder [26] (cognitive control) in 1975 and by Schiffrin and Schneider [27] (selective attention) in 1977. Later work by Norman and Shallice [19] in the mid-1980s helped define the frontal lobes in terms of a supervisory system, which attempts to explain how response to unique environmental stimuli leads to the activation of certain "schema" to guide behavior. Many competing theories arose in an attempt to explain frontal lobe *function*, but similar work at the time focused on frontal lobe dysfunction, which were termed "frontal syndromes."

Much of the investigation into frontal syndromes was driven by early descriptions of the clinical consequences of frontal damage. Studies by Milner, Benton, Logue, and Lhermitte were foundational in the understanding of these syndromes [28]. Symptoms arising from various frontal syndromes include abulia, apathy, aspontaneity, akinetic mutism, pseudodepressive state, lack of drive, poor motivation, euphoric state, distractibility, impulsivity, disinhibition, irritability, restlessness, moria, pseudopsychopathic state, anosognosia, indifference, confabulation, and perseveration [18]. As time passed by, 3 main "frontal lobe syndromes" were established, the neural circuitry for which was described by Cummings [28] in 1993.

As would be expected, given the wide range of symptomology associated with frontal syndromes, patients with these ailments often have diverse clinical presentations [18]. Briefly, each of these 3 syndromes corresponds with a distinct area of frontal lobe dysfunction, including dorsolateral prefrontal (i.e., dysexecutive), orbitofrontal, and medial frontal/cingulate areas. Damage to the dorsolateral prefrontal cortex was found to cause perhaps the most classic form of executive dysfunction, marked by poor problem solving, amotivation, and perseveration. Orbitofrontal syndrome was found to consist of disinhibited behavior, emotional lability, impulsivity, and lack of social graces, personality changes, and poor odor discrimination. Finally, medial frontal/cingulate syndrome, also known as akinetic/apathetic syndrome, consists of amotivation, akinesia, mutism, leg weakness, and urinary incontinence [4].

The term "frontal syndrome" was slowly replaced with "dysexecutive syndrome" because impairment leading to these symptoms is not always localized to the frontal lobes [18]. Nevertheless, modern neuropsychology has struggled to determine exactly what is meant by "executive dysfunction." Because there is no unitary definition of executive functioning, the numerous theories and models that exist, and continue to adapt, make a discussion at the construct level challenging.

As Daffner and Searl [3] described, there is more agreement on which areas fall under the umbrella of executive functioning than about what is at the core of executive functioning, though most models identify working memory and inhibition as essential components of executive functioning. They included these 2 areas, along with monitoring and initiation, to comprise what they referred to as "first-order executive functions" [3]. Barkley [29] contends that there are 4 types of executive functioning: nonverbal working memory, verbal working memory, emotion regulation, and planning/generativity. Barkley [29] stated that all of these functions share a common purpose to guide behavior to adapt in response to environmental changes. Lezak et al. [25] uses a simpler and broader definition of executive functioning, highlighting the capacity to "engage successfully in independent, purposive, self-directed, and self-serving behavior" (p 37). While it is difficult to subscribe to the notion of a "correct" theory or model of executive functioning, the mild but perpetual disagreement regarding just what executive functioning entails may detract from the remarkable scientific advances that have been made in understanding the frontal lobes.

The Future of Executive Function

So, then, what will the future hold for executive function? Scientific advancements have produced incredibly specific findings related to precise networks involving the frontal lobes and other areas of the brain. For example, one topic *du jour* related to executive functioning is the default mode network [30], which reignited a longstanding interest in the significance of the brain's ongoing or intrinsic activity. However, the lack of agreement on the definition combined with (and perhaps due to) the extremely broad array of symptoms comprising executive functioning may lead to a necessary fragmentation of executive functioning into subsections. This type of pattern may lead to a renaissance of sorts of the frontal or dysexecutive syndromes and provide more precise language to express "executive dysfunction."

References

1 Luria AR: Higher Cortical Functions in Man, ed 2. Moscow, Moscow University Press, 1980.
2 Goldstein S, Naglieri JA, Princiotta D, Otero T: Introduction: a history of executive functioning as a theoretical and clinical construct; in Goldstein S, Naglieri JA (eds): Handbook of Executive Functioning. New York, NY, Springer Science+Business Media, 2014.
3 Daffner KR, Searl MM: The dysexecutive syndromes. Handb Clin Neurol 2008;88:249–267.
4 Schoenberg MR, Scott J: The Little Black Book of Neuropsychology, 2011.
5 Sternberg RJ: The Nature of Cognition. Cambridge, MA, MIT Press, 1999.
6 Crivellato E, Ribatti D: Soul, mind, brain: Greek philosophy and the birth of neuroscience. Brain Res Bull 2007; 71:327–336.
7 Rapp B: The Handbook of Cognitive Neuropsychology: What Deficits Reveal about the Human Mind. New York, NY, Psychology Press, 2001.
8 Harlow J: Passage of an Iron Rod through the head. Boston Med Surg J 1848;39:389–393.
9 Grafman J: The structured event complex and the human prefrontal cortex; in Stuss DT, Knight RT (eds): Principles of Frontal Lobe Function. New York, NY, Oxford University Press, 2002.
10 Harlow JM: Recovery from the passage of an iron bar through the head. Publ Mass Med Soc 1869;2:327–347.
11 Finger S: Origins of Neuroscience: A History of Explorations Into Brain Function. New York, NY, Oxford University Press, 2001.
12 Jastrowitz M: Beiträge zur Localization im Grosshirn und über deren praktische Verwerthung. Dtsch Med Wochenschr 1888;14:81–83.
13 Bianchi L, Macdonald JH: The Mechanism of the Brain, and the Function of the Frontal Lobes. Edinburgh, E. & S. Livingstone, 1922.
14 Jackson J: Selected Writings of John Hughlings Jackson, vol 2. London, Hodder & Stoughton, 1932.
15 Goldstein K, Scheerer M: Abstract and concrete behavior. Psychol Monogr 1941;53:110–130.
16 Broadbent D: Neglect of the surroundings in relation to fatigue decrements in output; in Floyd WF, Welford AT (eds): Fatigue. London, Lewis, 1953, pp 173–178.
17 Milner B: Effects of different brain lesions on card sorting: the role of the frontal lobes. Arch Neurol 1963;9: 90–100.
18 Godefroy O: Frontal syndrome and disorders of executive functions. J Neurol 2003;250:1–6.
19 Norman DA, Shallice T: Attention to action; in Davidson RJ, Schwartz GE, Shapiro D (eds): Consciousness and Self-Regulation. Boston, MA, Springer, 1986, pp 1–18.

20 Shallice T: Specific impairments of planning. Philos Trans R Soc Lond B Biol Sci 1982;298:199–209.
21 Fuster JM, Alexander GE: Neuron activity related to short-term memory. Science 1971;173:652–654.
22 Luria AR: The Working Brain: An Introduction to Neuropsychology. New York, NY, Basic Books, 1973.
23 Pribram KH: The primate frontal cortex – executive of the brain; in Pribram KH, Luria AR (eds): Psychophysiology of the Frontal Lobes. New York, NY, Academic Press, 1974, pp 293–313.
24 Benton AL: The prefrontal region: its early history; in Levin HS, Eisenberg HM, Benton AL (eds): Frontal Lobe Function and Dysfunction. New York, NY, Oxford University Press, 1991.
25 Lezak MD, Howieson DB, Bigler ED, Tranel D: Neuropsychological Assessment, ed 5. New York, NY, Oxford University Press, 2012.
26 Posner MI, Snyder CRR: Attention and cognitive control; in Solso RL (ed): Information Processing and Cognition: The Loyola Symposium. Hillsdale, NJ, Lawrence Erlbaum, 1975, pp 55–85.
27 Schiffrin RM, Schneider W: Controlled and automatic human information processing: perceptual learning, automatic attending and a general theory. Psychol Rev 1977;84:127–190.
28 Cummings JL: Frontal-subcortical circuits and human behavior. Arch Neurol 1993;50:873–880.
29 Barkley RA (ed): Attention-Deficit Hyperactivity Disorder, Fourth Edition: A Handbook for Diagnosis and Treatment. New York, NY, The Guilford Press, 2014.
30 Raichle ME: The brain's default mode network. Annu Rev Neurosci 2015;38:433–447.

Jonathan DeRight, PhD
Private Practice
1390 Chain Bridge Rd, Box 85
McLean, VA 22101 (USA)
E-Mail jderightphd@gmail.com

Bogousslavsky J, Boller F, Iwata M (eds): A History of Neuropsychology.
Front Neurol Neurosci. Basel, Karger, 2019, vol 44, pp 108–117 (DOI: 10.1159/000494958)

History of Subcortical Cognitive Impairment

Christopher M. Filley

Behavioral Neurology Section, Departments of Neurology and Psychiatry, University of Colorado School of Medicine, Marcus Institute for Brain Health, Aurora, CO, USA

Abstract

The representation of cognitive function in the cerebral cortex has a long and cherished history, but much evidence also supports a critical role of subcortical structures in the operations of cognition. The idea of subcortical dementia, first proposed in 1932 and substantially expanded in the 1970s, is the most prominent formulation intended to capture the phenomenology of cognitive impairment attributable to subcortical involvement. Despite criticism highlighting its imprecision, subcortical dementia has endured as a useful general concept assisting the classification of dementia syndromes based on the primary site(s) of neuropathology. As neuroscientific knowledge expanded with the advent of modern structural and functional neuroimaging, a more detailed understanding of the contributions of specific subcortical regions emerged, such that the cognitive affiliations of the basal ganglia, thalamus, cerebellum, brainstem, and white matter are all better defined. Important advances have been made by the study of both neurodegenerative diseases and focal lesions. Today, the complex admixture of cortical and subcortical foundations of cognition is increasingly well appreciated, and has been conceptually organized within the broadly inclusive notion of distributed neural networks. These networks are thought to integrate cortical and subcortical gray and white matter structures throughout the brain into functional neuronal ensembles subserving various domains of cognition. In this light, specific disorders of subcortical regions produce cognitive sequelae that can be usefully analyzed within the context of networks that involve key cortical regions as well. The study of subcortical contributions to cognition has been highly informative in expanding neurobehavioral thinking to include regions beyond the cerebral cortex, adding nuance and sophistication to the conceptualization of brain-behavior relationships.

Introduction

The understanding of brain-behavior relationships is a central goal of neuroscience, and the cerebral cortex has traditionally been the major focus of research on the distinctive neurobehavioral capacities possessed by *Homo sapiens*. Much evidence supports this emphasis, from the importance of synaptic function in learning and memory to the role of cortical neurotransmitters in a wide variety of mental states. Yet the cortical gray matter occupies only a small percentage of brain volume, and most brain structures are subcortical in location. In this light, the subcortical regions – comprising all the gray and white matter structures lying subjacent to the cerebral cortex – merit attention as also contributing to the human behavioral repertoire. Indeed, these regions are increasingly appreciated as playing important roles in the organization of cognition and emotion. In this review, the history of investigation regarding cognitive impairment from damage to, or dysfunction within, subcortical regions will be summarized. To begin, the early studies of the subcortex as a whole will be reviewed, after which the specific contributions of the basal ganglia, thalamus, cerebellum, brainstem, and white matter will be considered (Tables 1, 2).

Subcortical Dementia

Neurologists of the 19th century recognized that diseases of the subcortical gray and white matter were often associated with cognitive impairment, but formal description of how subcortical neuropathology could disrupt cognitive function did not appear until the 20th century with the idea of subcortical dementia. The first proposal of this influential, albeit controversial notion was in 1932, when Franz Günther von Stockert used the descriptor "subcorticale demenz" to characterize the cognitive deterioration in a patient with postencephalitic parkinsonism [1]. In 1974, the first modern use of the term "subcortical dementia" appeared in a report of 5 patients with progressive supranuclear palsy, in whom the dementia syndrome was characterized by forgetfulness, slowing of thought processes, emotional or personality changes, and impaired ability to manipulate acquired knowledge [2]. A year later, a very similar profile was described in patients with Huntington's disease (HD; [3]). These studies proposed a largely qualitative cluster of neurobehavioral deficits, thought to be related to primary subcortical gray matter pathology [2, 3], in contrast to the traditional "cortical" features of amnesia, aphasia, apraxia, and agnosia that are seen in the prototype cortical dementia of Alzheimer's disease (AD; [4]). A tentative pathophysiological explanation of subcortical dementia was that the timing and activation of cognitive processes were impaired rather than the processes themselves [2].

By the early 1980s, the construct of subcortical dementia came to encompass many other disorders in which the cortex is not primarily involved, including Parkinson's disease (PD), Wilson's disease, spinocerebellar degeneration, idiopathic basal ganglia calcification, the lacunar state, and the dementia syndrome of depression [5]. As knowledge accumu-

Table 1. The clinical profile of the cerebellar cognitive affective syndrome

Executive function	Impaired planning, set-shifting, abstract reasoning, working memory
Language	Agrammatism, aprosodia, anomia
Spatial cognition	Visuospatial disorganization, impaired visuospatial memory
Personality	Blunting of affect, disinhibition, inappropriate behavior

Table 2. Prominent clinical features of cortical, white matter, subcortical dementia

Domain	Cortical	White matter	Subcortical
Cognitive speed	Normal	Slowed	Slowed
Sustained attention	Normal	Impaired	Impaired
Declarative memory	Amnesia	Retrieval deficit	Retrieval deficit
Procedural memory	Normal	Normal	Impaired
Executive function	Impaired	Impaired	Impaired
Language	Aphasia	Normal	Normal
Speech	Normal	Dysarthria	Dysarthria
Praxis	Apraxia	Normal	Normal
Visuospatial skills	Impaired	Impaired	Impaired
Recognition	Agnosia	Normal	Normal
Psychiatric status	Apathy, disinhibition	Depression, psychosis	Depression, psychosis
Extrapyramidal function	Normal	Normal	Hyperkinesia, rigidity

lated, the 2 most often mentioned entities in the subcortical dementia category came to be PD and HD, in both of which the most prominent neuropathology is found in the subcortical regions: the substantia nigra in PD and the striatum in HD (Fig. 1). Although criticism was raised, and remains alive today, because of the imprecision of clinical features and the neuropathological overlap of subcortical and cortical dementias [6], careful studies have lent support to the distinction between the 2 categories [7], and it has been contended that the subcortical dementias resemble each other more than they do AD [8].

The clinical similarity of subcortical dementia to frontal lobe disease was noted in the first modern report [2], and it became clear over time that frontal-striatal systems were intimately involved with subcortical dysfunction, leading to the alternative, and putatively more accurate descriptor of frontal-subcortical dementia [8]. Whatever terminology is preferred, there is substantial agreement that the subcortical-cortical dichotomy has validity. Although the presence of either pure subcortical or cortical neuropathology is clearly uncommon in dementia, and the categories of subcortical and cortical dementia may be best regarded as points on a continuum [8], the distinction between the 2 categories continues to find utility in both clinical and research settings, perhaps most visibly among neuropsychologists [7].

The widespread distribution of neuropathology in subcortical diseases, however, complicates the analysis of how any one area contributes to cognition, and it has long been apparent that more specificity in defining the role of subcortical structures in cognition is required. Recent research has proceeded to address this need, and the study of all major regions lying subjacent to the cerebral cortical mantle has been valuable in expanding the understanding of brain-behavior relationships.

Cognitive Impairment with Regional Subcortical Neuropathology

The structural and functional diversity of brain areas that lie below the cerebral cortex presents challenges in understanding their contributions to cognition and emotion, but investigators have adopted a range of innovative strategies to advance neurobehavioral research on specific subcortical regions. One influential idea informing this approach is that of frontal-subcortical circuits [9, 10], which are identified as integrated neuronal loops involving the frontal cortex, striatum, globus pallidus, thalamus, and connections between these regions that participate in a variety of neurobehavioral domains. These circuits highlight the importance of deep gray matter nuclei in the cerebrum that have extensive reciprocal connections with neocortical regions. In addition, the cerebellum has received major scrutiny in terms of its cognitive affiliations, and, related to this region, the brainstem has also been seen as important for cognition. Last, the white matter of the brain, which interconnects all gray matter areas within and between the hemispheres, and in the posterior fossa, has attracted long overdue attention in the organization of cognitive functions. These areas will each be covered in some detail.

Basal Ganglia

The basal ganglia are a group of large, gray matter nuclei that are traditionally regarded as having a major role in motor function, particularly motor planning and procedural learning. These functions continue to be vigorously studied, but the cognitive implications of the basal ganglia have attracted steady attention as well. Although the nuclei listed as basal ganglia varies in the literature, structures virtually always included in this group are the caudate and putamen (together known as the striatum), the globus pallidus, and the midbrain substantia nigra. Studies of patients with damage to these regions have come from both neurodegenerative diseases such as HD, PD, and progressive supranuclear palsy [11], and focal basal ganglia lesions, typically related to ischemic stroke [12]. Whereas the diversity of diseases studied precludes unifying statements that apply in every case, a general trend emerges suggesting that cognitive impairment from basal ganglia injury involves deficits in executive function, psychomotor speed, attention, memory retrieval, and visuospatial skills, with relative sparing of memory encoding and language [11, 12].

The striatum appears to be particularly well documented as a region associated with characteristic neurobehavioral dysfunction in disease states. Patients with HD, for example, whose most prominent neuropathology is typically in the caudate nucleus where dramatic atrophy can develop (Fig. 1a), show a profile of executive dysfunction, cognitive slowing, working memory deficits, attentional dysfunction, memory retrieval difficulty,

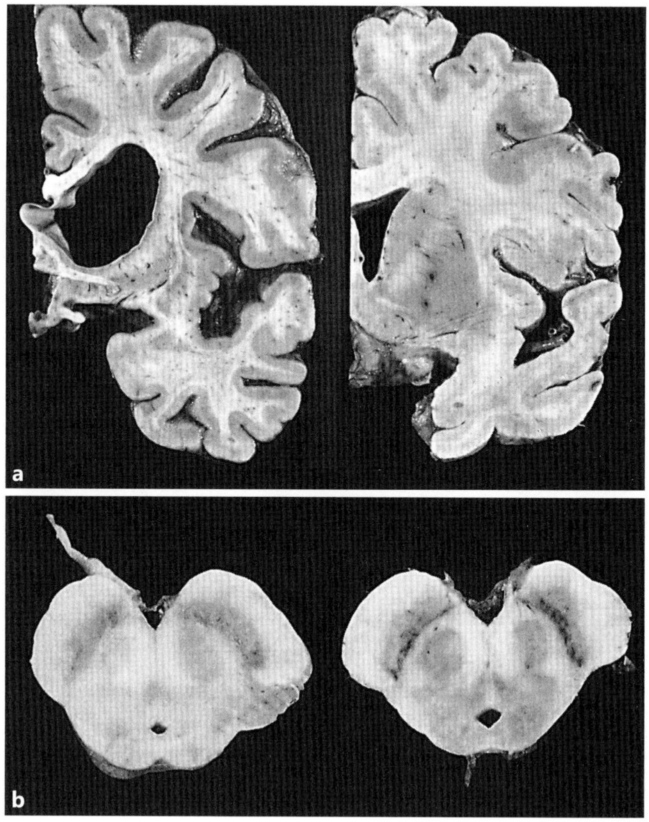

Fig. 1. a Gross neuropathology of the cerebrum in Huntington's disease. The coronal section on the left shows marked atrophy of the striatum, most prominently the caudate nucleus, compared to a normal post-mortem brain. **b** Gross neuropathology of the midbrain in Parkinson's disease. The horizontal section on the left shows bilateral loss of pigmented dopaminergic neurons in the substantia nigra, compared to a normal post-mortem brain. Reprinted from Filley CM: Neurobehavioral Anatomy, 3rd ed, 2011, with permission of the University Press of Colorado.

spared language, neuropsychiatric disturbances (depression, anxiety, irritability), and impaired procedural memory [11, 13, 14]. Thus, the original description of HD as a subcortical dementia [3] gathered additional support with further study. In later stages of the disease, the putamen, frontal cortex, and white matter connections are also affected [13], consistent with frontal-subcortical network involvement [9, 10].

In PD, definitive neuropathology is present in the midbrain substantia nigra (Fig. 1b), and dementia is well-known as a common non-motor manifestation of the disease. One of the classic subcortical dementias, PD was initially postulated to produce cognitive impairment by virtue of loss of dopaminergic input to the striatum, thus impairing the timing and activation of cortical operations such as memory, language, praxis, and gnosis [5]. This formulation, however, has been revised with the emergence of new data. Whereas some patients do indeed suffer from a traditional subcortical dementia pattern of deficits, with attentional, working memory, and executive dysfunction [11], others have a less specific profile that can be ascribed in part to Lewy bodies [15] and/or AD changes [16] in the neocortex and limbic cortices. Mirroring a trend frequently observed in other neurodegenerative diseases, most notably AD [17], detailed neuropathological observations of post-mortem PD brains have disclosed combined pathologies in many cases [15], rendering correlation of cognitive syndromes with specific regional neuropathology more challenging. Hallucinations and other psychotic features in PD, for example, may reflect combined subcortical and cortical involvement.

Thalamus

Together with the basal ganglia, the thalamus has been included on the list of major deep gray matter structures implicated in the operations of cognition and emotion [18]. Long appreciated as a crucial relay station of sensation that will be further processed in the cerebral cortex, and as a subcortical participant in motor function, this large collection of deep nuclei also has important neurobehavioral affiliations. The thalamus is increasingly included in discussions of distributed neural networks that can be studied in normal individuals with functional neuroimaging [18], but the clinical literature on cognitive correlates of the thalamus is somewhat limited by the rarity with which neurodegenerative diseases specifically target this region. Instead, the role of the thalamus has been elucidated to some extent by study of focal lesions, most notably neoplasms [19] and stroke [20].

A series of 8 patients with bilateral thalamic glioma disclosed that mental slowing, apathy, emotional lability, confusion, inattention, and memory loss were prominent, and that these changes were not explained by increased intracranial pressure [19]. In contrast to the dementia produced by neuropathology in both thalami, more specific cognitive deficits have been observed with unilateral thalamic lesions from ischemic infarcts. A comprehensive review of thalamic strokes found that anterior infarcts led to perseverations, apathy, and amnesia; paramedian infarcts to disinhibition, personality change, and amnesia; inferolateral infarcts to executive dysfunction; and posterior infarcts to neglect and aphasia [20]. It appears that a variety of neurobehavioral syndromes can be seen with thalamic lesions, in keeping with the emerging understanding of thalamic involvement in distributed neural networks devoted to cognition [20].

Cerebellum

The role of the cerebellum in the mediation of human behavior has been substantially investigated in recent decades [21], overturning the long-accepted appreciation of this structure being exclusively devoted to motor function. Although non-motor affiliations of the cerebellum had been suspected in the past, little study was devoted to this possibility until the contribution of the cerebellum to cognition was brought to light in the 1990s by detailed neurobehavioral study of a wide range of cerebellar disorders [22]. From this work, it was postulated that a "cerebellar cognitive affective syndrome" (CCAS) was clinically identifiable (Table 1) [21]. To explain the profile of deficits in the CCAS, the intriguing idea of "dysmetria of thought" was proposed, whereby a "universal cerebellar transform" facilitates the modulation of behavior as a result of specific functional interactions within cerebrocerebellar circuits [21]. The CCAS is thus a consequence of posterior cerebellar lesions that are mainly responsible for cognitive impairment and vermis lesions (of the limbic cerebellum) producing affective disturbances [21]. The linking of these cerebellar regions to allied cortical regions has been established by functional MRI studies demonstrating connections between the cerebellum and association and paralimbic cortices supporting cognition and emotion [22].

While still novel to many neurologists and neuroscientists who were educated in the tradition of the cerebellum as being dedicated to motor function, the idea of the CCAS is steadily gaining credibility as a clinical syndrome underscoring the contribution of a prominent subcortical structure to the human neurobehavioral repertoire. The consideration of the cerebellum in cognition also implicates the increasingly influential notion of connectivity, to be discussed more below.

Brainstem

As foreign as the idea may be that the cerebellum has neurobehavioral importance, still more unfamiliar is the notion that the brainstem has any role in the operations of cognition and emotion. This region, clearly subcortical in location, is well known to harbor many cranial nerve nuclei as well as numerous corticofugal and corticopetal tracts, but its importance for behavioral neurology has long been assumed to be limited to the pathogenesis of low-level states of altered consciousness such as stupor, coma, the minimally conscious state, and the vegetative state. This view, however, is currently undergoing revision. In a series of 30 carefully studied cases of focal brainstem strokes, a range of cognitive syndromes was found, including executive dysfunction, inattention, memory loss, aphasia, and visuospatial impairment, and nearly half of the patients presented with behavioral or affective changes [23]. The authors of this review concluded that whereas cognitive and affective symptoms with brainstem infarction are generally overlooked, neurobehavioral syndromes consistent with damage to networks involving higher cortical or limbic areas can occur, and these strokes can produce deficits closely resembling those of the CCAS [23]. More study is needed to extend these observations, but this report represents further recognition that all major brain regions below the cerebral cortex participate in higher functions.

White Matter

The last subcortical region to be considered, and the largest, is the brain white matter. This vast collection of myelinated fibers that course within and between the 2 cerebral hemispheres, and to and from posterior fossa regions, is highly developed in humans and serves to connect all gray matter regions into functionally coherent neural networks [24]. Although diseases of white matter were included in the original formulation of subcortical dementia [5], the preponderance of initial work on subcortical cognitive impairment was focused on subcortical gray matter structures as reviewed above. In the 1980s, however, white matter attracted much interest because of the advent of MRI, which permitted unprecedented imaging of myelinated fibers in vivo. Adding to prior knowledge of how white matter could be affected by various types of neuropathology, MRI offered an elegant modality to enable better characterization of old white matter diseases and the discovery of new ones.

The availability of MRI rapidly generated detailed investigations of the neurobehavioral sequelae of white matter disorders. While studies on classic focal disconnection syndromes of behavioral neurology, many of which follow focal white matter lesions [25]

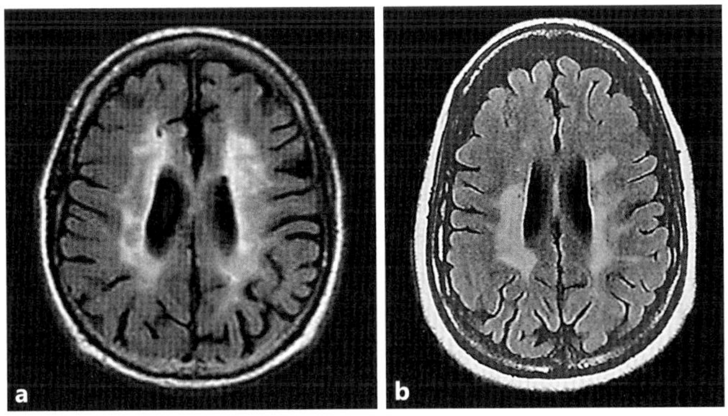

Fig. 2. a Axial MRI scan of an individual with Binswanger's disease, demonstrating widespread ischemic white matter disease in the cerebral hemispheres. **b** Axial MRI scan of an individual with multiple sclerosis, showing widespread white matter demyelination in the cerebral hemispheres.

continued, the concept of white matter dementia (WMD) was proposed in 1988 to highlight the potential for many diffuse or multifocal white matter disorders to cause cognitive dysfunction or dementia [26]. The most illustrative example of WMD is toluene leukoencephalopathy, in which long-standing toluene abuse from the intentional inhalation of spray paint leads to a characteristic dementia related to selective, diffuse leukoencephalopathy that spares both cortical and subcortical gray matter [27]. Toxic leukoencephalopathy [27] is one of ten neuropathological categories in which WMD can occur, the others being genetic, demyelinative, infectious, inflammatory, vascular, metabolic, traumatic, neoplastic, and hydrocephalic [26]. In each category, the primary or even exclusive damage can fall on white matter and produce dementia.

Although many unresolved issues remain about WMD in comparison to cortical and subcortical dementia, a growing body of evidence supports the clinical differentiation of WMD from its better-known counterparts. The 3 dementia categories have unique clinical features (Table 2), and the sharpest distinctions, such as those involving declarative and procedural memory dysfunction [24, 28], occur early in the dementia when neuropathology is most restricted to the primary regions involved. To illustrate WMD, 2 of the most commonly seen examples are Binswanger's disease (Fig. 2a) [29] and multiple sclerosis (Fig. 2b) [30]. While these diseases clearly affect the white matter and are capable of causing dementia, uncertainty persists about whether WMD is an appropriate term because co-existent gray matter damage may occur in both. However, the most consistent neuropathological feature of Binswanger's disease is widespread white matter ischemia that produces a unique type of vascular dementia [29], clinical features of which resemble dementia in other white matter disorders (Table 2). Moreover, in multiple sclerosis, MRI studies since the 1980s have consistently found that white matter lesions correlate with cognitive impairment, particularly slowed processing speed [30], a core feature of WMD (Table 2). Even if gray matter involvement occurs at some point in the disease course, the recognition of WMD has important clinical implications because many white matter disorders can be stabilized or even reversed, and treatment is most efficacious when initiated early [24, 26]. More work lies ahead to refine the idea, but WMD has helped broaden the scope of investigation into the neurobiological basis of cognition.

Distributed Neural Networks

The increasing knowledge of how gray and white matter neuropathology below the cerebral cortex contributes to cognitive impairment has led to another key concept of recent decades, the idea of distributed neural networks [31]. As the understanding of brain-behavior relationships expanded over the 20th century [25], both equipotentiality – the idea that all cerebral areas participate equally in mediating cognition – and strict localizationism – the assignment of one cognitive function to one specific brain region – gradually gave way to the notion that cognition is widely represented in distributed networks of structures dedicated to specific cognitive domains. These networks were first conceptualized in terms of the cerebral cortex and subcortical nuclei [9], and soon after the contributions of the white matter [26] and the cerebellum [21] were appreciated. Accordingly, it became commonplace to consider the operations of cognition as represented within ensembles of gray and white matter structures throughout the brain. These ideas have found their most recent expression in the notion of the connectome, a 21st century concept meaning a structural description of the human brain [32]. With methods now available to study distributed neural networks in vivo – most notably functional neuroimaging and diffusion tensor imaging – researchers and clinicians can now assess brain connectivity as never before; both the microconnectivity of synapses and the macroconnectivity of white matter can now be included in a complete account of the organization of behavior.

Conclusion

The history summarized in this review indicates that a wide range of neurobehavioral disorders have been found to be associated with subcortical involvement, and a secure link between acquired subcortical lesions and cognitive impairment and dementia has been established. These advances support the view that all regions of the brain subjacent to the cerebral cortex must be considered in a complete account of the neural origins of behavior. As much as neuroscience has steadfastly focused on the cortex as the essential mediator of cognition, such a perspective is inadequate for a full appreciation of how the brain subserves behavior. Indeed, the role of subcortical structures in behavioral neurology is closely associated with the unifying concept of connectivity, a concept not fully appreciated without considering how regions below the cortex contribute to the organization of cognition. As the study of subcortical regions continues to evolve, a deeper understanding of brain-behavior relationships can be anticipated.

References

1 Von Stockert FG: Subcorticale demenz. Arch Psychiatry 1932;97:720–722.
2 Albert ML, Feldman RG, Willis AL: The "subcortical dementia" of progressive supranuclear palsy. J Neurol Neurosurg Psychiatry 1974;37:121–130.
3 McHugh PR, Folstein MF: Psychiatric syndromes of Huntington's chorea: a clinical and phenomenologic study; in Benson DF, Blumer D (eds): Psychiatric Aspects of Neurologic Disease, vol. 1. New York, Grune and Stratton, 1975, pp 267–285.
4 Geldmacher DS, Whitehouse PJ: Evaluation of dementia. N Engl J Med 1996;335:330–336.
5 Cummings JL, Benson DF: Subcortical dementia. Review of an emerging concept. Arch Neurol 1984;41:874–879.
6 Whitehouse PJ: The concept of subcortical and cortical dementia: another look. Ann Neurol 1986;19:1–6.
7 Salmon DP, Filoteo JV: Neuropsychology of cortical versus subcortical dementia syndromes. Semin Neurol 2007;27:7–21.
8 Bonelli RM, Cummings JL: Frontal-subcortical dementias. Neurologist 2008;14:100–107.
9 Alexander GE, DeLong MR, Strick PL: Parallel organization of functionally segregated circuits linking basal ganglia and cortex. Annu Rev Neurosci 1986;9:357–381.
10 Cummings JL. Frontal-subcortical circuits and human behavior. Arch Neurol 1993;50:873–880.
11 Stout JC, Johnson SA: Cognitive impairment and dementia in basal ganglia disorders. Curr Neurol Neurosci Rep 2005;5:355–363.
12 Ward P, Seri S, Cavanna AE: Functional neuroanatomy and behavioural correlates of the basal ganglia: evidence from lesion studies. Behav Neurol 2013;26:219–223.
13 O'Callaghan C, Bertoux M, Hornberger M: Beyond and below the cortex: the contribution of striatal dysfunction to cognition and behaviour in neurodegeneration. J Neurol Neurosurg Psychiatry 2014;85:371–378.
14 Gabrieli JD, Stebbins GT, Singh J, Willingham DB, Goetz CG: Intact mirror-tracing and impaired rotary-pursuit skill learning in patients with Huntington's disease: evidence for dissociable memory systems in skill learning. Neuropsychology 1997;11:272–281.
15 Halliday GM, Leverenz JB, Schneider JS, Adler CH: The neurobiological basis of cognitive impairment in Parkinson's disease. Mov Disord 2014;29:634–650.
16 Boller F, Mizutani T, Roessmann U, Gambetti P: Parkinson disease, dementia, and Alzheimer disease: clinicopathological correlations. Ann Neurol 1980;7:329–335.
17 Schneider JA, Arvanitakis Z, Bang W, Bennett DA: Mixed brain pathologies account for most dementia cases in community-dwelling older persons. Neurology 2007;69:2197–2204.
18 Bell PT, Shine JM: Subcortical contributions to large-scale network communication. Neurosci Biobehav Rev 2016;71:313–322.
19 Partlow GD, del Carpio-O'Donovan R, Melanson D, Peters TM: Bilateral thalamic glioma: review of eight cases with personality change and mental deterioration. AJNR Am J Neuroradiol 1992;13:1225–1230.
20 Carrera E, Bogousslavsky J: The thalamus and behavior: effects of anatomically distinct strokes. Neurology 2006;66:1817–1823.
21 Schmahmann JD, Sherman JC: The cerebellar cognitive affective syndrome. Brain 1998;121:561–579.
22 Schmahmann JD: The role of the cerebellum in cognition and emotion: personal reflections since 1982 on the dysmetria of thought hypothesis, and its historical evolution from theory to therapy. Neuropsychol Rev 2010;20:236–260.
23 D'aes T, Mariën P: Cognitive and affective disturbances following focal brainstem lesions: a review and report of three cases. Cerebellum 2015;14:317–340.
24 Filley CM, Fields RD: White matter and cognition: making the connection. J Neurophysiol 2016;116:2093–2104.
25 Geschwind N: Disconnexion syndromes in animals and man. Brain 1965;88:237–294, 585–644.
26 Filley CM, Franklin GM, Heaton RK, Rosenberg NL: White matter dementia: clinical disorders and implications. Neuropsychiatry Neuropsychol Behav Neurol 1988;1:239–254.
27 Filley CM, Kleinschmidt-DeMasters BK: Toxic leukoencephalopathy. N Engl J Med 2001;345:425–432.
28 Lafosse JM, Corboy JR, Leehey MA, Seeberger LC, Filley CM: MS vs HD: can white matter and subcortical gray matter pathology be distinguished neuropsychologically? J Clin Exp Neuropsychol 2007;29:142–154.
29 Babikian V, Ropper AH: Binswanger's disease: a review. Stroke 1987;18:2–12.
30 Mollison D, Sellar R, Bastin M, Mollison D, Chandran S, Wardlaw J, Connick P: The clinico-radiological paradox of cognitive function and MRI burden of white matter lesions in people with multiple sclerosis: a systematic review and meta-analysis. PLoS One 2017;12:e0177727.
31 Mesulam MM: Large-scale neurocognitive networks and distributed processing for attention, language, and memory. Ann Neurol 1990;28:597–613.
32 Sporns O, Tononi G, Kötter R: The human connectome: a structural description of the human brain. PLoS Comput Biol 2005;1:e4.

Christopher M. Filley, MD
Behavioral Neurology Section, Departments of Neurology and Psychiatry
University of Colorado School of Medicine
12469 East 17th Place, Mail Stop F429
Aurora, CO 80045 (USA)
E-Mail christopher.filley@ucdenver.edu

Bogousslavsky J, Boller F, Iwata M (eds): A History of Neuropsychology.
Front Neurol Neurosci. Basel, Karger, 2019, vol 44, pp 118–126 (DOI: 10.1159/000494959)

History of Dementia

Frédéric Assal

Cognitive Neurology Unit, Neurology, Department of Clinical Neuroscience, Geneva University Hospital and Faculty of Medicine, Geneva, Switzerland

Abstract

The term dementia derives from the Latin root *demens*, which means being out of one's mind. Although the term "dementia" has been used since the 13th century, its mention in the medical community was reported in the 18th century. Even though the Greeks postulated a cerebral origin, the concept was not restricted to senile dementia and included all sorts of psychiatric and neurological conditions leading to psychosocial consequences. In the 19th century, individuals with dementia were recognized as patients, deserving medical care from specialists called alienists, and senile dementia became a medical disease. Subsequently, progresses in neuropathology allowed its fragmentation into different neuropathological conditions. Senile dementia was considered as a distinct entity from Alzheimer's seminal case published in 1906, and was first attributed to a vascular origin. However, from the late 1960s and for 20 subsequent years, Alzheimer's disease became the prototypical senile dementia. Only recently, the term dementia was abandoned for major neurocognitive disorder and the heterogeneity of the syndrome acknowledged again at the phenotypical and molecular levels. We hope a better understanding of this fascinating history will improve scientific research and impose humility towards the complex underpinnings of age-related cognitive decline.

Introduction

The history of dementia started centuries before Alois Alzheimer's seminal description in 1906. In this chapter, we will discuss the evolution of the concept of dementia from the Greco-Roman period up to the early 21st century, from morosis to senile dementia that recently became a major neurocognitive disorder, with particular focus on Alzheimer's

Table 1. Terms to describe senile dementia throughout history (for a review, see [1])

Before the 18th century	Amentia, dementia, imbecility, morosis, fatuitas, anoea, foolishness, stupidity, simplicity, carus, idiocy, dotage, senile debility, senility
Since the 18th century	Imbecility of the elderly, puerile sate, drivelling, senile madness, senile dementia
Since the 19th century	Aphrenia, mental impotence, presbyophrenia
Since the 20th century	Eponyms and dementia subtypes: Alzheimer's disease, Pick's disease, apoplectic, then arteriosclerotic then vascular dementia, etc.
Since the 21st century	Dementias abandoned for the term major neurocognitive disorders due to specific pathologies Molecular taxonomy (amyloïdopathies, tauopathies, syncleinopathies, …) including the concept of presymptomatic stage (MCI)

disease (AD). We will then briefly introduce major dementia subtypes from a historical perspective including vascular dementia (VaD), frontotemporal dementia (FTD), semantic dementia (SD), primary progressive aphasias, Lewy body dementia (LBD), and Parkinson's disease (PD) dementia.

From the Greco-Roman Period to the 18th Century: The Birth of a Concept

The term dementia (for a review, see Table 1 and [1]), derived from the Latin root *demens* for being out of one's mind, has been used since the 13th century and appeared in the medical community in the 18th century, in Blancard's *Physical Dictionary* in 1726 [2], meaning extinction of the imagination and judgment, and in the French *Encyclopédie* from Diderot and d'Alembert in 1754 where the clinical and the legal dimensions of the term in the broad sense were captured [3].

In fact, the concept of dementia including cognitive decline in the elderly had already been recognized in Ancient Egypt and in the Greco-Roman period (for reviews, see [4–6]). Pythagoras (570–495 BC) was probably one of the first physician to divide life into 5 stages, the last 2 belonging to a period of regression of mental capacities (the senium), where the system returns to the imbecility of the first epoch of infancy. According to Solon (500 BC), a Greek judge, judgment could be impaired by old age and incorporated in the laws and will procedures. Plato (428/7 or 424/3–348/7 BC) did not consider cognitive decline as an abnormality but as an unfortunate and inevitable consequence of aging due to the weakness of the brain. Hippocrates (460–370 BC) held that imbalance between 4 cardinal body fluids or humors (blood, phlegm, yellow bile, and black bile) explained different temperaments and considered that the aging brain would get dry and cold, predisposing the elderly to melancholy and mental decline. Aristotle (384–322 BC), unlike Hippocrates and Plato, did not attribute sensations, intelligence, and passions to the brain but to the heart (*sensorium commune*) and the function of the brain – called humid and cold – was to act as a refrigerator, humidifying the blood circulating through the heart. Interestingly, Aristotle defined memory as a perception of differences in sensations (between true sensation in the heart and the localized sensation in the body), and compared it with painting that could slip away in the infant and the elderly due to body growth or reduction, respectively. Later, the Roman Marcus Tullius Cicero (106–43 BC) coined the term senile debility (senile stultitia). Unlike the Greeks, he suggested that it was only present in individuals with weak will and claimed that an active mental life could prevent, or at least postpone cognitive decline. Claudius Galenus or Galen (150–200 AD) followed up on Hippocrates doctrine as opposed to Aristotle, and considered psychic pneuma, including representation, memory, and reasoning, localized in the brain and nerves. Obstruction of psychic pneuma due to humorous stagnation in the ventricles would cause movement, memory, and intelligence disorders. Galen introduced the term morosis to describe dementia ("when knowledge of letters and other arts are totally obliterated and people cannot even remember their own names") and considered this condition as an inevitable consequence of aging as well.

After Galen, due to the power of the clergy who disapproved and even prohibited autopsy, medical interest on cognitive decline significantly dropped in Europe unlike in the Middle East, where, among others, the Persian Avicenne (980–1037) perpetuated the Hippocratic-Galenical school. In Europe, the friar Roger Bacon (1214–1294) was one of the few intellectuals who studied the subject and was imprisoned for it. In his work *Methods of Preventing and Appearance of Senility*, he assumed old age was the home of forgetfulness and attributed memory to the posterior part of the brain, reasoning faculty to the middle, and imagination to the anterior parts, respectively (see [7]). Senile dementia was nevertheless recognized and accurately alluded to in European literature. Chaucer (1343–1400) and Shakespeare (1564–1616) described both cognitive and affective changes that accompany this condition: "I fear I am not in my perfect mind. Methinks I should know you, and know this man; Yet I am doubtful, for I am mainly ignorant. What place this is; and all the skill I have. Remembers not these garments; nor I know not. Where I did lodge last night." – *King Lear*, Act 4, scene 7 [8].

Around the discovery of the New World and during the Renaissance, medical research and interest came back although Galen's influence remained very strong. In the 17th century, as dissection of the human body became tolerated, physicians tempted to better capture the anatomical basis of mental disorders. Willis [9] (1621–1675), who named neurology the doctrine of the nerves, described patients with progressive cognitive decline accompanied by focal deficit, sometimes with recovery or partial resolution. He separated congenital mental retardation from acquired forms of dementia and listed aging, head injury, alcohol and opiate abuse, brain diseases, severe epilepsy, and strokes (apoplexy) as main etiologies, without finding any anatomical correlates [9].

In summary, at the end of the 18th century, it was recognized that dementia was a cognitive disorder, could affect any age group including the elderly, could cause behavioral and psychosocial incompetence, was chronic and not necessarily irreversible, and could complicate both psychiatric and neurological conditions – that were still intermingled at that time. Cerebral abnormalities were suspected but not clearly recognized yet.

The 19th Century: Medical Recognition of Dementia

The term *dementia* was coined by the famous alienist, Philippe Pinel (1745–1826). As a matter of fact, Arnulfe d'Aumont, introduced the term in the medical community in 1778, defined as a paralysis of spirit resulting from the abolition of reasoning faculty and insisted on its differentiation from delirium (see [10]). Up until the early 19th century, people suffering from dementia, including senile dementia, were imprisoned and lived in extremely poor conditions. A significant progress was made from very novel humanitarian reforms that were implemented by Philippe Pinel in 1806. He succeeded in establishing more appropriate asylums than prisons, and strongly advocated a scientific approach in the field of dementia in France and all over the world. He distinguished 4 mental disorders (melancholia, mania, idiotism, and dementia). He insisted on forgetfulness and memory loss including anterograde memory loss, and what became later Ribot's law (relatively preserved old memories compared to recent ones), lack of judgment, agitation, and rapid progression [11]. In 1812, the term dementia appeared in the US in the textbook of Rush [12] (1745–1813) who described a case, and suggested treatments to improve memory such as bleeding, purges, low diet, blisters, Java pepper, cardamom seeds, lavender and rosemary or cloves, cold bath and cold weather, and exercise. In France, Pinel's student Etienne Esquirol (1772–1840) expanded the classification of mental diseases and clearly differentiated dementia from congenital conditions [13]. "A man in a state of dementia is deprived of advantages which he formerly enjoyed; he was a rich man who has become poor. The idiot, on the contrary, has always been in a state of want and misery". He distinguished chronic dementia due to various causes (Table 2), and attributed senile dementia to ageing: "Senile dementia results from the progress of age." "Senile dementia commences with feebleness of memory, particularly recent memory…." "Dementia is a cerebral disease." He performed autopsies and specified that the arteries at the base of the brain were cartilaginous or ossified, especially in senile dementia, that the cerebral convolutions were atrophic, one gyrus separated from the next one, shallow, flattened, compressed, smaller, especially in the frontal region [13].

During the 19th century, dementia was considered as a syndrome and better understood at the morphological level. Vesanic dementia was used to refer to the cognitive deficits following mania and melancholia. Pseudodementia of Carl Wernicke described patients with chronic hysterical state mimicking dementia (for a review, see [14]). Dementia praecox appeared in 1893 in the fourth edition of Kraepelin's Textbook to describe a subgroup of patients with schizophrenia, considered at that time as a central nervous disease involving lesions of the cerebral cortex [15]. In parallel to this clinical fragmentation, anatomists searched actively for brain anomalies. In his brilliant medical thesis derived

Table 2. Causes of dementia, according to Esquirol [13]

Menstrual disorders
Severe weather conditions
Sequelae of delivery
Head injuries
Progression of age*
Ataxic fever
Hemorrhoids surgery
Mania and monomania
Paralysis
Apoplexy
Syphilis and mercury abuse
Dietary excesses and wine abuse
Masturbation
Unhappy love
Fears
Political upheavals
Unfulfilled ambitions
Poverty
Domestic problems
Unknown causes

* Corresponds to senile dementia and represented 20% of the 235 collected cases.

from the anatomopathological description of 6 cases, Antoine Laurent Jessé Bayle (1799–1858) claimed in 1822 that a chronic meningitis or "arachnitis" could cause both dementia and paralysis, and admirably described motor, cognitive, and neuropsychiatric signs of general paresis – that will be later called neurosyphilis [16]. Benedict Morel (1809–1873), a French alienist born in Vienna, stated in 1860 that loss of brain weight was a constant feature of dementia and present in aging [17], then British Samuel Wilks (1824–1911) defined cortical atrophy in 1864 [18]. He associated it with chronic alcoholism and syphilis first, then with senile dementia. At that time, syphilis contributed to 10% or more of all dementia cases and generated a lot of interest in the medical community. Decades before the discovery of the spirochete in 1905, the disease was shown to be associated with brain vessels narrowing explaining why research shifted from the cortex to cerebral vasculature and focal changes.

The 20th Century: From Dementia to Senile Dementia due to AD

By this time, arteriosclerotic brain atrophy was established as a predominant cause of senile dementia. Due to the significant improvement of histological techniques that allowed to better visualize the cortex, several researchers contributed to the understanding of new etiologies explaining dementia. Alzheimer [19] (1864–1915) observed neurofibrillary tangles and plaques in the brain of a woman with young-onset dementia and suggested a new and unique entity in 1905 and 1907. Several similar descriptions followed the seminal description, leading Kraepelin [20] to include AD eponym in the eighth edition of his Textbook of Psychiatry published in 1910. At that time, he postulated AD was a presenile dementia that was distinct from senile dementia. This dichotomy between AD and senile dementia, the former with prominent, the latter with less plaques and tangles and merely arteriosclerotic changes prevailed until the 1960s. The controversial significance of plaques and tangles in senile dementia even increased when it was published in 1933 that more than 80% of all non-demented subjects over 65 years of age had some plaques and tangles [21].

In 1966, Roth et al. [22] established quantitative methods in the study of post-mortem brain and published the first correlations between clinical scores and neuropathological changes in senile dementia – that became the classic and sporadic form of AD. The Diagnostic and Statistical Manual of Mental Disorders (DSM) clearly reflects both the confusion and the evolution of the concept: the first edition of 1952 rather mentioned organic brain syndrome and AD by name was absent [23]; the second edition introduced senile and presenile dementia under the heading of psychosis associated with organic brain syndromes [24]; the third edition defined dementia as a loss of intellectual abilities of sufficient severity to interfere with social or occupational functioning [25]. A conference held in 1977 concluded that both clinical and pathological findings of presenile and senile dementia were very similar and the first AD criteria were published in the 1980s by the NINCDS/ADRDA [26]. For 20 years, AD remained the dominant and prototypical form of dementia centered around prominent memory disturbances. In the 1990s, due to advancements in neuropsychological testing, longitudinal follow-up of patients from the presymptomatic stage to autopsy, the use of in vivo neuroimaging and molecular biomarkers, both the clinical heterogeneity of AD at the dementia stage, and its presymptomatic and preclinical stage (MCI for mild cognitive impairment) were acknowledged in the new AD criteria [27]. Last but not least, in 2013, the DSM5 abandoned the stigmatized term dementia for major neurocognitive disorder [28].

Vascular Dementia

As previously mentioned, in 1672, Willis [9] reported, VaD following stroke, called apoplexy. In subsequent years, brain congestion, or cerebral hyperemia was considered the main cause of apoplexy explaining the recommended venesection to alleviate it. Binswanger (1852–1929) in 1894 [29], then Alzheimer [30] separated VaD from neurosyphilis, and described dementia post-apoplexy (post-stroke dementia), arteriosclerotic brain degeneration (lacunar state), vascular cortical atrophy (granular atrophy), and subcortical encephalopathy (Binswanger disease). Kraepelin [20] even used an illustration of Binswanger in his textbook in the chapter "Senile and Presenile Dementia" [20] then, as mentioned earlier, arteriosclerotic dementia, cerebral arteriosclerosis, and senile dementia became almost synonymous, or at least their distinction became fuzzy. In 1974, Hachinski et al.

[31] coined the term multi-infarct dementia and that term became synonymous with VaD. In 1991, consensus diagnostic criteria included a new VaD subtype due to small vessel disease [32] and in 1995, mild cognitive impairment of vascular origin or vascular cognitive impairment no dementia was proposed [33]. In recent years, research shifted to pathophysiological mechanisms of strokes and small vessel disease as illustrated by the molecular underpinning of cerebral autosomal-dominant arteriopathy with subcortical infarcts and leukoencephalopathy CADASIL [34].

SD, Primary Progressive Aphasia, and the FTD Spectrum

The clinical phenotype of SD was reported by Arnold Pick in 1892 who described a case with the so-called progressive amnesic aphasia with loss of memory for words due to focal cerebral atrophy [35]. A British group recently reported an unpublished case of Macdonald Critchley from 1938 of a patient who disclosed early severe anomia, surface dyslexia, and loss of semantic impairment in object recognition [36]. The seminal paper appeared in 1975 where Elisabeth Warrington described the loss of semantic knowledge in 3 patients with left temporal atrophy [37]. Mesulam [38] coined the term primary progressive aphasia in 1982, representing a wider spectrum of language disorders in the absence of generalized dementia and concluded that most cases were due to non-Alzheimer pathology. In 1989, Snowden et al. defined what they called SD in 3 patients with fluent, empty speech, and impaired naming and single word comprehension [39]. SD and progressive aphasias reunified in the 2011 Diagnostic criteria that distinguished a semantic, a logopenic, and a non-fluent variant [40]. In his 1892s case [35], Arnold Pick also reported behavioral symptoms and further expanded the clinicopathological description [41] of what became Pick's disease for decades. In the 1980s, the Swedish group introduced the term *frontal lobe dementia of the non-Alzheimer's type* [42] and the British group *dementia of the frontal type* [43]. Both groups published the first consensus clinical and neuropathological criteria for FTD in 1994, modified in 1998, and used the term frontotemporal lobar degeneration to encompass FTD, progressive non-fluent aphasia, and SD [44]. Frontotemporal spectrum further fragmented into various phenotypical conditions including FTD, and syndromes with motor signs (motor neuron disease, corticobasal, and supranuclear palsy syndromes), resulting from non-specific protein aggregations including tau, TDP-43 or FUS pathologies (for a review, see [45]).

PD and LBD

In 1976, Kosaka et al. [46] published the first case of an *unclassifiable presenile dementia* that will be later called LBD. The patient presented with abnormal movement of the neck and memory disturbances that progressed to severe dementia, rigidity of the extremities, and walking difficulties. The autopsy found AD, Picks' disease, and idiopathic PD pathologies, the latter consisting of Lewy bodies and Lewy-like bodies in the brainstem and the cortex. Lewy bodies were actually described by Fritz Jakob Heinrich Lewy in PD in 1912 [47], and Konstantin Nikolaevich Trétiakoff first employed its eponym in 1919 [48]. The composition of Lewy bodies remained unknown till the alpha-synuclein protein was discovered in 1997 in families with PD [49], then the link made with the sporadic form of PD and LBD (for a review see [50]).

Conclusion

We moved from a broad phenomenological concept with legal consequences to a heterogeneous disease due to various molecular conditions. First, dementia needed to be acknowledged as a cerebral condition and disentangled from major psychiatric diseases. Then, syphilis, vascular disease, and Alzheimer's pathology were described at the microscopical level. Due to its high prevalence and phenotypical overlaps with other diseases, AD dominated the field for decades and influenced research and classifications. Dementia is now an obsolete term that has been replaced by the less stigmatized major neurocognitive disorder, and research is shifting towards the detection at a presymptomatic level of complex and heterogeneous molecular pathways.

References

1 Berrios G: Dementia: historical overview; in Burns A, O'Brien J, Ames A (eds): Dementia, ed 3. London, Hodder Arnold, 2005, pp 3–15.
2 Blancard S: The Physical Dictionary, Wherein the Terms of Anatomy, the Names and Causes of Diseases, Chirurgical Instruments, and Their Use, are Accurately Described, ed 7. John&Benj Sprint, Edw. Symon, 1726.
3 Diderot D, d'Alembert JBLR, Fauche S: Encyclopédie ou Dictionnaire Raisonné des Sciences, Des Arts et Des Métiers. Paris, Briasson, 1756.
4 Berchtold NC, Cotman CW: Evolution in the conceptualization of dementia and Alzheimer's disease: Greco-Roman period to the 1960s. Neurobiol Aging 1998;19: 173–189.
5 Soury J: Système Nerveux Central, Carré et Naud, 1899.
6 Halpert BP: Development of the term "senility" as a medical diagnosis. Minn Med 1983;66:421–424.
7 Torack RM: The Early History of Senile Dementia. New York, NY, The Free Press, 1983.
8 Nagarajan S: Shakespeare's King Lear: An Edition with New Insights. Newcastle upon Tyne, Cambridge Scholars Publishing, 2017.
9 Willis T: The London Practice of Physick. Boston, MA, Longwood Press, 1977.
10 Schwab RN, Rex WE: Inventory of Diderot's Encyclopédie, Studies on Voltaire and the Eighteenth Century. Norwich, Voltaire Foundation, 1971.
11 Pinel P: A Treatise on Insanity (1806). Translation by Davis DD. New York, NY, Hafner Publishing, 1962.
12 Rush B: Medical Inquiries and Observations Upon the Diseases of the Mind. New York, NY, Kimber, Richardson, Philadelphia Hafner Press, 1962.
13 Esquirol É: Des Maladies Mentales Considérées Sous les Rapports Médical, Hygiénique et Médico-Légal, vol. 1. Paris, Jean-Baptiste Baillière, 1838.
14 Bulbena A, Berrios G: Pseudodementia: facts and figures. Br J Psychiatr 1986;148:87–94.
15 Kraepelin E: Psychiatrie: Ein Lehrbuch für Studierende und Ärzte, ed 4. Leipzig, Barth, 1893.
16 Bayle ALJ: Recherches sur les Maladies Mentales: Thesis, De l'imprimerie de Didot le jeune, 1822.
17 Morel BA: Traité des Maladies Mentales, Victor Masson, 1860.
18 Wilks S: Clinical notes on atrophy of the brain. Br J Psychiatr 1864;10:381–392.
19 Alzheimer A: Über eine eigenartige erkrankung der hirnrinde. Allgemeine Zeitschrife Psychiatr 1907;64: 146–148.
20 Kraepelin E: Das Senile und Prasenilar Irrsein. Psychiatrie, Ein Lehrbuch für Studierende und Ärzte, 1910.
21 Gellerstedt N: Zur Kenntnis der Hirnveränderungen bei der Normalen Altersinvolution. Inaug. Diss, Uppsala Läkareförenings Förhandlingar NF, 1933.

22 Roth M, Tomlinson BE, Blessed G: Correlation between scores for dementia and counts of 'senile plaques' in cerebral grey matter of elderly subjects. Nature 1966; 209:109–110.
23 American Psychiatric Association: Diagnostic and Statistical Manual of Mental Disorders. Washington, American Psychiatric Association, 1952.
24 American Psychiatric Association: Diagnostic and Statistical Manual of Mental Disorders (DSM II), ed 2. Washington, American Psychiatric Association, 1975.
25 American Psychiatric Association: Diagnostic and Statistical Manual of Mental Disorders (DSM-III), ed 3. Washington, American Psychiatric Association, 1980.
26 McKhann G, Drachman D, Folstein M, Katzman R, Price D, Stadlan EM: Clinical diagnosis of Alzheimer's disease report of the NINCDS-ADRDA work group under the auspices of Department of Health and Human Services Task Force on Alzheimer's Disease. Neurology 1984;34:939–944.
27 McKhann GM, Knopman DS, Chertkow H, Hyman BT, Jack CR, Kawas CH, Klunk WE, Koroshetz WJ, Manly JJ, Mayeux R: The diagnosis of dementia due to Alzheimer's disease: recommendations from the National Institute on Aging-Alzheimer's Association workgroups on diagnostic guidelines for Alzheimer's disease. Alzheimers Dem 2011;7:263–269.
28 American Psychiatric Association: Diagnostic and Statistical Manual of Mental Disorders (DSM-5). Washington, American Psychiatric Association, 2013.
29 Binswanger O: Die Abgrenzung des allgemeinen progressiven Paralysie. Klin Wochenschr 1894;31:1103–1105, 1137–1139, 1180–1186.
30 Alzheimer A: Die Seelensto (...) rungen auf arteriosklerotischer Grundlage. Allg Z Psychiat Psych Gericht Med 1902;59:695–711.
31 Hachinski VC, Lassen NA, Marshall J: Multi-infarct dementia: a cause of mental deterioration in the elderly. Lancet 1974;304:207–209.
32 Román GC, Tatemichi TK, Erkinjuntti T, Cummings J, Masdeu J, Garcia JA, Amaducci L, Orgogozo JM, Brun A, Hofman A: Vascular dementia diagnostic criteria for research studies: report of the NINDS-AIREN International Workshop. Neurology 1993;43:250–260.
33 Bowler J, Hachinski V: Vascular cognitive impairment: a new approach to vascular dementia. Baillieres Clin Neurol 1995;4:357–376.
34 Joutel A, Corpechot C, Ducros A, Vahedi K, Chabriat H, Mouton P, Alamowitch S, Domenga V, Cécillion M, Maréchal E, Maciazek J, Vayssière C, Cruaud C, Cabanis E-A, Ruchoux MM, Weissenbach J, Bach JF, Bousser MG, Tournier-Lasserve E: Notch3 mutations in CADASIL, a hereditary adult-onset condition causing stroke and dementia. Nature 1996;383:707–710.
35 Pick A: Über die Beziehung der senilen Hirnatrophie zur Aphasie. Prag Med Wochenschr 1982;17:165–167.
36 Witoonpanich P, Crutch SJ, Warren JD, Rossor MN: The undiscovered syndrome: Macdonald Critchley's case of semantic dementia. Neurocase 2015;21:408–412.
37 Warrington EK: The selective impairment of semantic memory. Quart J Exp Psychol 1975;27:635–657.
38 Mesulam M: Slowly progressive aphasia without generalized dementia. Ann Neurol 1982;11:592–598.
39 Snowden JS, Goulding PJ, Neary D: Semantic dementia: a form of circumscribed cerebral atrophy. Behav Neurol 1989;2:167–182.
40 Gorno-Tempini ML, Hillis AE, Weintraub S, Kertesz A, Mendez M, Cappa SF, Ogar JM, Rohrer JD, Black S, Boeve BF, et al: Classification of primary progressive aphasia and its variants. Neurology 2011;76:1006–1014.
41 Pick A: Zur Symptomatologie der linksseitigen Schläfenlappenatrophie. Eur Neurol 1904;16:378–388.
42 Brun A: Frontal lobe degeneration of non-Alzheimer type. I. Neuropathology. Arch Gerontol Geriatr 1987;6: 193–208.
43 Neary D, Snowden J, Northen B, Goulding P: Dementia of frontal lobe type. J Neurol Neurosurg Psychiatr 1988; 51:353–361.
44 Neary D, Snowden J, Gustafson L, Passant U, Stuss D, Black S, Freedman M, Kertesz A, Robert PH, Albert M, Boone K, Miller BL, Cummings J, Benson DF: Frontotemporal lobar degeneration: a consensus on clinical diagnostic criteria. Neurology 1998;51:1546–1554.
45 Warren JD, Rohrer JD, Rossor MN: Frontotemporal dementia. Br Med J 2013;347:f4827.
46 Kosaka K, Oyanagi S, Matsushita M, Hori A, Iwase S: Presenile dementia with Alzheimer-, Pick- and Lewy-body changes. Acta Neuropathol 1976;36:221–233.
47 Lewy F: Paralysis agitans. I. Pathologische anatomie. Handbuch der Neurologie 1912;3:920–958.
48 Trétiakoff C: Contribution à l'étude de l'anatomie pathologique du locus niger de Soemmering avec quelques déductions relatives à la pathogénie des troubles du tonus musculaire et de la maladie de Parkinson. Doctoral Dissertation, 1919.
49 Polymeropoulos MH, Lavedan C, Leroy E, Ide SE, Dehejia A, Dutra A, Pike B, Root H, Rubenstein J, Boyer R: Mutation in the α-synuclein gene identified in families with Parkinson's disease. Science 1997;276:2045–2047.
50 Goedert M, Spillantini MG, Del Tredici K, Braak H: 100 years of Lewy pathology. Nature Rev Neurol 2013;9: 13–24.

Dr. Frédéric Assal
Unité de Neurologie générale et cognitive, Service de Neurologie
Département de Neurosciences cliniques, HUG
Gabrielle Perret Gentil 4
CH–1211 Geneva 11 (Switzerland)
E-Mail Frederic.Assal@hcuge.ch

Bogousslavsky J, Boller F, Iwata M (eds): A History of Neuropsychology.
Front Neurol Neurosci. Basel, Karger, 2019, vol 44, pp 127–140 (DOI: 10.1159/000494960)

Neurology versus Psychiatry? Hallucinations, Delusions, and Confabulations

Antonio Carota[a] Julien Bogousslavsky[b]

[a]Clinique de Genolier, Genolier, Switzerland; [b]Neurocenter, Swiss Medical Network, Clinique Valmont, Montreux, Switzerland

Abstract

Hallucinations, delusions, and confabulations are common symptoms between neurology and psychiatry. The neurological diseases manifesting with such symptoms (dementia, epilepsy, Korsakoff's disease, brain tumors, Parkinson's disease, migraine, right hemisphere stroke and others) would be the key to understand their biological mechanisms, while the cognitive sciences, neuropharmacology and functional neuroimaging would be the tools of such researches. It is possible to understand the perceptive rules of the mind and the mechanisms of the human consciousness based on these symptoms. However, hallucinations and delusions manifest with extraordinary vehemence with psychiatric disorders such as psychosis and schizophrenia, with which there is no evidence of brain lesions. Furthermore, they are subjective symptoms, and they do not have biological markers. Hence, they are prone to high inter-individual variability and depend on other variables (such as education, history of trauma), and are therefore difficult to reduce to unequivocal constructs. Causative mechanisms are probably multiple. For understanding these symptoms, a common framework between neurology and psychiatry is still missing. The psychopathology of French alienists over the 19th century, of S. Freud, and of Henry Ey over the 20th century gave way, in the second half of the 20th century, to the adoption of the DSM and neurosciences, to pursue a pure neurological perspective. However, although psychodynamic models seem nowadays (in a technological era) less influential, detailed clinical evaluations focusing on emotional-cognitive paradigms are probably the only way to lead to new neurobiological researches.

Introduction

Hallucinations, delusions, and confabulations are symptoms that belong to the border zone between neurology and psychiatry.

The neurological diseases manifesting with such symptoms (dementia, epilepsy, Korsakoff's disease, brain tumors, Parkinson's disease, migraine, stroke and others) would be the key to understand their biological mechanisms, while the cognitive sciences, neuropharmacology and functional neuroimaging would be the tools of such researches. We can understand the perceptive rules of the mind and the mechanisms of the human consciousness from these symptoms. This is the reason why such phenomena have been studied many centuries before Christ's birth, with almost all religions being permeated by histories of hallucinations, delusions, and confabulations; the most important philosophers, writers, and artists tried to deal with them in their works. In the 19th century, French alienists established the constructs of psychiatric diseases and psychopathology. However, the conceptual-clinical models of psychiatric diseases, together with the Freudian psychoanalysis and the orgodynamism of Henry Ey found a conclusion in the second half of the 20th century with the publication of the Diagnostic and Statistic Manual of Mental Disorders (DSM) (a "psychiatric utensil") and the advances of neurology and neurosciences. However, hallucinations and delusions manifest with extraordinary vehemence in psychiatric disorders such as psychosis and schizophrenia, where there is no evidence of brain lesions. Furthermore, they are subjective symptoms and not biological markers. They are prone to high inter-individual variability and depend on factors such as education and history of trauma. Thus, they are difficult to reduce to unequivocal constructs.

For these reasons, the neurological and psychiatric frameworks of these symptoms did not and do not fit together in the same puzzle. The Capgras syndrome (CS) is probably a history apart.

Hallucinations

A list of neurological, psychiatric diseases and other conditions associated with these phenomena (occurring in the 5 senses, but also in the dimensions of thought, memory, and imagination) is reported in Table 1. It should be noted that hallucinations (mostly auditory) can occur in otherwise healthy people.

In 1646 (according to the English Oxford Dictionary), the doctor, writer and scientist Sir Thomas Browne gave the first "medical" definition of "hallucination," intended as a distorted vision of the real. The term derived from the Latin "allucinari" (related to the Greek "aluo," wandering in the mind) included the idea of madness and insanity. At that time, on the stage, Shakespeare's Macbeth became insane by hearing voices and seeing visions.

However, the category of the real (or the reality) was already firmly questioned by Plato, Kant, Schopenauer, and Gestalts psychologists. For all of them the human being could

Table 1. Conditions associated with hallucinations

Sleep phenomena/parasomnia	
	Hypnagogic/hypnopompic hallucinations
	Dreams
Sleep deprivation	
Sensory deprivation/changes (visual or auditory) with release phenomena	
	Charles-Bonnet Syndrome with ophthalmologic diseases and severe visual loss (most commonly with macular degeneration)
	Musical ear syndrome with progressive deafness
Synesthesia	
Toxic/substances	
	Natural or synthetic hallucinogens (LSD, DMT, DXM, Cocaine, Methamphetamine, Alcohol, Mescaline, Psilocybin, Butofenines, Atropa, Datura, *Herba apollinaris*, *Salvia divinorum*, *Mandragora officinarum*, Cannabinoids, Peyote, Ketamine, Phencyclidine)
	Psychotropic drugs
	Alcohol, barbiturate, and benzodiazepine withdrawal
Migraine	
	With brainstem aura
	With "sensorial" aura
Epilepsy	
	Temporal lobe epilepsy and other "focal" epilepsy
Dementia	
	Alzheimer's disease
	Lewy body disease
	Parkinson's disease (hallucinations increased by dopaminergic treatments)
	Frontotemporal dementia
Brain lesions	
	Tumor, stroke, brain injury
	Peduncular hallucinosis
Right hemisphere stroke	
	Anosognosia of hemiparesis, illusory limb movements, misoplegia, somatoparaphrenia, Asomatognosia
Corticobasal degeneration	
	Alien hand and leg
Delirium and encephalopathies	
	For example: zoopsy with delirium tremens
Encephalitis of various origin (immunologic or infectious)	
	Anti-NMDAR encephalitis, herpes encephalitis
	Creutzfeldt-Jacob disease
Psychiatric conditions	
	Schizophrenia spectrum disorder (voices, command hallucinations), psychoses, bereavement, bipolar disease, dissociative identity disorder, borderline personality disorders
Near to death experiences	
	Autoscopic phenomena
Healthy subjects with no specific diagnosis	
Hallucinatory "professionists"	
	Swamies, Sciamans, Medium
	Meditators (Yogi, Buddhists)

have only a subjective understanding of the real (corresponding to "ideas" for Plato, "categories" for Kant, "dream-likes creations" for Schopennauer, "units" for the Gestalts psychologists).

The human consciousness is that brain function which creates a representation of the external world to keep it distinct from the self. Thus, self-consciousness, reality, and hallucinations are all non-measurable subjective experiences.

The definition of Esquirol (1817, French Dictionary of Medical Sciences) is phenomenologically more accurate: the hallucination is a perception without the object. On this basis, Esquirol separated hallucinations from illusions.

The link between madness and hallucinations was initially discussed by the 19th century French alienists. The treaty of Pinel on mental alienation (1801) was their manifest. According to their "romantic" ideas, hallucinations and insanity were symptoms of the imaginative mind, passions, and politics of the time. For most of them, at least in the first half of the 19th century, emotions could modify the structure of the brain or the body but cerebral lesions could not be the mechanisms of hallucinations and alienation. Indeed, the phrenologist-alienist Luis-Francisque Lélut (1804–1877) underlined that the genius and madness of Socrates and Pascal were the result of auditory hallucinations (an inner voice).

Despite these premises, alienists attempted to fit psychiatric symptoms and diseases into models (psychopathology). It was the first tentative of madness medicalization, the birth of modern psychiatry [1]. The alienist Alexandre-Jacques-François Brierre de Boismont (1797–1881) described in his scholastic books (1845 and 1853) the connection among moralism, hallucinations, and psychiatric diseases. For him, epidemic hallucinations, vampirism, ecstasy could be transmitted only by "ideas." Thus, hallucinations should be cured (in accordance with Pinel), by "ideas" or "reasoning with the patient" (the dawning of psychotherapy) together with "water irrigation." The so-called "douche" was probably a purge rather than a cure.

However, in the 18th century, the Genevan philosopher, botanist and scientist Charles Bonnet (1720–1792), was the first to provide in an essay (1760) a biological explanation for the complex visual hallucinations of his 87-year-old grandfather who, surprisingly, was not demented. Indeed, Bonnet thought that hallucinations, in a cognitively normal person, were due to cataracts and anomalous optic nerves stimulation. This was the first description of the "release" hallucinations. The Charles Bonnet syndrome (CBS) was named after him only later in the 1930s by the Swiss neurologist Georges de Morsier (1894–1982). The CBS still remains underdiagnosed [2].

The alienist Jean-Etienne Esquirol (1772–1840) already indicated (1817) that all hallucinatory experiences should be accounted for by similar perceptual phenomena. In 1840, one of his pupils, Jules Baillarger (1809–1890), tried to effectuate the first clinical studies (1842–1844) on the physiological causes of hallucinations (fever, delirium tremens, mania, ecstasy, hysteria and so on). He made a clear demarcation between hallucinations and symptoms due to their interpretation.

Jules Séglas (1856–1839) further enriched the semiology of hallucinations, indicating their link with the faculty of language. He described the "psychomotor non auditory verbal hallucinations" (subvocalization or motor verbal acts), the "syndrome d' influence" (delusion of being directed), and the psychomotor hallucinations (in case of lesions of the Broca's area). Clérambault classified the sensorial hallucinations as mental automatisms, emphasizing their histological origin. The British neurologist, John Hughlings Jackson (1835–1911), described brain functions in terms of hierarchical systems of control and input, and he considered hallucinations as a "release" phenomenon due to a loss of cortical control.

Thus, already in the 19th century, a "neurologic" concept of hallucinations emerged at the side of the "psychiatric" theories of the alienists. According to this new concept, hallucinations were not mediated by the stress or trauma but were the result of brain changes or inflammation (the neurosyphilis was the prototype of these disorders). Antoine Laurent Jessé Bayles (1799–1858), who provided the first description of the "general paralysis of the insane," was an influential precursor of this "neurologic" doctrine. However, his conclusions were vehemently confuted by the majority of alienists of his time.

According to a neurologic construct, a parallelism (Maury, 1848; Baillarger, 1846) was traced between hallucinations and some conditions of the sane, such as dreams, hypnotism [3] somnambulism and the effects of substances, such as cannabis (Moreau de Tours – 1845, "folies haschischiques").

As it concerns hallucinations (as it happened before for the neurosyphilis), some clash was inevitable between the neurological and psychiatric perspectives. In 1855 and 1856, at the meeting of the French medico-psychological association (reports in the annals of the association), the main question was whether hallucinations had biological or psychologic causes. These debates introduced the several antinomies which were pervasive until now in the era of neurosciences (true versus pseudo-hallucinations, hallucinations with or without insight, hallucinations in the sane and the insane, voice auditory hallucinations versus visual hallucinations, dream versus non-dream hallucinations, body misperceptions – synesthesia, eidetic imagery, palinacousis and palinopsia, tinnitus, hypnagogic states, autoscopy, Ekbom states – versus visionary states such as trance, somnambulism, illusions).

The psychodynamic approach was again empowered by Freud in the first half of the 20th century. He indicated that dreams and hallucinations stem from a timeless psychotic state whereas traumatic memories are converted into thoughts, images, and words. At that time, on May 16, 1920, Joan of Arc (1412–1431) was canonized Saint by Pope Benedict XV because she heard the voice of God saying how to liberate France from the English domination.

In 1930, Georges de Morsier criticized the psychodynamic account of hallucinations, suggesting that they are neurological symptoms, due to aberrant activity of the visual regions of the brain. Lhermitte (1922) and Van Bogaert (1924) described patients with peduncular hallucinosis due to brainstem lesions, of which the unreal nature was recognized by the same patients.

In the 20th century, a new psychodynamic approach made some resurgence with the monumental treaty (1973, 1,540 pages) of Henri Ey (1900–1977 on hallucinations). He utilized the hallucinations to provide a new global concept of cerebral functions (organo-dynamism). In this new doctrine, the consciousness (due to superposed levels of brain functions) and not the unconscious had the primacy.

He reported that the dissolution of the conscience opens the door to hallucinations. Ey describes meticulously all the forms of hallucinations, the ones derived by a global disintegration of the conscience (generally occurring with psychiatric diseases), and the others (eidolia) which manifests with a circumscribed cerebral dysfunction as it is the case with the neurologic diseases. Examples of eidolia are the CBS or the body schema illusions ("somato-éidolia"). A case of peduncular hallucinosis corresponding to fantastic "distorteidolias" has been recently reported with a paramedian thalamic stroke [4].

Finally, after Ey's death, psychiatry definitely turned towards neurosciences and, the adoption of the American DSM (1952), a sort of a mere "psychiatric utensil" more than a doctrine, was a sort of tombstone of all the psychopathological constructs.

Indeed, in the second half of the 20th century, the description of neurologic diseases associated with hallucinations such as narcolepsy, peduncular hallucinosis, Lewy body dementia, Parkinson's disease (and related dopaminergic treatments) [5], and Alzheimer's diseases [6], took hold.

Cholinergic, serotoninergic, and dopaminergic dysfunction together with Lewy bodies were identified as the neurobiological mechanisms of visual hallucinations and delusions in dementia with Lewy bodies [7], Parkinson-related dementia [8], and Alzheimer's disease [9]. Somatic spatial and sensorial hallucinations (reduplication of body parts, surnumerary body parts, misoplegia, phantom limb movements, asomatognosia) were recognized to manifest with right frontal and parietal stroke [10]. Alien hand and leg phenomena were reported with corticobasal degeneration [11]. In the 20th and 21st centuries, neurologic theories of hallucinations were further supported by studies with EEG, brain cartography, electrode stimulation, sensory deprivation, neurochemical, neuroimaging, and genetic analyses.

Lilly [12] and Walters et al. [13] conducted experiments on healthy volunteers floating in barrels of saline liquids and deprived of lights, sound, and gravity. In these conditions, all the subjects presented hallucinations. Hallucinations appear after 2 or 3 days of sleep deprivation together with some personality disorganization [14] Devillières et al. [15]. Trained subjects, could have enlightened experiences with meditation (Yogi, Buddhists) [16] or leave their bodies with the hypnosis.

Hallucinogens (typified by LSD) have been extensively studied in the 20th century, but they went down because of the risk of a persistent perception disorder [17].

In the 20th century, all the possible hallucinations in all the sensory modalities (visual, auditory verbal and musical, olfactory and gustatory, hallucinations of bodily sensations – tactile, somatic and visceral, proprioceptive, kinesthetic, vestibular, hallucinated central pain, sexual, thermal hallucinations, phantom limb, phantom body phantom-self hallucinations, sensed presences, autoscopic phenomenon) have been described and investigated.

Once again, it was evident that all these phenomena manifest either with neurological (tumor, migraine, epilepsy, and delirium) or psychiatric disorders. However, primary delusions accompany hallucinations, especially in the case of psychosis and schizophrenia.

Cognitive studies of auditory hallucinations of psychotic patients demonstrated anomalous language lateralization, intrusive thoughts, metacognitive believes, deficits of mental imagery, familiar and non-familiar voices recognition, episodic and source memory, reality monitoring, top-down, executive control and inhibitory functions, deficits that are more pronounced than in healthy voice-hearers [18–20].

PET and fMRI studied showed that musical hallucinations occurring with deafness (musical ear syndrome) are associated with the activation of the same brain network of the normal musical perception (auditory areas, visual cortex, basal ganglia, brainstem, pons tegmentum, cerebellum, hippocampus, amygdala) [21].

Structural MRI and VBM studies of schizophrenic patients with auditory hallucinations, demonstrated reduced volumes of the superior temporal gyrus, prefrontal cortex, and regions involved in emotional processes (insula, amygdala, anterior cingulate cortex, parahippocampal, and hippocampal gyrus) [22].

FMRI and PET studies showed that hippocampus and para-hippocampal region and language areas (primary auditory cortex) are activated with auditory hallucination [23, 24]. The consequent hypothesis is that schizophrenic subjects fail in recognizing verbal memories or self-generated inner speech (that they attribute to external agents) released by the homologous language areas of the right hemisphere. Neuroimaging studies found other relevant areas for hallucinations, involved in language, memory, and reward-punishment (anterior cingulate, the insula, the cerebellum, the thalamus, and the orbitofrontal cortex).

One of the most recent hypothesis conceives consciousness as the result of an oscillatory resonance of a cholinergic thalamo-cortical network, which integrates inputs ascending from the brainstem [25]. This network is active during dreams and paradoxical sleep although, at that time, it is impermeable to external sensory stimuli.

In case of schizophrenia and auditory hallucinations, the network activity disengages and does not reflect reality any more (as during sleep). Deficient gabaergic transmission and NMDA-receptor hypofunction in the hippocampus and basolateral amygdala may contribute to the formation of aversive memories and delusions. Antipsychotic treatment with risperidone can reduce cerebral metabolism in the left hippocampus with a gradual reduction in hallucinations and delusions.

Delusions

The term has Latin origin and means lying and to fraud. However, the French term delire ("going out from the lira") indicates "going out" from the reality. Thus, since the beginning, delusions have been associated with mental illness. In the first half of the 19th century, French alienists Esquirol and Pinel (1838), the fathers of psychiatry, identified paranoia and delusions as fixed ideas (monomania), deriving from passions, ideas that could be removed by the mind or cured ("disalienation"). Later, Morel (1860) and Magnan in France refused the concept of partial insanity and placed paranoia among the degenerative states. However, most of the actual first-rank symptoms of schizophrenia, were already reported by the French alienist Jules Séglas (1856–1939). De Clérambault (1885) described the "erotomania" (delusion of being loved) and other passional delusions. Lasègue (1852) and Legrand du Saulle (1871) described the paranoiac delusions, Trélat (1861) the pathological jealousy, Foville (1869) the grandiose delusions, and Lasègue et Jules Flarte la folie à deux.

At the turn of the 19th century, the German physician Kraepelin (1887) and the Swiss psychiatrist Bleuer (1911) described schizophrenia as an independent disease and delusions and hallucinations as its main symptoms (positive symptoms). Schneider (1939) described in his monography specific delusions and hallucinations (audible thoughts, voice arguing, voices commenting on one's action, influence playing on the body-somatic passivity, thought withdrawal, thought insertion, thought broadcasting, made feelings, made impulses, made volitional acts, delusional perception), occurring with schizophrenia (first-rank symptoms) which had diagnostic value per se. In 1954, chlorpromazine was first approved by the US Food and Drug Administration and then rapidly and extensively used in patients with delusions and schizophrenia.

Finally, delusions are false and persistent beliefs, sustained with extraordinary vehemence, despite every incontrovertible evidence of the contrary. Normal thoughts and logic are invaded by fantastic ruminations, which have negative valence and induce invalidating affects.

As for hallucinations, the antinomy is created between the mental (subjective, phenomenological) and biological (organic) dimensions, that is, once again, between psychiatry and neurology. Indeed, delusions manifest with psychotic disorders, schizophrenia, schizoaffective disorders, delusional disorders, substance-induced psychotic disorders, bipolar disorder, major depressive disorder with psychotic features, but also with neurologic diseases such as delirium, dementia, Parkinson's disease [26] right hemisphere stroke [10, 27, 28], autoimmune encephalitis Herken and Prüss [29]. The prevalence rate of delusions is about 30% in patients with Alzheimer's disease [30].

However, in comparison to hallucinations, delusions have a less unequivocal meaning.

Thus, primary delusions should be differentiated from secondary delusions, delusion-like or overvalued ideas. Primary delusions occur with psychosis and schizophrenia but not with mood disorders. The primary delusion is an autochthonous idea according to Wernicke (1906), non-mediated by thoughts or interpretations. According to Jasper (1963), primary delusions are not understandable by cultural background, education, personality, and circumstances of life. Jasper indicated that delusion is not a judgment but rather a direct experience of its meaning.

Primary delusions can be classified on the basis of their phenomenology in delusional mood, delusional perception, delusional memory, delusional ideas or awareness, and, on the basis of their content, into delusions of control, delusions of mind being read, delusions of thought insertion, delusions of references, persecution, identity, infidelity and jealousy, love (erotomania), grandiose delusions (supernatural, science-fictional or religious events), religious, delusions of guilt, sin and unworthiness, nihilist delusions (such as the Cotard syndrome [31]), somatic delusions (Ekbom states), delusions of poverty. The severity of delusions is determined by the strength of conviction, extension to the patient's life, bizarreness, disorganization, psychological pressure, affective response, and deviant behavior (the degree to which the patient acts according to delusions).

The psychoanalytical approach (Freud and his scholars) considered delusions as the result of unconscious conflicts, which are projected to the external world with the goal of removing guilt. Freud indicated that latent homosexual tendencies were specifically related to paranoid delusions.

In contrast, the cognitive approach, after 1990, attributed delusions to decision-making false paradigms ("jumping to conclusions" [32]), lowered decision threshold [33], assessment of certainty [34], wrong memory source attribution [35], dysfunction of the theory of mind [36], disruption of conscious access with unimpaired unconscious processing [37].

On a neurological perspective, since the 1960, the clinical efficacy of antipsychotics (D2 receptor antagonists) in reducing delusions suggested the etiologic role of dopaminergic hyperactivity in mesolimbic and mesocortical circuits.

Despite the difficulty of psychotic or primary delusions to be amendable to neurological frameworks, the CS (a delusional misidentification syndrome) Barrelle and Luauté [38] is a history apart.

The patients with CS (first description by Capgras and Reboul-Lachaux on 1923) are convinced that impostors, counterparts, aliens, or robots have replaced one or several intimate persons and feel in danger. The attribution of a false identity may also concern inanimate objects, voices, and domestic animals. Reduplicative paramnesia (Pick, 1903) is a similar misidentification but it concerns places. The CS can occur with schizophrenia but also with right frontal and parieto-occipital stroke or lesions [39], although often in the context of diffuse cortical atrophy or bilateral frontal dysfunction. Bogousslavsky suggested in 1981 that a cerebral lesion should be always researched in the case of a patient with CS [40].

The CS has been interpreted in the context of a model of face recognition constituted by 2 pathways [41]. The first is determinant of face identification and the second mediates the affective response, which is usually associated to that face when it is identified. Failure of the first pathway engenders prosopagnosia (a cognitive syndrome of face non-recognition); the damage of the second pathway generates the delusion of the CS, which is a mismatch between a correctly recognized face and an incongruous (or non-recognized) emotional reaction. The evidence that psychiatric patients with CS, compared with patients with prosopagnosia, do not show normal skin conductance responses to famous faces [42] supports the theory of a mismatched emotional reaction to a known face.

Regarding anatomoclinical correlations, there are sufficient clinical and experimental data supporting the idea that the fusiform gyrus of the right temporal lobe is determinant for face recognition (the first pathway). However, brain regions involved in face emotional recognition remain uncertain. They could be located on a dorsal system (parieto-occipital junction, inferior parietal lobule, superior temporal sulcus, cingular gyrus, amygdala) or on a ventral system, located in the temporal lobe, which parallels circuitries of the face recognition system. In a recent case series studies of CS, the retrosplenial cortex and the right frontal lobe have been found as the neuroanatomical correlate, respectively, for impaired familiarity perception and belief evaluation [43].

A complementary hypothesis conceives that working memory dysfunction, secondary to right frontal damage, may be responsible for difficulty in negotiating simultaneously cognitive and emotional data relative to an identity. The disconnection hypothesis supposes that misidentification syndromes derive from a disturbed integration of the 2 hemispheres as each hemisphere may have a different role in processing identities. Another theory conceives a disconnection from frontal areas implicated in self/other discrimination and a parietotemporal or occipitotemporal region involved in sensorial analysis of identity features. This theory gives relevance to feelings of alienation, depersonalization or unreality that are manifest with misidentification syndrome, and that resemble "dejà-vu" or other similar phenomena of temporal lobe epilepsy. The common thread to all the forms of misidentification might be the loss of the sense of uniqueness in experience [44, 45].

The role of dopaminergic transmission should be the object of further investigations because misidentification syndromes respond to neuroleptic drugs. Research on these disorders can bring novel insights into the neurobiology of paranoid schizophrenia.

Confabulations

The confabulation consists of the production of statements and actions that are unintentionally incongruous to the subject's history, background, present and future situation. The patient seems to ignore the falsity of his statements. Nevertheless, it is always very difficult to understand completely what the truth and the falsehood and the degree of consciousness is (or the intent) of the confabulators.

There is an evident clinical overlap between confabulations and delusions and, conceptually, the distinction could be difficult [46]. However, the presence of amnesia and a brain lesion with the MRI would make the difference between confabulations related to neurological disorders and those associated with psychosis or schizophrenia. The epidemiology of confabulation is unknown, they are probably a rare or temporary phenomenon. The etymology is from the Latin "fabulare," that means telling tales or histories. The term was currently used in clinical contexts only during the second part of the 19th century.

The Korsakoff's syndrome (the prototypical neurological disease with confabulations) was named after the Russian neurologist, Sergei Korsakoff, who provided, first, between 1887 and 1891, a detailed clinical description of that syndrome (that he called "polyneuritic psychosis"). He underlined the association of memory dysfunction and confabulations with polyneuropathy and alcohol consumption. Few years before, the German psychiatrist Carl Wernicke described the disease ("polioencephalitis superior hemorrhagica"), named later upon him (Wernicke's encephalopathy), which usually associates and precedes the symptoms of the Korsakoff's disease. Only in the 20th century thiamine was isolated and synthesized (1936) and related to the Korsakoff syndrome in 1952.

Wernicke specified that the confabulations of his disease corresponded to the "pseudoreminiscences" (pseudomemories), of the Kraepelin classification (1886) of "paramnesias."

In 1901, Bonhoffer distinguished embarrassment or "momentary" confabulations of the Korsakoff's syndrome (which were filling a memory gap), and spontaneous or fantastic confabulations, related to dream-like states or psychosis. The association of memory disturbance and confabulations was also supported by Gregor and Roemer (1932) and Liepmann (1910).

Van der Holst (1932) pointed to the role of the disturbance of time sense [46].

Confabulations were reported in prisoners or soldiers with brain trauma during the WWII. Since 1970, spontaneous confabulations have been significantly associated with ruptured aneurysms of the anterior communicating artery [47]. However, confabulations could be also a symptom of herpes encephalitis, nicotinic acid deficiency, multiple sclerosis, frontotemporal dementia, frontal lobe epilepsy and inter-ictal psychosis, vascular dementia, and Alzheimer's disease. Lesion sites are orbitofrontal, the basal forebrain, amygdala, cingulate gyrus, the dorsomedial nucleus of the thalamus, and medial hypothalamus [48].

Lafora (1935) already indicated the role of arteriosclerotic changes in the frontal lobes. However, during the 1970s, with the advent of the clinicopathological studies based on CT scan, the frontal lobe theory of confabulations took place [49].

Kopelman emphasized the distinction of confabulations in "provoked" and "spontaneous" [50]. The first type (with the Korsakoff syndrome) are created by questioning the patient and seems to have some truthful or plausible autobiographic content. They could be elicited also in normal controls with memory tests specifically designed to induce false responses. On the contrary, the spontaneous confabulations are unprovoked, grandiose, manifestly impossible. According to Kopelman, spontaneous confabulations are due to the combination of memory and frontal lobe dysfunction.

Over the last 30 years, several cognitive theories of spontaneous confabulations were elaborated, such as the deficit of memory temporal ordering, deficit of temporal consciousness [51], deficit at memory consolidation or strategic retrieval [52, 53], source memory deficits, dysfunction of the constructive memory framework [54], frontal lobe dysfunction [49, 55], loss of inhibiting inappropriate responses, loss of reality checking, confusion between unique and repeated events, habits, and routine [53, 56–58]. According to Schnider, the behavior of patients with spontaneous confabulation is guided by memory traces that are founded (real autobiographical events), but that do no longer belong to the ongoing reality [59, 60]. For example, these patients would quit the hospital to return to professions that they exerted many years before. In contrast to patients with other amnesic disorders, Schnider indicated as diagnostic the fact that patients with spontaneous confabulations believe their confabulations and act consequently with behaviors and emotions. Other authors insisted on the "narrative" "myth-telling" functions of confabulations, or their value of brain symptom as a "strong belief" or "pathological certainty" (or pre-conscious feeling of rightness). "Psychological" theories (unconscious mechanisms to avoid catastrophic reactions, motivational factors, and pre-existing personality traits [61], emotion dysregulation hypothesis [62], have more sparse evidence. Finally, confabulations, as hallucinations and delusions are probably not a unitary phenomenon.

Conclusions

Although the progress of the investigational methods in neurosciences spans over the last 50 years, the biological underpinnings of psychiatric symptoms still remain elusive. Auditory hallucinations and primary delusions are the main symptoms of psychosis and schizophrenia. They are related to language areas, neural networks of memory, executive functions, and emotions and are induced by dopaminergic, cholinergic, and serotoninergic dysfunctions.

Visual hallucinations associate mostly with neurological diseases such as Lewy body disease and Parkinson disease-associated dementia, REM-sleep behavior disorder and with cholinergic and dopaminergic hypoactivities.

Confabulations are generally associated with neurological disease and brain lesions, with an amnesic syndrome in case of provoked confabulations (as in Korsakoff's disease) and with amnesia and frontal dysfunction in case of fantastic or spontaneous confabulations.

Although hallucinations, delusions, and confabulations are at the border zone of neurology and psychiatry, a common framework is still missing. Causative mechanisms are probably multiple. In the second half of the 20th century, the psychopathology of the French alienists, S. Freud and Henry Ey disappeared under the tombstone of the DSM and with the advancement of neurosciences. However, although psychodynamic models seem nowadays (in a technological era) less influential, detailed clinical evaluations focusing on emotional-cognitive paradigms are probably the only way to lead to new neurological and neurobiological researches.

References

1 Poirier J, Clarac F, Barbara JG, Broussolle E: Figures and Institutions of the neurological sciences in Paris from 1800 to 1950. Part IV: Psychiatry and psychology. Rev Neurol (Paris) 2012;168:389–402.

2 Schadlu AP, Schadlu R, Shepherd JB 3rd: Charles Bonnet syndrome: a review. Curr Opin Ophthalmol 2009;20: 219–222.

3 Sommer A: Professional heresy: Edmund Gurney (1847–88) and the study of hallucinations and hypnotism. Med Hist 2011;55:383–388.

4 Delgado MG, Bogousslavsky J: "Distorteidolias" – fantastic perceptive distortion. A new, pure dorsomedial thalamic syndrome. Eur Neurol 2013;70:6–9.

5 Jellinger K: New developments in the pathology of Parkinson's disease. Adv Neurol 1990;53:1–16.
6 Perry EK, McKeith I, Thompson P, Marshall E, Kerwin J, Jabeen S, et al: Topography, extent, and clinical relevance of neurochemical deficits in dementia of Lewy body type, Parkinson's disease, and Alzheimer's disease. Ann N Y Acad Sci 1991;640:197–202.
7 Pezzoli S, Cagnin A, Bandmann O, Venneri A: Structural and functional neuroimaging of visual hallucinations in Lewy body disease: a systematic literature review. Brain Sci 2017;7:pii:E84.
8 Nishio Y, Yokoi K, Uchiyama M, Mamiya Y, Watanabe H, Gang M, et al: Deconstructing psychosis and misperception symptoms in Parkinson's disease. J Neurol Neurosurg Psychiatry 2017;88:722–729.
9 Factor SA, McDonald WM, Goldstein FC: The role of neurotransmitters in the development of Parkinson's disease-related psychosis. Eur J Neurol 2017;24:1244–1254.
10 Bartolomeo P, de Vito S, Seidel Malkinson T: Space-related confabulations after right hemisphere damage. Cortex 2017;87:166–173.
11 Schaefer M, Heinze HJ, Galazky I: Alien hand syndrome: neural correlates of movements without conscious will. PLoS One 2010;5:e15010.
12 Lilly JC: Mental effects of reduction of ordinary levels of physical stimuli on intact, healthy persons. Psychiatr Res Rep Am Psychiatr Assoc 1956;5:1–9, discussion 10–28.
13 Walters C, Shurley JT, Parsons OA: Differences in male and female responses to underwater sensory deprivation: an exploratory study. J Nerv Ment Dis 1962;135: 302–310.
14 Babkoff H, Sing HC, Thorne DR, Genser SG, Hegge FW: Perceptual distortions and hallucinations reported during the course of sleep deprivation. Percept Mot Skills 1989;68:787–798.
15 Devillières P, Opitz M, Clervoy P, Stephany J: [Delusion and sleep deprivation]. Encephale 1996;22:229–231.
16 Lindahl JR, Kaplan CT, Winget EM, Britton WB: A phenomenology of meditation-induced light experiences: traditional buddhist and neurobiological perspectives. Front Psychol 2014;4:973.
17 Orsolini L, Papanti GD, De Berardis D, Guirguis A, Corkery JM, Schifano F: The "Endless Trip" among the NPS Users: Psychopathology and Psychopharmacology in the Hallucinogen-Persisting Perception Disorder. A Systematic Review. Front Psychiatry [Internet]. https://www.ncbi.nlm.nih.gov/pmc/articles/PMC5701998/ (November 20;8, 2017).
18 Waters F, Allen P, Aleman A, Fernyhough C, Woodward TS, Badcock JC, et al: Auditory hallucinations in schizophrenia and nonschizophrenia populations: a review and integrated model of cognitive mechanisms. Schizophr Bull 2012;38:683–693.
19 Baumeister D, Sedgwick O, Howes O, Peters E: Auditory verbal hallucinations and continuum models of psychosis: a systematic review of the healthy voice-hearer literature. Clin Psychol Rev 2017;51:125–141.
20 Alderson-Day B, Lima CF, Evans S, Krishnan S, Shanmugalingam P, Fernyhough C, et al: Distinct processing of ambiguous speech in people with non-clinical auditory verbal hallucinations. Brain J Neurol 2017;140: 2475–2489.
21 Kumar S, Sedley W, Barnes GR, Teki S, Friston KJ, Griffiths TD: A brain basis for musical hallucinations. Cortex 2014;52:86–97.
22 Kim GW, Kim YH, Jeong GW: Whole brain volume changes and its correlation with clinical symptom severity in patients with schizophrenia: a DARTEL-based VBM study. PLoS One 2017;12. https://www.ncbi.nlm.nih.gov/pmc/articles/PMC5435302/.
23 Kompus K, Falkenberg LE, Bless JJ, Johnsen E, Kroken RA, Kråkvik B, et al: The role of the primary auditory cortex in the neural mechanism of auditory verbal hallucinations. Front Hum Neurosci 2013;7. https://www.ncbi.nlm.nih.gov/pmc/articles/PMC3633947/.
24 Cui LB, Chen G, Xu ZL, Liu L, Wang HN, Guo L, et al: Cerebral blood flow and its connectivity features of auditory verbal hallucinations in schizophrenia: a perfusion study. Psychiatry Res Neuroimaging 2017;260:53–61.
25 Orliac F, Delamillieure P, Delcroix N, Naveau M, Brazo P, Razafimandimby A, et al: Network modeling of resting state connectivity points towards the bottom up theories of schizophrenia. Psychiatry Res Neuroimaging 2017;266:19–26.
26 Ffytche DH, Creese B, Politis M, Chaudhuri KR, Weintraub D, Ballard C, et al: The psychosis spectrum in Parkinson disease. Nat Rev Neurol 2017;13:81–95.
27 Gurin L, Blum S: Delusions and the right hemisphere: a review of the case for the right hemisphere as a mediator of reality-based belief. J Neuropsychiatry Clin Neurosci 2017;29:225–235.
28 Martinaud O, Besharati S, Jenkinson PM, Fotopoulou A: Ownership illusions in patients with body delusions: different neural profiles of visual capture and disownership. Cortex 2017;87:174–185.
29 Herken J, Prüss H: Red flags: clinical signs for identifying autoimmune encephalitis in psychiatric patients. Front Psychiatry 2017;8:25.
30 Lai L, Lee PE, Chan P, Fok MC, Hsiung G-YR, Sepehry AA: Prevalence of delusions in drug-naïve Alzheimer disease patients: a meta-analysis. Int J Geriatr Psychiatry 2017, Epub ahead of print.
31 Sahoo A, Josephs KA: A neuropsychiatric analysis of the cotard delusion. J Neuropsychiatry Clin Neurosci 2017; 30:58–65.
32 Ward T, Garety PA: Fast and slow thinking in distressing delusions: A review of the literature and implications for targeted therapy. Schizophr Res 2017;pii: S0920-9964(17)30521-2.
33 Moritz S, Pfuhl G, Lüdtke T, Menon M, Balzan RP, Andreou C: A two-stage cognitive theory of the positive symptoms of psychosis. Highlighting the role of lowered decision thresholds. J Behav Ther Exp Psychiatry 2017; 56:12–20.

34 Broyd A, Balzan RP, Woodward TS, Allen P: Dopamine, cognitive biases and assessment of certainty: a neurocognitive model of delusions. Clin Psychol Rev 2017;54:96–106.
35 Griffin JD, Fletcher PC. Predictive processing, source monitoring, and psychosis. Annu Rev Clin Psychol 2017;13:265–289.
36 Phalen PL, Dimaggio G, Popolo R, Lysaker PH: Aspects of theory of mind that attenuate the relationship between persecutory delusions and social functioning in schizophrenia spectrum disorders. J Behav Ther Exp Psychiatry 2017;56:65–70.
37 Berkovitch L, Dehaene S, Gaillard R: Disruption of conscious access in schizophrenia. Trends Cogn Sci 2017;21:878–892.
38 Barrelle A, Luauté JP: Capgras syndrome and other delusional misidentification syndromes. Front Neurol Neurosci 2018;42:35–43.
39 Darby R, Prasad S: Lesion-related delusional misidentification syndromes: a comprehensive review of reported cases. J Neuropsychiatry Clin Neurosci 2016;28:217–222.
40 Bogousslavsky J, Salvador A: [Capgras syndrome. Clinical aspects and organic problems: a re-evaluation]. Ann Med Psychol (Paris) 1981;139:949–964.
41 Ellis HD, Young AW: Accounting for delusional misidentifications. Br J Psychiatry 1990;157:239–248.
42 Ellis HD, Young AW, Quayle AH, De Pauw KW: Reduced autonomic responses to faces in Capgras delusion. Proc Biol Sci 1997;264:1085–1092.
43 Darby RR, Laganiere S, Pascual-Leone A, Prasad S, Fox MD: Finding the imposter: brain connectivity of lesions causing delusional misidentifications. Brain J Neurol 2017;140:497–507.
44 Cutting J: Delusional misidentification and the role of the right hemisphere in the appreciation of identity. Br J Psychiatry Suppl 1991;14:70–75.
45 Margariti MM, Kontaxakis VP: Approaching delusional misidentification syndromes as a disorder of the sense of uniqueness. Psychopathology 2006;39:261–268.
46 Berrios GE: Confabulations: a conceptual history. J Hist Neurosci 1998;7:225–241.
47 DeLuca J, Cicerone KD: Confabulation following aneurysm of the anterior communicating artery. Cortex 1991;27:417–423.
48 Fischer RS, Alexander MP, D'Esposito M, Otto R: Neuropsychological and neuroanatomical correlates of confabulation. J Clin Exp Neuropsychol 1995;17:20–28.
49 Stuss DT, Alexander MP, Lieberman A, Levine H: An extraordinary form of confabulation. Neurology 1978;28:1166–1172.
50 Kopelman MD: Two types of confabulation. J Neurol Neurosurg Psychiatry 1987;50:1482–1487.
51 Dalla Barba G, La Corte V: A neurophenomenological model for the role of the hippocampus in temporal consciousness. Evidence from confabulation. Front Behav Neurosci 2015;9:218.
52 Moscovitch M, Melo B: Strategic retrieval and the frontal lobes: evidence from confabulation and amnesia. Neuropsychologia 1997;35:1017–1034.
53 Gilboa A, Alain C, Stuss DT, Melo B, Miller S, Moscovitch M: Mechanisms of spontaneous confabulations: a strategic retrieval account. Brain J Neurol 2006;129:1399–1414.
54 Schacter DL, Norman KA, Koutstaal W: The cognitive neuroscience of constructive memory. Annu Rev Psychol 1998;49:289–318.
55 Johnson MK, O'Connor M, Cantor J: Confabulation, memory deficits, and frontal dysfunction. Brain Cogn 1997;34:189–206.
56 Metcalf K, Langdon R, Coltheart M: Models of confabulation: a critical review and a new framework. Cogn Neuropsychol 2007;24:23–47.
57 Nahum L, Bouzerda-Wahlen A, Guggisberg A, Ptak R, Schnider A: Forms of confabulation: dissociations and associations. Neuropsychologia 2012;50:2524–2534.
58 Serra M, La Corte V, Migliaccio R, Brazzarola M, Zannoni I, Pradat-Diehl P, et al: Confabulators mistake multiplicity for uniqueness. Cortex 2014;58:239–247.
59 Schnider A, von Däniken C, Gutbrod K: The mechanisms of spontaneous and provoked confabulations. Brain J Neurol 1996;119:1365–1375.
60 Schnider A: Spontaneous confabulation, reality monitoring, and the limbic system – a review. Brain Res Brain Res Rev 2001;36:150–60.
61 Fotopoulou A, Conway MA, Solms M: Confabulation: motivated reality monitoring. Neuropsychologia 2007;45:2180–2190.
62 Turnbull OH, Salas CE: Confabulation: Developing the 'emotion dysregulation' hypothesis. Cortex 2017;87:52–61.

Antonio Carota
Clinique de Genolier
Route du Muids 3
CH-1272 Genolier (Switzerland)
E-Mail a.carota@bluewin.ch

Bogousslavsky J, Boller F, Iwata M (eds): A History of Neuropsychology.
Front Neurol Neurosci. Basel, Karger, 2019, vol 44, pp 141–163 (DOI: 10.1159/000494961)

Developmental Cognitive Deficits: A Historical Overview of Early Cases

Paul Eling

Donders Institute for Brain, Cognition and Behaviour, Radboud University, Nijmegen, The Netherlands

Abstract

In this chapter, I will present an overview of early case descriptions of specific isolated cognitive deficits in children for which no clear brain impairment could be demonstrated and which were therefore considered to be congenital or developmental in nature. Three kinds of syndromes will be discussed. First, more general deficits like the attention and hyperactivity disorder and congenital aphasia will be presented. The second category relates to the more specific cognitive deficits, like developmental prosopagnosia, that have been reported, especially from the early 1980s onwards. In particular, early reports of specific congenital deficits in the areas of attention, language, perception, and memory will be presented. And finally, I will briefly discuss early case descriptions of individuals with autism and savant syndrome. Instead of suffering from a specific cognitive deficit, the latter show a special talent.

Introduction

Neuropsychology is primarily seen as a field of science dealing with the cognitive and behavioral consequences of brain damage. In addition, neuropsychologists have also studied "deficits" that seemed to be inborn, present from birth, or at least not easily attributable to an incident shortly after birth. When core concepts like aphasia, agnosia, and apraxia had been developed in the second half of the 19th century and people began to think of the brain as a collection of centers with connecting pathways, some physicians began to use the neuropsychological framework for understanding some phenomena observed in children. Probably the best example here is (developmental) dyslexia, being modeled after (acquired) alexia following brain disorder in adults.

In this chapter, I will focus on the early case descriptions of specific isolated cognitive deficits in children for which no clear brain impairment could be demonstrated and therefore were considered to be congenital or developmental in nature. Three kinds of syndromes may be distinguished. First, more general deficits like the attention and hyperactivity disorder and congenital aphasia will be discussed. The second category relates to the more specific cognitive deficits that have been reported, especially from the early 1980s onwards, like developmental prosopagnosia and various types of developmental dyslexia. And finally, I will briefly discuss early case descriptions of individuals with autism and with savant syndrome. Instead of suffering from a specific cognitive deficit, the latter show a special talent.

I will not systematically discuss acquired brain disorders in children. However, as will become clear in this chapter, in some cases a serious incident probably caused functional or structural damage, likely related to the cognitive deficit, as for instance in the case of developmental amnesia. In addition, while in some early studies on developmental cognitive deficits no brain abnormalities could be detected, even when computer tomography and magneto-resonance-imaging had been introduced, it cannot be concluded that better procedures underlying anatomical or functional abnormalities can explain these specific deficits. But the crucial point is that the fact that such specific deficits can occur, may tell us about the underlying cognitive architecture.

Although the study of congenital disorders and talents may be of even more relevance for our understanding of the functioning of the brain than that of acquired deficits, at least in the eyes of Gall, it has received relatively little attention. Only few studies examining congenital deficits in various cognitive domains are available. Temple ([1]; Fig. 1), a pioneer in this field and producing case studies in different cognitive domains, published a monograph on these developmental cognitive deficits. Tranel and De Haan [2] edited a special issue of the journal Cortex on this issue in 2007. There are also special issues from the journal Cognitive Neuropsychology, one on developmental prosopagnosia (2012, issue 5–6), and one on developmental dysgraphia (2017, issue 3–4). These articles, of course, all relate to current investigations. To the best of my knowledge no overview of early studies on congenital deficits has been prepared before.

Tranel and De Haan [2] provide special reasons for studying developmental deficits. First of all, brains and cognitive functions develop and it is not only important to understand the more or less stable adult state, but also understand how cognitive processes evolve over time, which is a topic of interest for its own sake. Second, developmental cases may constitute additional evidence for the modular structure of the adult brain. Third, plasticity, the capacity to adapt to "external" conditions appears to be different during development than in the adult state. Fourth, developmental neuropsychology forms a basis for connecting to neurogenetics. Last, but not the least, there is a clinical reason: we need to understand these deficits for understanding, assessing and, if necessary and possible, treating these disorders.

In this chapter, I will provide an overview of early descriptions of specific congenital deficits, or talents, in the areas of attention, language, perception, and memory. I will also

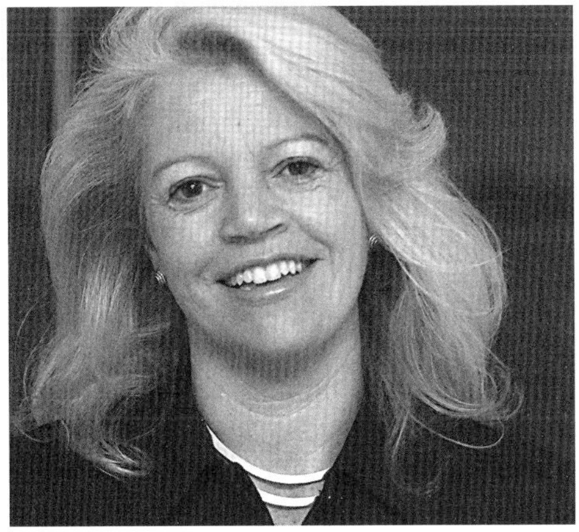

Fig. 1. Christine Temple, University of Essex, a pioneer in the study of developmental cognitive deficits. Courtesy Alexander Temple.

discuss autism, even though this syndrome seems to involve 3 different areas of cognitive processes (social cognition, communication, and repetitive behavior). I have no intention to make it exhaustive. Early here means tracing reports of "first" cases with a specific deficit or talent. In addition, it is not my intention to settle theoretical issues. Scientists may differ in opinion with respect to the fundamental nature of a given deficit or whether a specific underlying biological cause can account for the behavior. Much recent research has provided new insights into observations and interpretations of similar cases in the past, but these will not be analyzed here. With these preliminaries in mind, I will now proceed with discussing early cases with what is by some assumed to be attention deficit and hyperactivity disorder (ADHD).

Attention

Since the introduction of the ADHD label in the early 1980s, the number of children receiving a psychiatric diagnosis indicating that they suffer from an attention deficit has increased tremendously. But a long history preceded this event. As Foley [3] indicates, stories of unruly and intransigent children have been told at all times and it is hardly (if at all) possible to determine when a child stops being hard to handle and becomes pathological. Consequently, we cannot say which case description may be regarded as the first of a child with what we now regard as ADHD.

Russell Barkley, a leading ADHD expert, and his coauthors Barkley and Peters [4] maintain that Melchior Adam Weikard (1742–1803) produced the first description of ADHD. Weikard was a German physician who published numerous works, among them a medical textbook *Der Philosophische Arzt* in 1775. The third chapter of this book is devoted to lack of attention and the English translation can be found in Barkley and Peters [4]. Weikard first described the features of individuals who lack the ability to concentrate. An important cause, he argued, is the distraction of children by a hundred things at the same time. He also mentioned an example, not coming from his own experiences. King Carl II was said, by the Duke of Buckingham, to have a quick and vibrant mind. Weikard also argued that the youth is less attentive than the old, the girl less than the man, a sanguine less than a choleric person. Weikard's chapter hinted at attention problems as a problem per se. He even claimed that the problem can be treated by a physician. But it seems a matter of interpretation whether he described ADHD and whether the case he presented may be regarded as the first example of ADHD.

Palmer and Finger [5] stated that the Scottish-born physician Alexander Crichton (1763–1858) described ADHD, in particular the inattentive type, in 1798 in his *Inquiry into the nature and origin of mental derangement*, consisting of 3 books. In the second chapter of Book II, he dealt with attention and attention disorders. He defined attention as the capacity to focus on one thing while excluding others. He distinguished 2 kinds of attention disorders. One state of inattention is a "morbid diminution of its power or energy," and he defined the second as "the incapacity of attending with a necessary constancy to any one object." He argued that the latter is due to an "unnatural or morbid sensibility of the nerves." According to Palmer and Finger, Crighton's description of the disorder meets the criteria of what is currently diagnosed as ADD. However, Crichton did not provide information on individuals he (or others) had examined in detail.

This brings us to the lectures of the English pediatrician George Still (1868–1941; [6]) that for a long time have been considered the first description of attention disorder as a specific disorder. Still gave three lectures to the Royal College of Physicians of London, titled *On some abnormal psychical conditions in children*. He specifically wanted to draw attention to a behavioral problem that he had observed in children, not just in mentally retarded children, but also in children with a normal intelligence. The nature of the problem, Still argued, is a *lack of moral control*. They do not control their activities "in conformity with the idea of the good of all." This category of children with intact intelligence and lack of control can be split up into children also suffering from other physical disease that is associated to this lack of control, and children showing this lack of control without having an intellectual impairment or any other medical disorders. He observed 20 children that fell in this latter category, 15 boys and 5 girls, ranging in age from almost 5 until 13.5 years. Notably, symptoms were not observed until the age of 2 or 3 years, sometimes even later. In some children, the loss of moral control seemed to be developmental in nature while in other children loss of control disappeared after it had been acquired. Still described nine different forms of behavior in which this lack of control could be expressed but the major feature seemed to be impulsivity. He provided concrete examples of these kinds of uncontrolled behaviors that he himself had observed. He also mentioned that these children cannot sustain attention for a longer period of time, which he also regarded as a problem of attention, be it somewhat different in nature than moral loss of control.

Perhaps somewhat surprisingly, even though Still's description of a very impulsive child seems easily recognizable, the disorder was not "recognized" as such by his contemporaries. Around the 1950s and 1960s, the concept of hyperactivity began to dominate the literature, originally observed in children with congenital brain disorders and subsequently applied to hard-to-handle children without brain disorder. Only after a new formal definition had been adopted in the Diagnostic and Statistical Manual, combining attention problems and hyperactivity as defining features, ADHD as a syndrome resembling Still's description of the disorder, began to be recognized broadly (see for a detailed historical overview [3]).

Language

As in the acquired forms of aphasia, various different forms of developmental language disorders may be distinguished. I will first deal with congenital aphasia, word deafness and anomia. Subsequently, types of dyslexia and dysgraphia will be discussed.

Congenital Aphasia
From a cognitive neuropsychological point of view, the most important (in terms of theory development) form of language disorder in aphasia are Broca's and Wernicke's aphasia, defined in respectively 1861 and 1874, shortly followed by a number of other aphasia syndromes. Around 1900, physicians also began to look more specifically at language disorders in children.

Weiner [7] mentioned that Delius in his book *De Alalia* (no details on the person or the book could be retrieved by me) described the condition of children who do not know how to speak, but do not suffer from an intellectual impairment and they can understand almost as good as other children that do speak. Unfortunately, his essay is not available in an accessible form to see whether he actually investigated cases with this condition. Franz Joseph Gall ([8] vol 5, p 39) also mentioned this phenomenon, but did not provide a concrete case. He complained that he had been unable to get a cranium of such an individual.

Weiner [7] listed a number of publications that may be considered to touch upon the issue. The fact that it is almost impossible to establish whether or not a child was intellectually intact and/or had problems with articulation rather than language, makes it difficult to determine whether these articles indeed were dealing with a condition for which Léon Vaïsse (1807–1881), specialized in deaf children, introduced the notion of congenital aphasia in 1866.

Towards the end of the 19th century, speech doctors (*Sprachärzte*) began to see children with language development disorders that were also referred to as *Hörstummheit* (hearing mutism or audimutism). An early extensive description was produced by the Croatian-Viennese physician Rafael Coën (1839–1904), who in fact suggested the notion of *Hörstummheit* [9]. He began his description by noting that it often begins with parents who visit the doctor with the complaint that the child still has not begun to speak. The child hears very well, understands all that is within his scope of intelligence, and is in good health. The basic deficit, according to Coën, is the complete incapacity to form articulate sound. He assumed it was a functional problem rather than the result of a lesion. The problem seems analogous to that of the adult patient with Broca's aphasia.

Coën apparently was familiar with children suffering from the disorder but he did not provide examples. He also developed bodily and mental gymnastics as a form of treatment as the condition did not improve spontaneously. He published a second account [10] in which he stated that he had seen 81 children and treated 29 children. Shortly after Coën's publications, Berlin physicians Hermann Gutzmann (1865–1922), Albert Liebmann (1865–1924), and Leopold Treitel (1845–1931), all active as speech doctor, followed up on Coën ideas on congenital aphasia (for a detailed analysis of their contributions, see [7]).

Apparently independent from these developments in Austria and Germany, the topic of congenital aphasia was "discovered" in London as well, in particular at Great Ormond Street Hospital for Sick Children [11]. In 1891, three papers were published dealing with this topic. One was written by Walter Baugh Hadden (1856–1893) [12] discussing three cases with speech problems without other intellectual or medical problems. The first, Charles M, an 11-year-old boy, seemed bright but could only utter a few words. Hadden mentioned a variety of tests he applied to examine his language capacities. The two other cases, boys aged 7 and 4 years, respectively, and coming from a family with more reports of language developmental problems, are described more succinctly.

Hadden assumed that the nature of the problem had to do with the process of combining speech sounds into a word, that is, at the level of phonology rather than semantics or syntax if we translate it in current terminology. Language perception also seemed to be impaired and Hadden argued that apparently the process of learning the language, essentially dependent on the interaction with a mother, did not initiate properly.

A meeting was organized by the Royal Medical and Chirurgical Society 2 months after Hadden's paper appeared in press and here several other cases were presented, presumably suffering from the same deficit. William Hale White (1857–1949) and Cuthbert Hilton Golding-Bird (1848–1939) presented their observations on 2 brothers, 9 and 10 years old [11]. The younger boy's only problem seemed to be that he could not speak. He was intelligent, could calculate, and even write to dictation. When discussing the case, Hale White and Golding-Bird did not think the problem was analogous to a form of acquired aphasia. They considered it to be a problem of language development and suggested the term idioglossia for this "new" disorder.

At that same meeting, another case was presented by Fredrick Taylor, an assistant of Golding-Bird. The case concerned a boy of 8 years who according to Taylor resembled the one described before, but he rejected the term idioglossia for several reasons. An important barrier for finding an appropriate term was the fact that at the time no clear distinction could be made between language and speech. In fact, while the main deficit in these children with idioglossia perhaps were linked to speech production than language in general, the term survived for some time and became even more strongly linked to language development rather than to speech.

Word Deafness

In a series of studies, Worster-Drought and Allen [13–15] presented the case of a boy, 12 years old, who showed a special kind of auditory agnosia, a difficulty in recognizing auditory words as the most prominent symptom. They argued that the term *word deafness* was perhaps the first that would come to mind, but it did not properly describe the nature of the deficit as the boy could not distinguish a range of nonverbal sounds as well. On the contrary, auditory agnosia was too broad as he could distinguish some sounds. They therefore concluded that the proper term would be *auditory imperception*. In addition, they call it congenital as the deficit appeared to be one that is developmental in nature rather than resulting from a lesion. In the last of the three papers, Worster-Drought and Allen discuss a long list of preceding case descriptions. It is very difficult to determine the exact nature of the language and/or speech deficit of these cases, and whether or not it is valid to group all these cases under the same umbrella. Generally, cases were not systematically investigated and the terminology was not yet crystallized making distinctions we now consider crucial, for instance between dysarthria, apraxia of speech and higher levels of language processing, difficult to detect in these early descriptions. Moreover, language comprehension may impress as more intact than it actually is, if a person can compensate by using nonverbal cues. Statements about the quality of language comprehension in these early cases are difficult to interpret given the lack of systematic language tests.

Anomia

Anomia, also referred to as amnestic aphasia, is a mild form of acquired aphasia, where an individual has a specific problem of retrieving words from memory.

Van Hout [16] studied two children with naming problems not due to an acquired disorder. The first child was 7 years of age but performed at the level of a 3-year-old child, and the second was 9 years old and performed at the level of a 5-year-old. The kind of error produced most often (around 50%) was a semantic paraphasia (e.g., producing dog instead of cat). It should be noted that its passive receptive vocabulary was not impaired, as was demonstrated in a multiple choice pointing task and a task in which the child was presented with a noun and had to describe its meaning. Furthermore, the pattern of responses in the two developmental anomic children resembled that of children with an acquired anomia.

Temple [17] described a 12-year-old boy with a developmental deficit that she characterized as anomia. At the age of 3 and 5, he had suffered a generalized epileptic fit and the EEG then showed frequent high voltage spikes and sharp waves confined to the right central area. Neurological examination showed no abnormality. He sometimes experienced sudden problems in expressing himself while at other moments he was clearly able to function at a reasonable intellectual level. Neuropsychological assessment suggested a specific problem with naming pictures. This was more systematically investigated and it appeared that his naming of animals was particularly impaired, while his performance on indoor objects seemed even better than that of control children. Temple argued that the pattern reminds of the category-specific agnosia, where patients with brain lesions may show a specific impairment for animate objects but not for inanimate objects.

Very Early Descriptions of Dyslexia

Perhaps the earliest description of a congenital cognitive disorder based on 19th century models of language and the brain relates to reading problems in children with no obvious neurological damage. The German ophthalmologist Rudolph Berlin (1833–1897) introduced the term dyslexia in 1887 [18]. He had examined several patients experiencing reading problems without an obvious reason for that. His first case was "Herr B," a civil servant 66 years of age, claiming that he had reading problems affecting his work. Moreover, he complained that he could read the first few words but then could not continue. Ophthalmologic investigations did not reveal any disturbances. B could read letters and indicated that words did not appear blurred. In a period of 23 years, Berlin collected six cases and in all cases he observed the same phenomenon: they could read three to five words and then could not proceed. His patients did show some additional deficits, suggesting there could be a brain lesion in the left hemisphere. He used the term dyslexia, defining it as an incomplete isolated word blindness. While no obvious brain disorder causing the reading problem was demonstrated, Berlin did assume that a lesion was responsible.

Pringle Morgan (1861–1934) [19] published a case of congenital word blindness in Percy F., a boy of 14 years. He had always been a bright and intelligent boy, quick at games. However, he was unable to learn to read. He could read and write isolated letters. In writing to dictation he made many spelling errors, also producing nonwords. Reading a short text from a children's book, he did not read a single word correctly except for some short (highly frequent!) words such as "and," "the," or "that." Morgan claimed that the basic deficit was an incapacity to store and preserve visual word images. Hinshelwood (1859–1919) [20] maintained that Morgan's study was in fact inspired by an earlier note by Hinshelwood on dyslexia.

Hinshelwood, surgeon in the Glasgow Infirmatory and lecturer in ophthalmology, produced case studies in a series of articles between 1996 and 1910 and compiled them in his monograph [20]. These also included studies on children from the same family, and Hinshelwood suggested that the disorder may have a familial or even a hereditary basis. Furthermore, he described cases suffering from letter dyslexia, while other cases appeared to have no problems with reading letters but with reading words.

Dual Route Model and Variants of Dyslexia and Dysgraphia

Marshall (1939–2007) and Newcombe's (1925–2001) [21] dual route model for reading and writing [21], in particular in patients with brain lesions, triggered a new interest in searching for cases with specific forms of reading and writing problems that might be associated with specific components of this model.

Temple and Marshall [22] studied the case of HM, a 17-year-old girl with an IQ of around 110 and no medical problems. She was extensively investigated with neuropsychological tests. The main finding was a severe reading and spelling problem. Her reading was at the level of a 9-year-old. HM could not read nonwords. In reading words, she made many visual errors and derivational errors. She had no specific problem with irregular spelled words. This pattern is similar to that of *phonological dyslexia* in acquired cases of dyslexia. Her spelling was at the level of a 10-year-old child. Her spelling errors were often phonologically accurate. She produced no semantic paragraphias and her ability to spell phonologically regular nonwords was fair. This pattern matched that of patients with acquired *phonological dysgraphia* and HM's deficit may be characterized as a developmental variant.

Temple (1958–2014) [23] presented two cases with developmental reading and spelling disorders, RB and AH who suffered from qualitatively different forms of dyslexia and dysgraphia. Their error patterns resembled those of then newly defined acquired forms of dyslexia, in particular *surface* and *phonological dyslexia.*

RB was a 10-year-old girl, showing a perfectly normal development and a full scale IQ of 115. She appeared to be somewhat slow in learning to read. Upon examination no neurological abnormalities were found. Her speech was fluent and normal in all respects. She read words equally well as nonwords, but was significantly better in reading regular words than irregular words. Her errors tended to be neologisms. They were phonologically plausible. Temple classified RB as a *developmental surface dyslexic.*

The pattern of spelling errors of RB mirrored that of her reading errors. No difference between words and nonwords was observed, but there was a significant difference between orthographically regular and irregular words. Errors were often phonologically plausible. Consequently, apart from being a developmental surface dyslexic, she was also a *developmental surface dysgraphic.* This mirror image pattern in reading (input) and writing (output) raises interesting questions about the commonality of cognitive processes for input and output that I will not examine here. However, these observations do point to the relevance of such cases for theorizing about cognition and the brain.

As a kind of double dissociation, Temple also described the case of AH, a 10-year-old boy. Developmental milestones and speech development were within normal limits. Hearing and vision were normal. Handwriting was poor and his drawing seemed immature. No abnormalities were found on neurological examination. IQ scores were relatively high. AH was significantly poorer at reading nonwords than words. He read orthographically regular and irregular words equally well. His errors could be seen as paralexias. He made morphological and visuo-semantic errors. AH can be classified as a *developmental phonological dyslexic.*

Like RB, AH's spelling problems resembled those observed in his reading of words: a more severe problem with nonwords but no difference between regular and irregular words. Moreover, spelling errors were mostly not phonologically plausible. Consequently, AH suffered from a *developmental phonological dysgraphia*, characterized by a problem of segmentation and using phoneme-grapheme correspondence rules as the only route for reading and writing.

Investigations of acquired reading disorders in the 1980s, stimulated by the dual route model, also revealed a remarkable syndrome called deep dyslexia. And it appears there is a developmental analogy as well. Stuart and Howard [24] investigated KJ, a 13-year-old girl, with a reading age of about 6 years. Her reading of single words and nonwords was examined, and a remarkable number of responses was incorrect but was semantically related to the target words. She also produced morphological errors and visual errors. This pattern clearly matches that of acquired deep dyslexia.

KJ's spelling of words and nonwords was also tested. Her writing of nonwords was clearly more impaired than that of regular words. She made occasional semantic errors and function word substitutions, writing "the" for "is." Clearly, KJ had problems with grapheme-phoneme correspondence rules, but in addition she also experienced other problems causing semantic errors and the substitutions. Taken together, Stuart and Howard concluded that KJ represented a case of *developmental deep dyslexia.*

Friedmann and Nachman-Katz [25] presented the case of a Hebrew reading (from right to left) boy, NT, 10-years-old, showing left neglect in reading. He developed quite normally. Teachers in the classroom noted some problems with concentration. Reading single words, his error percentage was 96%, mostly due to omitting left-sided, final letter(s) of a word. No neglect was observed in reading numbers or symbols. Nor did he show neglect symptoms on clinical tests for neglect. Friedmann and Nachman-Katz [25] concluded that this was the first case of *developmental neglect dyslexia.*

Yet another form of developmental dyslexia was observed by Friedmann et al. [26]. By presenting a reading test battery they selected a group of 10 individuals, 1 being an adult and 1 child suffering from a brain lesion. The nature of the errors in word reading in this group consisted of "migration" of letters between neighboring words, for instance, *fig tree* is read as *fig free.* This type is called *developmental attentional dyslexia* and has also been observed in acquired dyslexia.

Dyscalculia

Children often show problems with calculation in school, just as they may show reading problems. However, the amount of research devoted to dyslexia is immensely larger than that on calculation problems or dyscalculia. This is also true for the historical background of the two kinds of disorders. Perhaps an important reason for this difference resides in the nature of the disorder of dyscalculia. There may be many different factors that contribute to problems in calculation and it seems there is no underlying core deficit, functional or anatomical, that can be held responsible. These factors may relate to, for instance, visuospatial abilities, number processing, and abilities to handle arithmetic procedures [26, 27].

A more systematic investigation of potential sources of developmental dyscalculia was stimulated by a cognitive analysis of acquired acalculia by McCloskey et al. [28]. Temple [29] described a case of what she called *digit dyslexia.* A boy, Paul, was examined first at the age of 11 years. His medical record appeared uneventful and he attended a normal school. From the beginning difficulties with arithmetic were reported. When reading and writing Arabic numerals, the syntactic component was processed accurately, but the lexical processing resulted in incorrect digit selection. For example, he would read 88 as "Eighty-two." Reading of words and texts was normal except for reading numeral words, where the same kind of error would be produced: digits were replaced by other digits. The same pattern of errors was observed for writing numbers to dictation.

Temple [30] used the same theoretical framework to describe two cases of developmental dyscalculia, presenting a double dissociation with respect to number facts and number processing. SW was a 17-year-old boy. He suffered from tuberous sclerosis, but his medical history indicated that his arithmetic problems dated from before and have not ameliorated since. Therefore, it is likely that his calculation deficit is developmental in nature. He had no problems in reading numbers and numeral words, and the understanding of the numbers appeared intact. Knowledge of number facts was also intact: he could recall tables and define arithmetic operations. In contrast, procedures for calculation were impaired for multiplication, division, and subtraction. Adding numbers was intact. Temple concluded that SW suffered from *procedural dyscalculia*.

The mirror image type of dyscalculia is presented by Temple's second case HM, 19-years-old, with a normal intelligence and no known neurological abnormality. HM read numbers and word numerals well. Her performance on addition and subtraction did not differ from normal controls. However, she made much more errors on multiplication problems, while taking the same amount of time as controls. Division was also very difficult although she could explain the steps required. Temple concluded that HM had specific problems in mastering the arithmetic tables and her condition could be characterized as *number fact dyscalculia*.

Perception

In this section, a number of different disorders related to perception will be discussed, in particular difficulties in perceiving and identifying objects, faces, color, music, and voices.

Object Agnosia

A person may fail to recognize objects without having any problems with sensory processing. Lissauer [31] showed that cortical lesions may produce two kinds of agnosia: apperceptive and associative agnosia. Children with developmental agnosia have been reported, although the number is very limited indeed. While in some of them the deficit may be limited to a special kind of stimuli, there are also cases with mixed forms.

The 8-year-old boy LG was presented by Ariel and Sadeh [32]. He had a high IQ and intact basic perceptual skills. He could read and write and do math at age level or above. Extensive testing of his object recognition skills suggested that he showed symptoms resembling those of apperceptive agnosia. Visual memory and visual imagery were normal. He also showed face recognition problems. However, he could not recognize photos of familiar persons, could not match unfamiliar faces and could not correctly infer age or gender from photos of faces. Identifying emotions on faces was also very difficult for him. He had no real problem with remembering faces in a face learning task, but he indicated that he recognized faces using remarkable features like hair style, color or extra-facial features.

LG suffered from both object recognition and prosopagnosia. But pure developmental object agnosia, without prosopagnosia, has been reported as well. Germine et al. [33] described this selective developmental deficit. It concerned a 19-year-old woman, AW, who they found through a web-based screening test. She did not suffer from low-level perceptual problems and showed no general memory problems. She had severe problems on tests requiring within-class visual recognition memory for 6 categories: guns, horses, scenes, tools, doors, and ears. However, she performed normal on the categories of houses and glasses as well as on tests for memory of visual shapes. The authors claim this is the first case of *developmental agnosia* for objects without prosopagnosia and that the case provides evidence for category-specific dissociations in visual recognition.

Face

While cases of *developmental prosopagnosia* may also show problems with object recognition, some cases with pure prosopagnosia have also been reported in the literature. A relatively early case was AB, studied by McConachie [34]. AB's development was uneventful from a medical point of view. She was first studied when she was 12-years-old. Her EEG showed abnormalities in the right posterior hemisphere. She indicated that she recognized people by marking their voice, clothing, and mannerisms. She could recognize familiar people, but never recognized unfamiliar persons. Basic perceptual skills appeared intact and there was no sign of a more global agnosia.

AB was tested again when she was 27-years-old [35]. Color vision, contrast sensitivity, and judgment of line orientation were intact. A battery of face perception and matching tests suggested that AB seemed to have problems with encoding the structural features of a face. AB could tell that a face is a face and to some extent could match faces on expression, but she could not identify, expressions, gender or age.

Temple [36] reported on Dr. S, a highly intelligent female physician, 60 years of age at the time of testing, but suffering from face recognition problems from early childhood on. No problems were observed for basic perceptual skills, judgment of line orientation, and mental rotation. The Mooney face test, requiring judgment of gender and age of black and white drawings, was performed normally. Face matching, as assessed with Benton's Face Recognition test, was intact. She had no difficulties with Warrington's Recognition Memory test, assessing memory for words and faces. Her real problem was recognizing familiar and famous people. Apparently, Dr. S's structural encoding capacities were intact and she appeared to have problems in accessing identity information.

In conclusion, pure developmental prosopagnosia has been documented. Surprisingly, individuals with this condition seem to be able to cope with it and live a more or less normal life. More importantly, as much research on face perception has demonstrated, face perception is a complex process and may be impaired for different reasons. Like in cases with acquired agnosia, there may be problems at the level of processing of the visual pattern and there may be problems accessing relevant information stored in memory.

Color

Agnosia for stimulus features like color and motion have been described in patients with brain lesions. However, to my knowledge, no developmental case with a problem in motion perception has been described and only one individual with developmental color agnosia. Van Zandvoort et al. [37] studied MAH, a 43-year-old man, who had been hospitalized because of a right cerebellar stroke. In a neuropsychological assessment, it was discovered that he could not name color patches. Additional tests revealed that he had no problem in discriminating colors. He had severe problems in naming and pointing to colors. Naming colors of common objects was intact, suggesting that object-color knowledge is intact. Coloring in line drawings with the appropriate color (for instance a cherry) appeared to be impossible. MAH claimed that he had had this problem all his life and the authors therefore argued that this is the first case of developmental color agnosia. Covert color processing appeared to be intact in MAH, like in acquired cases of color agnosia [38]. Subsequently, it was established that his mother and one of his daughters had similar problems, although less severe [39].

Location Orientation

Individuals may experience problems with recognizing objects, faces or words. This kind of perception may relate to what is now commonly referred to as the "what" system in perception. There is an additional perceptual route, characterized as the "where" or "how" route. This latter processing stream appears to be involved in spatial processing, in particular in actions. McCloskey et al. [40] investigated a case, AH, a 20-year-old female university student. During elementary school, she experienced problems with spelling and arithmetic, but otherwise her academic performance was good. Her medical history was unremarkable and a neurological examination, including an EEG and MRI-scan, also revealed no abnormalities.

Scores on tests for visual acuity, perimetry, and contrast sensitivity were normal. She appeared substantially impaired on a test for phoneme discrimination. Direct copying of a complex figure was severely impaired. For instance, parts of the Rey Figure were copied correctly, but she made numerous errors with the location and orientation of parts. Copying from memory was significantly impaired. A more controlled test for visual localization was given to AH: an X was presented on a computer screen and she had to indicate the place by moving the computer mouse. She made many errors, reversing up and down or left and right. In another task, she had to reach for an object under visual guidance. She could name the object correctly but when reaching for the object she also produced left-right reversals. She made no errors when reaching for objects directly in front of her. Moreover, she also showed no deficits at all when tested for localization in the auditory and tactile modality. McClosky et al. [40] argued that AH suffered from a specific *developmental deficit in visual object localization*. They also maintained that the early spelling and arithmetical problems observed at school may be associated with this specific deficit as well.

Music

It is common knowledge that individuals vary in their talent for music. For Gall, the observation of a young girl with an exceptional talent for music was a crucial moment [41]. He realized that the traditional view of the mind having a general memory for all sorts of materials, could not fully explain human behavior, in particular differences in talent among individuals. However, in our society lacking a sense for music is not regarded as a troublesome feature, let alone a cognitive deficit. This may explain that the first case of *developmental amusia* was not thoroughly investigated until 2002.

Peretz et al. [42] presented the case of Monica. The kind of disorder she presented is commonly referred to as tone deafness. The woman was in her forties. She had responded to a newspaper advertisement, seeking individuals with problems in music perception. She was extensively tested on aspects of music perception as well as other cognitive abilities. She appeared to have above average intellectual, language, and memory capacities. Audiometric tests were normal. The basic deficit was characterized by Peretz et al. [42] as a problem with fine-grained discrimination of pitch, and they labeled her as congenital amusia. Neuroimaging procedures could not reveal any functional or structural brain deficits that could explain the behavioral deficit.

Lebrun et al. [43] examined AS, a 10-year-old girl. Using the Montreal Battery for the Evaluation of Amusia revealed the severe problems of AS with melodic, rhythmic discrimination, and memory for melodies. Detecting small pitch changes also appeared to be difficult for her. Lebrun et al. [43] concluded that her deficit is comparable to the adult form of congenital amusia and that AS can be considered to be the first case of congenital amusia in childhood.

Voice

We usually recognize individuals from their appearance, especially their faces. But as was mentioned above, if the capacity to recognize people from their face is lost, like in cases suffering from prosopagnosia, a person can often still be recognized by hearing the voice. Van Lancker et al. [44, 45] published early reports of an acquired disorder in which a patient no longer can identify a person from hearing the voice. They introduced the term phonagnosia for this disorder. In particular lesions, to the temporal lobes appear to interfere with voice discrimination, while parietal lesions are associated with recognizing familiar voices.

Presumably the first case of *developmental phonagnosia* was presented by Garrido et al. [46]. They described the case of KH, a 60-year-old woman who reported to always having experienced severe problems with voice recognition. Her hearing abilities were normal. No abnormalities were seen on MRI scans in regions associated with voice or auditory perception. A battery of tests aiming to assess aspects of voice perception and recognition, face perception and recognition, as well as processing of emotional characteristics of voice and face was presented to KH. A selective deficit was observed for recognition of famous voices and the learning of new voices. Garrido et al. [46] concluded that recognizing the identity of a person on the basis of the sound of the voice may require a specific mechanism that is not required for recognizing non-voice auditory stimuli.

Memory

Arguably the best known case with an acquired selective cognitive deficit is HM, who lost his memory after resection of parts of the medial temporal lobes for relief of epileptic convulsions [47]. Various dissociations have been reported regarding declarative and nondeclarative memory. There also appear to be developmental memory problems, although brain lesions seem to always play a role here.

Developmental Dysmnesia

While many children may have problems with learning and remembering, this is usually not regarded as a specific developmental syndrome. Often these deficits are associated with more general problems in cognition or intelligence. However, some cases have been described in which a specific problem with memory was observed without a general decline in cognition. Ostergaard [48] described a child of 10 years who developed a severe amnesia following an incident of diabetic ketoacidosis, clearly an acquired form of amnesia. As in other domains of developmental deficits, it is sometimes very difficult to demonstrate that a functional deficit is purely functional and not due to an abnormal structural or functional organization of the brain.

De Renzi and Lucchelli [49] described the case of MS, a 22-year-old man. He suffered from a moderate dyslexia but he had always experienced memory problems. There were no remarkable incidents in his development. No medical abnormalities were observed and a CT scan also showed no abnormalities. Despite a normal intelligence, a battery of memory tasks showed a moderate deficit of verbal and visual memory, as reflected in learning names, mathematical formulae, poems, and songs. However, his spatial memory appeared intact.

Casalini et al. [50] reported on a 9-year-old girl suffering from a severe and specific verbal memory disorder, without a definite etiology. The deficit concerned episodic and semantic memory, both short-term and long-term memory. Visuospatial memory was intact.

Even though in these early cases no structural brain abnormalities were observed, no functional imaging was performed and functional brain deficits cannot be excluded. Dzieciol et al. [51] showed that in a group of 18 individuals with developmental amnesia, two-thirds showed a marked degree of atrophy of the mammillary bodies, which suggests that in developmental dysmnesia a brain disorder is likely to be the cause of the deficit.

Topographical Disorientation

Topographical disorientation as a result of a brain lesion has been documented for a long time. Aguirre and D'Esposito [52] reviewed the extensive literature on this disorder and concluded that different variants can be discriminated, based on the main behavioral deficit and lesions in specific brain areas. More particularly, they distinguished between egocentric disorientation (posterior parietal lesions), heading disorientation (posterior cingulated lesions), landmark agnosia (lingual gyrus lesions), and anterograde disorientation (parahippocampus).

Surprisingly, no case of developmental disorientation had been described by then. The first case was reported by Iaria et al. [53] in 2009. The case concerned a 43-year old left-handed woman, Pt1. She had experienced topographical orientation problems during her entire life, but otherwise she was intellectually intact. Alarmed by an announcement that the office where she worked would move, she decided to seek help, anticipating problems in finding her way to the new office. A thorough neuropsychological assessment revealed the remarkable deficit. Medical examinations including structural imaging revealed no abnormalities. She seemed to be the first case of developmental topographical disorientation (DTD). Her navigation skills were tested in real and virtual environments. She had no problems in both route-based navigation and landmark-based navigation, and also finding her way using a set of verbal instruction appeared to cause no problems. Map-based navigation in essence caused no problems as well.

In contrast, drawing a map of her house revealed part of her problem: the number of rooms was correct but the spatial relations were not. In a similar way, a drawing of the route to her office, one that she knew very well, showed severe spatial distortions. The authors concluded that the fundamental deficit underlying this specific pattern of intact and disturbed functions was a problem in constructing a cognitive map, a representation of an environment. The cognitive problems Pt1 showed in a virtual reality experiment supported this interpretation.

In addition, fMRI measures were collected during the virtual reality task. These data revealed a remarkable lack of activation in the hippocampal complex and the retrosplenial cortex. Healthy control participants did reveal clear activations in these regions during this task, suggesting that this lack of activation is relevant for the nature of the cognitive deficit of Pt1.

The next year, Bianchini et al. [54] reported another case of DTD: FG, a healthy 32-year-old man. An extensive neuropsychological assessment revealed a severe DTD and problems with cognitive functions that directly or indirectly seemed to play a role in spatial orientation. In contrast to Pt1, FG seemed to suffer from a complete lack of navigation skills. He was also unable to process spatial relations of parts of a whole (e.g., Picture Completion, Block Design and Object Assembly subtests of the WAIS). Structural imaging did not show any abnormalities. Unfortunately, no functional imaging data were collected.

That same year, Iaria and Barton [55] published a study, claiming to have detected now 120 new cases of DTD. Following reports of their earlier study on the first case with DTD in various public media, they were contacted by many individuals from all over the world. Having developed an online battery, they could screen these individuals. Apparently, the condition is not that rare but has up to recently not been considered as one that may require attention of medically or psychologically trained professionals.

DTD may be due to very subtle functional brain abnormalities that may not be detected with structural imaging. Nevertheless, it is now clear that the developmental disorientation disorder illustrates that specific neural mechanisms are involved in spatial orientation and can be disrupted without affecting cognition in general.

We now turn to a developmental disorder, autism, that in recent years has been detected in a relatively large proportion of children. It also differs from most of the disorders discussed above in the sense that it is considered to be a syndrome characterized by a triad of cognitive deficits.

Autism

Autism was clinically defined in the early 1940s, but knowing the symptoms, one may look back and search for case description that might fit the criteria. Perhaps the oldest case that may be considered as a child with autism is, according to autism-expert Utah Frith, Hugh Blair who in 1747 at the age of 39 appeared in court for a decision on his mental capacity to contract a marriage [56]. Blair had problems with social relations, he was retarded and his language was abnormal, as indicated by, for instance, echolalia, and the repetition of simple phrases. He showed obsessive and repetitive behavior and mannerisms and was described as lacking common sense.

Another early case was described by the English physician John Haslam (1764–1844) in his *Observations on madness and melancholy* [57]. He mentioned a boy 7-years-old with infantile convulsions, severe measles, and small pox inoculation. He began to speak rather late. He was solitary, watching other boys playing but never joining in. He also showed some obsessive behavioral patterns.

Yet another early case might be the wild boy of Aveyron, Victor. He was found in the woods in 1798, at the age of about 11 or 12 years. The French physician, Jean Itard (1774–1838), took care of the boy. At first the boy seemed indifferent to noises and smells. He looked expressionless. He seemed melancholic, but also showed outbursts of laughter. He had a good memory and a good sense of order. His speech never progressed beyond the production of some monosyllables. Utah Frith assumes that Victor was autistic. These early cases are anecdotal, and the lack of systematic collection of observations makes it difficult to establish a diagnosis [58].

The first "official" description of the syndrome came from 2 physicians, Leo Kanner (1894–1981) in 1943 and Hans Asperger (1906–1980) in 1944. The Hungarian-Austrian Leo Kanner immigrated in 1924 to the United States and there became the first child psychiatrist and head of the Child Psychiatry department of the Johns Hopkins Hospital in Baltimore. Since 1938, he collected observations on children with what he called *Autistic Disturbance of Affective Contact* [59]. Kanner described in a systematic way 11 cases: Donald, Frederick, Richard, Paul, Barbara, Virginia, Herbert, Alfred, Charles, John, and Elaine. He described for each child its preoccupations with objects, repetitious behavior, and language problems. He also provided details about the family background.

Analyzing the symptoms of this new syndrome, he stressed the emotional basis as well as the presence of these symptoms from birth, indicating that the syndrome differed from schizophrenia. He also recognized the desire of the children for sameness and aloneness and their communication problems.

One year later, Hans Asperger, director of the Orthopedagogic Unit of the Vienna University Child Clinic, published his view on this disorder in a paper *Die "Autistischen Psychopathen" im Kindesalter.* Asperger [60] aimed to describe a group of children with a common disorder, expressed in body and behavior, namely a problem in social interaction. However, he also pointed out that it is sometimes accompanied by very original ways of thinking. Asperger gave quite elaborate descriptions of his four cases: Fritz V., Harro L., Ernst K., and Hellmuth L., and he summarized findings of similar children. Their emotional and social relationships were poor. They showed stereotypic behavior and pervasive special interests. According to Asperger, parents often showed similar character traits.

For a long time, it was generally thought that the publication of these 2 reports by 2 colleagues was accidental. Recently, it has been argued that it was not so accidental and that there are arguments to think that in fact Asperger made the discovery and Kanner learned of it via Asperger's assistant who joined Kanner.

Fitzgerald [61] discovered that Asperger's chief diagnostician Georg Frankl and his psychologist Anni Weiss, who both immigrated to the United States to escape the Nazi's, had been rescued by Leo Kanner. Chown and Hughes [62] made a convincing case that Kanner must have heard from them about Asperger's work. However, he nowhere refers to Asperger's ideas. But if Kanner indeed began to collect his observations in 1938, then the riddle of how these two Austrians produced similar descriptions of this new disorder independently from each other has not been solved completely yet.

Originally, these 2 attempts to define a new syndrome were interpreted as relating to the same disorder: autism. Wing [63] argued that Asperger's syndrome may be regarded as a separate syndrome, specifically characterized by higher intelligence than that observed in regular autistic children. The syndrome that Kanner described, was characterized by rather severe behavioral problem and was assumed to occur very rarely. The children Asperger had in mind seemed to behave less abnormally.

The term autism spectrum disorder has been introduced and covers both the more severe form of autism and the less severe form of Asperger syndrome. This approach explains why currently a relatively large group of individuals is regarded to be autistic.

Autism has also been associated with a very special condition, savant syndrome, although it is clear that only about 10% of people with autism show signs of this syndrome and the syndrome is also observed in individuals that are not considered to be autistic (see chapters in [64], for recent studies on this topic).

Savant Syndrome

Savant syndrome is a rare condition in which a person with developmental disabilities has some exceptional "islands of genius," as Darold Treffert, an experienced researcher of this phenomenon, characterized the specific talents observed in some individuals. Franz Joseph Gall (1758–1728) admitted that isolated deficits following focal lesions could be informative, but he regarded this kind of evidence as very difficult to interpret. Instead, he preferred to look at individuals performing extremely or surprisingly well in a specific behavioral or cognitive area, while being (sub)normal in other areas. And in an attempt to provide various pieces of evidence for the faculties he claimed to have discovered, he mentioned a number of individuals with special talents. Of course, he realized that excellence could be reached by practice and in the "cases" he mentioned in support of the 27 faculties he distinguished, he always attempted to ascertain that performance level was not due to heavy practice and, consequently, should be considered as an inborn talent. In my view, this category of individuals has been neglected in the study of the cognitive architecture of the brain.

The talent of an individual with savant syndrome may be present from birth, but it may also develop later in life following a CNS injury. Males are affected 4–6 times more often than females. Typically, only a single skill seems to be exceptionally well developed, but in some cases more than one skill can be performed at a high level. Extraordinary memory skills seem to be involved in all cases [65]. Savants may vary in their specific capacity: calculation, art (in particular, playing music, drawing), Treffert distinguished between a savant with a splinter, a savant with a talent and a prodigious savant, showing a talent that would even be exceptional for an individual without an intellectual disability. He does not indicate whether these are merely differences in degree, or whether these differences also imply qualitative differences in cognitive structure of these savants.

Treffert [65] and many others maintain that the notion of "idiot savant" was introduced by British physician John Langdon Down (1828–1896) in 1887, but the well-known French-American physician Edouard Séguin (1812–1880) used the term "savant" in 1866 and the notion "idiot savant" in 1870 [66, 67]. The English physician, George Grabham (1836–1912) introduced the term in England [68].

Perhaps the earliest person that we now can recognize as having savant syndrome was the Derbyshire born Jedediah Buxton (1707–1772), a mathematical genius, who was poor on other subjects. Apart from the fact that he earned himself drinks in the local pub with his special talent, we know very little of him. The American physician Benjamin Rush (1746–1813) wrote a short account of a slave, Thomas Fuller, also referred to as Blind Tom, who was gifted with an exceptional talent for arithmetic [69].

Down [70] published his experiences with mentally retarded children. He devoted a short section to "idiot savants," describing 10 children he had observed himself. He noted that these individuals may excel in a variety of skills (music, drawing, arithmetic, time keeping, memory for a given kind of facts) and they also showed a phenomenal memory for this skill. He also observed that even though the fundamental talent must have been inborn, these individuals perfected it by much practice and if they did not practice, they would become less proficient.

The notion of savant syndrome tends to be associated with individuals that show a special talent or skill, in combination with a below average intelligence. However, some children with a special talent are called prodigies, Mozart being the prototypical example.

They show this talent at a young age, below 10 years is the common but arbitrary limit. The question can be asked: what is the essential difference between a prodigy and an individual with savant syndrome? At the moment, there is no good and generally accepted answer to this question.

Perhaps the first systematic study of prodigies was performed by the French psychologist Alfred Binet (1857–1911), who had a great interest in memory. Stimulated by Jean Martin Charcot (1825–1893), who also had a special interest in the workings of memory, Binet investigated a number of individuals with a savant-like syndrome. Two of these were Jacques Inaudi (1867–1950) and Périclès Diamandi (b. 1868). There are no indications that either of them was autistic or mentally retarded. Inaudi was an Italian shepherd who did not go to school and only learned to read and write at the age of 20. His exceptional arithmetic skills were discovered by an impresario who sent him to Paris, where Broca met him in the Anthropological Society in Paris [71]. Diamandi was of Greek origin and also an excellent calculator. The French Academy of Sciences named a special committee to study Inaudi's exceptional qualities and not much later Inaudi and Diamandi ended up in Binet's laboratory for some experimental studies on their calculations skills. Charcot and Binet [72] argued that they used rather different cognitive strategies, one relying on verbal representations of numbers while the other used visual representations.

Older prodigy cases are commonly presented in a rather anecdotal way and no systematic evaluation of cognitive functioning is performed. They are therefore much less informative with respect to the underlying cognitive architecture that enables these kinds of specific talents. More importantly, the relevance of the phenomenon has hardly been discussed in terms of a memory theory or of a modularity view of the mind.

What Can We Learn?

In this chapter, I have presented an overview of early descriptions of developmental or congenital cognitive deficits. In some cases, the deficit could not be attributed to a structural or functional brain disorder. However, at the time most of these early case descriptions were produced, no adequate methods were available to detect such abnormalities, if they would have been there. In some cases, like for instance in children with congenital dysmnesia, a brain disorder appears to be the most likely cause of the deficit. But irrespective of the question whether or not the deficit was purely developmental (that is, resulting from a natural development of the brain of that specific person) or caused by an interruption of the normal development by an "external" cause, the mere fact that such a cognitive deficit can be limited to a special category of cognitive processes, should be informative with respect to our understanding of the functioning of the brain, and in particular with the functional development of cognition. Unfortunately, in most studies on these specific deficits only one or a limited numbers of individuals are investigated. They have not been designed to test specific models of the development of cognition.

Many of the studies discussed here were triggered by the discussion on the modular mind, started in the early 1980s by the American philosopher Jerry Fodor (1935–2017) [73]. According to Fodor's view, not all cognition is performed by modular systems. Modularity is specifically realized at a more peripheral level of processing input or output. Central processes like thinking or conscious processing, are not modularly organized. Looking at the clinical pictures discussed here, in particular those in the perception section, it seems that many of these may comply with this basic assumption. With respect to congenital aphasia, ADHD and autism, it is less clear that they fit with Fodor's modularity view. One may ask the question whether we indeed have a precise understanding of the nature of the cognitive disorder, or indeed disorders as in the case of autism, underlying these syndromes. For instance, arguing that ADHD results from an inhibition problem requires also a cognitive process model detailing at what level this inhibition problem occurs. With respect to autism, it seems that the three symptoms characterizing this syndrome may have independent genetic causes, raising the question what actually binds these three causes? Are there also individuals with just 2 of these features and should they also get a label?

Focusing on cases with a deficit that seems to be limited to a very special kind of materials, such as faces, letters or objects, it has been argued that these cases fit with the modular theory of mind and that they point to the presence of modules specialized in specific kinds of information. In contrast, others have argued that this is not necessarily so. Connectionist models, not having a modular architecture, may also explain what seem to be examples of a double dissociation (see for an extensive discussion of this issue [74] and commentaries). But again, irrespective of whether one looks at these cases from a modularity or connectionist point of view, these observations are very significant for furthering our understanding of the functioning of the developing brain.

In comparison to investigations of acquired disorders, the area of developmental disorders has been neglected too long. Clearly, a variety of specific phenomena have been observed and it may require special ways of detecting individuals with these limited deficits. However, more time and energy spent on these phenomena may help in our overall attempt to understand the brain.

Another issue that arises, looking at these various cases, is the question whether we are dealing with a deficit or a normal variation in capability. Not all men are equal and we do not all possess the same capacities. The notion of intelligence may, incorrectly, suggest that all faculties are, under normal circumstances, developed to the same degree. However, in daily life, we do know, and accept without any problem, that some people have a talent for math or for music. In a similar way, an individual may lack a specific "talent," not due to a disorder, but as a naturally occurring pattern of cognitive faculties. In some cases, clearly a brain disorder seemed to be the underlying cause, but in others no obvious disorder could be detected. This may be due to limited technical capacities, but we should also consider that the pattern observed is a normal pattern, just deviating from what we observe in a majority of individuals. But that is a typical feature of a normal distribution.

References

1 Temple CM: Developmental Cognitive Neuropsychology. Hove, East Sussex, Psychology Press, 1997.
2 Tranel D, De Haan E: Selective developmental neuropsychological disorders. Cortex 2007;43:667–671.
3 Foley PB: Sons and daughters beyond your control: episodes in the prehistory of the attention deficit/hyperactivity syndrome. Atten Defic Hyperact Disord 2014;6: 125–151.
4 Barkley RA, Peters H: The earliest reference to ADHD in the medical literature? Melchior Adam Weikard's description in 1775 of "attention deficit" (Mangel der Aufmerksamkeit, attentio volubilis). J Atten Disord 2012;16:623–630.
5 Palmer ED, Finger S: An early description of ADHD (inattentive subtype): Dr Alexander Crichton and 'mental restlessness' (1798). Child Psychol Psychiatry Rev 2001;6:66–73.
6 Still GF: The Goulstonian lectures. On some abnormal psychical conditions in children. Lancet 1902;159:1008–1112, 1077–1082, 1163–1168.
7 Weiner P: The study of childhood language disorders: nineteenth century perspectives. J Commun Disord 1986;19:1–47.
8 Gall FJ: Sur les Fonctions du Cerveau et sur Celles de Chacune de ses Parties (6 vols). Paris, J-B Baillière, 1822–25.
9 Coën R: Pathologie und Therapie der Sprachanomalien. Vienna, Urban & Schwarzenberg, 1986.
10 Coën R: Die Hörstummheit und ihre Behandlung. Wiene Klin 1888;7:201–230.
11 Lorch M, Hellal L: The 'idioglossia' cases of the 1890s and the clinical investigation and treatment of developmental language impairment. Cortex 2012;48:1052–1060.
12 Hadden WB: On certain defects of articulation in children with cases illustrating the results of education on the oral system. J Ment Sci 1891;37:96–105.
13 Worster-Drought C, Allen IM: Congenital auditory imperceptions (congenital word-deafness): with report of a case. J Neurol Psychopathol 1929a;9:193–208.
14 Worster-Drought C, Allen IM: Congenital auditory imperceptions (congenital word-deafness): investigation of a case by Head's method. J Neurol Psychopathol 1929b; 9:289–319.
15 Worster-Drought C, Allen IM: Congenital auditory imperceptions (congenital word-deafness) and its relation to idioglossia and other speech defects. J Neurol Psychopathol 1930;10:194–236.
16 Van Hout A: Acquired aphasia in childhood and developmental dysphasias: are the errors similar? Analysis of errors made in confrontation naming tasks. Aphasiology 1993;7:525–531.
17 Temple CM: Anomia for animals in a child. Brain 1986; 109:1225–1242.
18 Wagner R: Rudolf Berlin: originator of the term dyslexia. Ann Dyslexia 1973;23:57–63.
19 Pringle Morgan W: A case of congenital word blindness. Br Med J 1896;2:1378.
20 Hinshelwood J: Congenital word blindness. London, H.K. Lewis, 1917.
21 Marshall JC, Newcombe F: Patterns of paralexia: a psycholinguistic approach. J Psycholinguist Res 1973;2: 175–199.
22 Temple CM, Marshall JC: A case study of developmental phonological dyslexia. Br J Psychol 1983;74:517–513.
23 Temple CM: Developmental dysgraphias. Quart J Exp Psychol 1986;38A:77–110.
24 Stuart M, Howard D: KJ: a developmental deep dyslexia. Cogn Neurops 1995;12:793–824.
25 Friedmann N, Nachman-Katz I: Neglect dyslexia in a Hebrew-reading child. Cortex 2004;40:301–313.
26 Friedmann N, Kerbel N, Shvimer L: Developmental attentional dyslexia. Cortex 2010;46:1216–1237.
27 Ardila A, Rosselli M: Acalculia and dyscalculia. Neuropsychol Rev 2002;12:179–231.
28 McCloskey M, Caramazza A, Basili A: Cognitive mechanisms in number processing and calculation: evidence from dyscalculia. Send to Brain Cogn 1985;4:171–196.
29 Temple CM: Digit dyslexia: a category-specific disorder in development dyscalculia. Cogn Neurops 1989;6:93–116.
30 Temple CM: Procedural dyscalculia and number fact dyscaiculia: double dissociation in developmental dyscalculia. Cog Neurops 1991;8:155–176.
31 Lissauer H: Ein fall von seelenblindheit, nebst einem beitrag zur theorie derselben. Arch Psychiat Nervenkr 1888;21:222–270.
32 Ariel R, Sadeh M: Congenital visual agnosia and prosopagnosia in a child: a case report. Cortex 1996;32:221–240.
33 Germine L, Cashdollar N, Düzel E, Duchaine B: A new selective developmental deficit: Impaired object recognition with normal face recognition. Cortex 2011;47: 598–607.
34 De Haan EH, Campbell R: A fifteen year follow-up of a case of developmental prosopagnosia. Cortex 1991;27: 489–509.
35 McConachie HR: Developmental prosopagnosia. A single case report. Cortex 1976;12:76–82.
36 Temple CM: Developmental memory impairment: faces and patterns; in Campbell R (ed): Mental Lives: Case Studies in Cognition. Oxford, Blackwell, 1992, pp 199–215.
37 Van Zandvoort M, Nijboer T, de Haan E: Developmental colour agnosia. Cortex 2007;43:750–757.
38 Nijboer T, van Zandvoort M, de Haan E: Covert colour processing in colour agnosia. Neuropsychologia 2006; 44:1437–1443.
39 Nijboer T, van Zandvoort M, de Haan E: A familial factor in the development of colour agnosia. Neuropsychologia 2007;45:1961–1965.
40 McCloskey M, Rapp IB, Yantis IS, Rubin G, Bacon IWF, Dagnelic G, Gordon B, Aliminosa D, Boatman DF, Badecker W, Johnson DF, Tusa RJ, Palmeri E: A developmental deficit in localizing objects from vision. Psychol Sci 1995;6:112–117.

41 Eling P, Finger S, Whitaker H: On the origins of organology: Franz Joseph Gall and a girl named Bianchi. Cortex 2017;86:123–131.
42 Peretz I, Ayotte J, Zatorre R, Mehler J, Ahad P, Penhune V, Jutras B: Congenital amusia: a disorder of fine-grained pitch discrimination. Neuron 2002;33:185–191.
43 Lebrun MA, Moreau P, McNally-Gagnon A, Mignault Goulet M, Peretz I: Congenital amusia in childhood: a case study. Cortex 2012;48:683–688.
44 Van Lancker D, Canter G: Impairment of voice and face recognition in patients with hemispheric damage. Br Cogn 1982;1:185–195.
45 Van Lancker D, Kreiman J, Cummings J: Voice perception deficits: neuronanatomical correlates of phonagnosia. J Cl Exp Neurops 1989;11:665–674.
46 Garrido L, Furl N, Draganski B, Weiskopf N, Stevens J, Tan GC, Driver J, Dolan RJ, Duchaine B: Voxel-based morphometry reveals reduced grey matter volume in the temporal cortex of developmental prosopagnosics. Brain 2009;132:3443–3455.
47 Corkin S: Permanent Present Tense. The Unforgettable Life of the Amnesic Patient, H. M. New York, Basic Books, 2013.
48 Ostergaard AL: Episodic, semantic and procedural memory in a case of amnesia at an early age. Neuropsychologia 1987;25:341–357.
49 De Renzi E, Lucchelli F: Developmental dysmnesia in a poor reader. Brain 1990;113:1337–1345.
50 Casalini C, Brizzolara D, Cavallaro MC, Cipriani P: "Developmental dysmnesia": a case report. Cortex 1999;35: 713–727.
51 Dzieciol AM, Bachevalier J, Saleem KS, Gadian DG, Saunders R, Chong WKK, Banks T, Mishkin M, Vargha-Khadem F: Hippocampal and diencephalic pathology in developmental amnesia. Cortex 2017;86:33–44.
52 Aguirre G, D'Esposito M: Topographical disorientation: a synthesis and taxonomy. Brain 1999;122(pt 9):1613–1628.
53 Iaria G, Bogod N, Fox CJ, Barton JJ: Developmental topographical disorientation: case one. Neuropsychologia 2009;47:30–40.
54 Bianchini F, Incoccia C, Palermo L, Piccardi L, Zompanti L, Sabatini U, Peran P, Guariglia C: Developmental topographical disorientation in a healthy subject. Neuropsychologia 2010;48:1563–1573.
55 Iaria G, Barton JJ: Developmental topographical disorientation: a newly discovered cognitive disorder. Exp Brain Res 2010;206:189–196.
56 Houston R, Frith U: Autism in History: the Case of Hugh Blair of Borgue. Blackwell, Oxford, 2000.
57 Vaillant GE: John Haslam on early infantile autism. Am J Psychiatry 1962;119:376.
58 Wolf S: The history of autism. Eur Child Adolesc Psychiatry 2004;13:201–208.
59 Kanner L: Autistic disturbances of affective contact. Nervous Child 1943;2:217–250.
60 Asperger H: "Autistischen Psychopathen" im Kindesalter. Arch Psychiatr Nervenkr 1944;117:76–136.
61 Fitzgerald M: Autism: Asperger's syndrome – history and first descriptions; in Rausch JL, Johnson ME, Casanova MF (eds): Asperger's Disorder. New York, Informa Healthcare, 2008.
62 Chown N, Hughes L: History and first descriptions of autism: asperger versus kanner revisited. Autism Dev Disord 2016;46:2270–2272.
63 Wing L: Asperger's syndrome: a clinical account. Psychol Med 1981;11:115–129.
64 Happé F, Frith U (eds): Autism and Talent. Oxford, Oxford University Press, 2010.
65 Treffert D: The savant syndrome: an extraordinary condition. A synopsis: past, present, future. Philos Trans R Soc Lond B Biol Sci 2009;364:1351–1357.
66 Séguin E: Idiocy and Its Treatment by the Physiological Method. New York, W. Wood and Company, 1866.
67 Séguin E: New Facts and Remarks Concerning Idiocy: Being a Lecture Delivered before the New York Medical Journal Association, October 15, 1869. New York, Wood & Co., 1870.
68 Grabham GW: Remarks on the origin, varieties and terminations of idiocy. Br Med J 1875;1:73–76.
69 Rush B: Account of a wonderful talent for arithmetical calculation in an African slave, living in Virginia. Am Mus 1789;5:62–63.
70 Down JL: On Some of the Mental Affections of Childhood and Youth. London, Churchill, 1887.
71 Nicholas S, Gounden Y, Levine Z: The memory of two great mental calculators: Charcot and Binet's neglected 1893 experiments. Am J Psychol 2011;124:235–242.
72 Charcot JM, Binet A: Un calculateur du type visuel et un calculateur de type auditif. Revue Phil de la France et de l'Étr 1893;35:590–594.
73 Fodor J: The Modularity of Mind. Cambridge, MIT Press,1983.
74 Thomas M, Karmiloff-Smith A: Are developmental disorders like cases of adult brain damage? Implications from connectionist modeling. Behav Brain Sci 2002;25: 727 788.

Paul Eling
Department of Psychology, Donders Institute for Brain, Cognition and Behaviour
PO Box 9104
NL–6500 HE Nijmegen (The Netherlands)
E-Mail p.eling@donders.ru.nl

Bogousslavsky J, Boller F, Iwata M (eds): A History of Neuropsychology.
Front Neurol Neurosci. Basel, Karger, 2019, vol 44, pp 164–178 (DOI: 10.1159/000494963)

History of Neuropsychological Assessment

Paul Eling

Donders Institute for Brain, Cognition and Behaviour, Radboud University, Nijmegen, The Netherlands

Abstract

This chapter presents a historical overview of observations, instruments, and approaches in the area of neuropsychological assessment. In the 17th and 18th century literature dealing especially with language disorders following a brain disorder, one finds observations of physicians of striking dissociations of mental faculties that were impaired while others remained intact. Around the middle of the 19th century, neuropsychiatrists like Carl Wernicke began to develop procedures for assessing more specific components of mental functioning. German physicians, Conrad Rieger and Theodor Ziehen, seem to have developed the first neuropsychological test batteries. Kurt Goldstein, inspired by the rising Gestalt theory, argued that not the test score but the strategy used by a patient to perform a task is important. Alexander Luria also promoted an approach to assessment that was mainly based on subjective judgment. Studies on individual differences led to the development of an intelligence test battery by Alfred Binet. This battery was later transformed into the Army Alpha and Army Beta tests for selecting soldiers. Components of these intelligence tests have survived in the test kit of the modern neuropsychologist. This tradition also stimulated the development of psychometric analysis of tests. Two pioneers in the field of neuropsychological assessment were Shepherd Ivory Franz, favoring a clinical approach, and Ward Halstead, stimulating a strongly psychometric-based approach. The evaluation of language disorders has always been a specific area, requiring its own set of tests. The first comprehensive language battery was compiled by Bastian. Around the middle of the 20th century, when the localization of function approach had been rejected, neurologists preferred to examine language disorders clinically, using a battery that evaluated speech, comprehension, reading, and writing.

Assessment: Observation, Test, and Measurement

Modern neuropsychology developed in the 1960s. Boston (Norman Geschwind; 1926–1984), Cambridge (GBr; Oliver Zangwill; 1913–1987), and Paris (Henri Hécaen; 1912–1983) were crucial centers. However, long before this "new" rise of neuropsychology, neurologists, psychiatrists, and also psychologists, investigated patients, suspected of brain impairments, with various procedures.

In this chapter, roots of 3 aspects of neuropsychological assessment will be examined. We will first look at observations made by physicians and noted in case reports. At first, only the "naked eye" was used. Later, doctors developed bed-side tests, often the origins of current neuropsychological tests. As we will see, many tests and test batteries were developed by European "neuropsychologists" from around 1900 (see also Barr [1])! The *psychometric* approach, stemming from intelligence testing, introduced a more formal assessment of deficits within neuropsychology.

Observation

Every clinician knows how crucial observations are. Assessment often starts when the patient enters the room and introduces himself and describes his complaints. A clinician may quickly develop ideas about the nature of the problem and possible causes. Already in the famous Edwin Smith papyrus, used many centuries before Christ, instructions are given to look for specific symptoms, and conclusions are formulated that can be drawn from those concerning the nature of the disorder and of the treatment: no treatment possible or a disease that can be treated [2]. Hippocrates (460–370 BC) and Galen (130–210) also left their instructions for assessment and treatment, and these have been taught and used until approximately the 18th or even the 19th century.

At the beginning of the renaissance, a new spirit inspired physicians. Doubt was raised about the accuracy of some classical observations and rules. Andreas Vesalius (1514–1564) demonstrated that Galen was not infallible. Some physicians began to collect their own observations and produced written case descriptions [3]. They sometimes published bundles of such case descriptions in the form of books with the Latin term *Observationes*; we would now speak of case studies. Doctors were not specialized in a specific discipline at that time, and among those observations one could find all sorts of diseases and disorders. Two of these bundles are of special interest for neuropsychologists. The first is that of Johannes Schenk (1530–1598): *Observationes medicae de capite humano* from 1584 (see for a more complete overview, Eling and Whitaker [4]). The second is by Johannes Jacob Wepfer (1620–1695). *Observationes anatomicae ex cadaveribus eorum quos sustulit apoplexia*, published posthumously in 1727.

Schenk's book includes descriptions of 568 authors, mostly from old sources, as well as 64 previously unpublished cases of contemporaries. According to Luzzatti and Whitaker, the book is a gold mine for neuropsychologists because of the neuropsychological descriptions, but unfortunately the text is in Latin [5]. Also 16 cases with language disorders are described and the French physician Armand Trousseau (1801–1867), who introduced the notion of "aphasia" in 1864, referred to Schenk's book as the first clear description of aphasia patients. In the days of Schenk, such a disorder was regarded as a memory disorder, a disorder of memory for words!

Wepfer's book contains vivid and structured case descriptions with at least 13 cases with a specific language disorder. They were, in comparison with Schenk's collection, more systematically selected to demonstrate certain symptoms. In many cases, a post-mortem examination was also carried out. Wepfer's observations are interesting because of the assumptions made about the underlying cognitive processes.

Some of the very old case descriptions are still mentioned in contemporary aphasia literature because they show striking patterns of deficits, such as Johann Schmidt's (1624–1690) patient that could write but not read, a case of pure alexia that was only recognized as a syndrome by Jules Dejerine in 1892. Peter Rommel (1634–1708) described a patient in 1683 under the title "aphonia rara." The man could not speak spontaneously but he could give his prayers. It is an early description of the dissociation between spontaneous and automatic speech.

These physicians were traveling doctors who had no specific scientific purpose. They often wanted to show that they were competent and that one did not necessarily have to deal with complex theories at the universities. The situation changed in the 19th century.

First Steps

Until the mid-19th century, psychiatrists diagnosed patients on the basis of behavioral symptoms [6]. No systematic examination was performed; a psychiatrist simply relied on what he saw. Over time, increasingly more tests were devised to examine potential deficits. The Belgian psychiatrist Joseph Guislain (1797–1860) pointed out the importance of the way in which patients were interviewed: when one poses a "why" question, the answer may reveal something about a patient's judgment qualities; questions about "when" and "how long" assess his memory faculty, and questions that begin with "how many" may tell something about his calculation capacity [7].

The German neuropsychiatrist Carl Wernicke (1848–1905) assumed that the severity of a disorder was reflected in the "size" or extension of concepts [8]. A concept (meaning associated with a word image), Wernicke argued, "consists" essentially of the collection of images (representations) associated with a word image and is scattered throughout the cerebral cortex, in sensory and motor areas. For instance, the concept "dog" is represented by the shape, smell, and sound representations of dogs that we have perceived before. If a larger portion of the cortex is disrupted, more parts of a conceptual representation will be affected and thus disturb the concept associated with that word image. Patients thus become impaired in their thinking about certain concepts, in determining similarities and differences among concepts, or they can differentiate (*Differenzierung*) and generalize

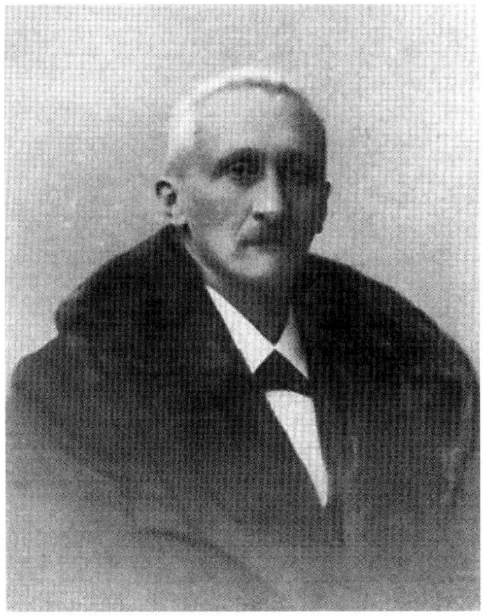

Fig. 1. Conrad Rieger (1855–1939). From Gaupp R: Konrad Rieger. Z f d g Neur u Psych 1939;166:309. https://doi.org/10.1007/BF02896085. Springer Nature, with kind permission.

(*Generalisation*) less well, as Wernicke would say. To investigate this capacity, he developed a list of questions such as: what is the difference between a ladder and stairs, between a hill and a mountain, between a bull and a cow? Or a more difficult question: what is the difference between church, religion, and belief; or between a nation, a people, and a state? The subtest Similarities of the Wechsler Adult Intelligence Scale looks very similar to this test of Wernicke.

Diagnostic tests are normally used for evaluating a potential deficit, but sometimes it is used to establish that there are no problems, while the patient insists that he has a serious illness. At the end of the 20th century, neuropsychologists began to develop specific procedures to detect this kind of behavior that originally was referred to as malingering and later with the more neutral term underachievement [9]. Such tests are sometimes called symptom validity tests. However, such a test was already developed in 1881 by German psychiatrist Ludwig Snell (1881), of whom not much is known. He developed some very easy tasks and showed that simulants made mistakes on these. This principle is still used today in so-called "symptom validity tests" [10].

Towards a Neuropsychological Battery

Conrad Rieger (1855–1939; Fig. 1), a psychiatrist from Würzburg, developed a method that he claimed "is generally suitable for intelligence research" [11]. The concept of intelligence had not yet been linked to the idea of inter-individual differences in test scores and intelligence quotient (IQ). Rieger's intelligence appears to reflect what we now would call

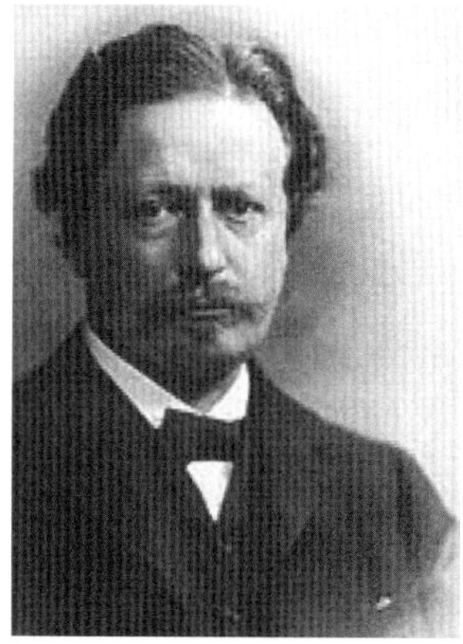

Fig. 2. Theodor Ziehen (1862–1950). https://de.wikipedia.org/wiki/Datei:T._Ziehen.jpg (public domain).

cognition. He used a series of tests to examine intelligence. He applied this battery only to brain-damaged patients and he had not collected observations from healthy individuals for comparison. His battery consisted of 8 subtests evaluating apperception and perception, memory (short and long term), imitation, recognition, reading aloud, and combining individual words in a sentence. The latter subtest was used in 1897 by the German memory investigator Hermann Ebbinghaus (1850–1909) for his *Sentence Completion* test for measuring intelligence [12]. Rieger determined himself, with his "clinical eye" whether performance on a test indicated a disorder. In this respect, his method differed from that of Ebbinghaus and the French psychiatrist Alfred Binet, who compared scores to the average of a standard group.

The German psychiatrist and philosopher Theodor Ziehen (1862–1950; Fig. 2) published a manual of a test battery [13]. He discussed various procedures for investigating psychological (cognitive) process. He distinguished among various aspects of cognition, such as memory, formation of associations, and concept formation. He examined memory (*Retention*) quite extensively. He warned that one should not examine "school knowledge" but "knowledge of life," which seems to correspond to what we would call semantic memory. He also asked about issues from a person's past (we would say, autobiographical memory). He asked a patient to generate sequences (days of the week, months) and examined storage of information by presenting series of digits, from 1 to 6 (or sometimes more). The reproduction of such a short series of digits in the reverse order is also described by Ziehen. In another test, he presented a series of 10, 15 or 20 individual words which the subject then had to recall (word list learning). He examined visual memory using simple geometric figures. These were presented for 15 s, and after a 15 s interval, the patient had to reproduce these pictures. This may be regarded as a precursor of the Memory for Design Test [14]. In the final part of the memory section, Ziehen gave the patient 2, 3 or 4 tasks simultaneously and these had to be executed sequentially. This part of the battery is reminiscent of the Wechsler Memory Scales and the Rivermead Behavioural Memory Test (Lezak et al. [14], 2012).

The next section of Ziehen's manual dealt with concept learning, the description of which resembles that of Wernicke (see above). It concerns reasoning about concepts, for instance the isolation of the color of the concept sugar or the combination of the elements thunder and rain for the concept storm.

Another test used, Ziehen, adapted from a test developed by the English educational psychologist Whipple [15] (1876–1941). A patient was asked to produce within 2 min as many words as possible containing the letter O or A (In Whipple's version, words had to begin with the letter). Here we recognize the forerunner of today's fluency tests.

The final section in the manual concerned the formation of associations. The patient had to select from a set of pictures those that were associated to each other. The backwards recall of a series of digits Ziehen put in this section as the association of the digits are new (not in the normal order), requiring the formation of new associations. This section also contained a test for arithmetics. Finally, he mentioned the *method of Masselon*, a doctor from Paris: the patient was presented with 3 words and he had to produce a sentence with these.

Ziehen warned that speed of thought also can play a role. He furthermore believed that emotion is important arguing that an apathic patient may score low because of a lack of interest. Ziehen mentioned almost nothing about how subtests should be evaluated or scored. Presumably, common sense will tell the doctor which behavior is abnormal.

Russian neurologist Grigory Rossolimo (1860–1928 [28]) developed a test battery for examining children and adults. He also developed a method to make a psychological profile, to which he referred as psychograph. That was not a machine but a graph showing the scores (on a scale of 0–10) of 9 subtests in a circle: attention, will, perception, memory, comprehension, construction, mechanical problem solving, imagination, and observation. Rossolimo did compare the psychographs of a number of individuals, but he never collected normative data for this battery.

Observation Is the Rule!

It is now almost taken for granted that a neuropsychologist formulates his findings as much as possible using objective scores, but at the beginning of the 20th century, not everyone thought like that! Two pioneering neuropsychologists, Kurt Goldstein (1878–1965) and Alexander Luria (1902–1977), claimed that one had to carefully observe how a patient performed a particular task, and that simple scores essentially could not say anything about the underlying problem. One can arrive at a certain outcome in so many ways and there may be so many reasons why somebody fails; this cannot be deduced from a single number.

Kurt Goldstein (Fig. 3) in 1914 was in charge of a newly founded clinic for soldiers with brain injuries in Frankfurt am Main, Germany [16]. He distinguished *general* (screening especially cognitive functions) examination from a special investigation. If a severe impairment was found in the areas of oral language, reading, writing or math, a special investigation was conducted.

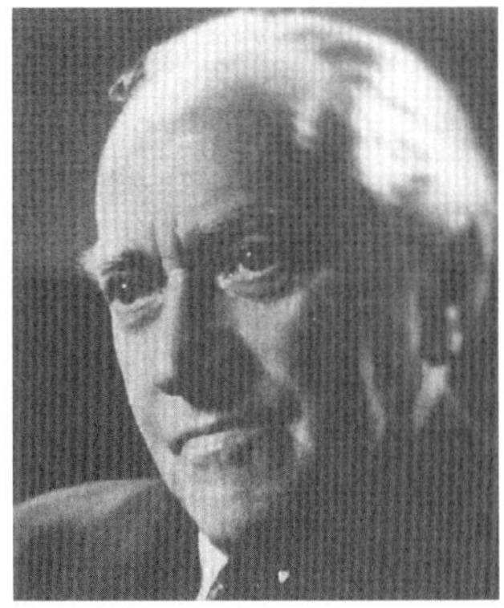

Fig. 3. Kurt Goldstein (1878–1965) (public domain).

General screening began with tachistoscopic tests, followed by several other experimental psychological tasks. Thus, it was established whether a patient was suffering from a general impairment of mental processes, memory problems, attention problems, perseveration, various types of visual disorders, alexia, agnosia, visual field defects, amnestic aphasia, a learning disability, a color vision disorder, or arithmetic problems. In addition, Goldstein used a complex task, which is reminiscent of working in an office. On a large board, attached to the wall a number of instruments were mounted with a lamp under each instrument. The patient had to operate an instrument under which a light came on. According to Goldstein, this test was more ecologically valid than the experimental tasks. To measure sustained attention, Kraepelin's calculation test was used. A series of numbers was presented on a piece of paper and the patient had to count 2 consecutive digits as fast as possible for an hour! This test can be seen as the (albeit visual) precursor of the Paced Auditory Serial Addition Test either, which is still widely used in neuropsychological assessment. Goldstein also used a specific kind of sorting tasks, which formed the basis of the Wisconsin Card Sorting Test [17]. The German psychologist, Narziss Ach (1871–1946), wrote his dissertation on the effects of the will on perception to demonstrate that there is top-down control. He used sorting tasks to demonstrate that task instruction has an effect on how an individual perceives. Goldstein, attracted to the then rising Gestalt psychology, used these tasks, which led him to formulate his theoretical framework of the concrete and abstract attitude.

He also included some performance tests (*Leistungsprüfungen*), which focused on fine motor skills, such as pulling strength of a finger and its susceptibility to motor fatigue. Muscle activity was measured with an "ergograph," attached to the finger. In addition, Goldstein used a test evaluating physical power (lifting), important for determining whether an individual would be able to perform labor, for instance in a factory.

Goldstein considered the more "traditional" (still quite young at the time) ergograph measurement (fine motor skills) as an abstract laboratory test (*lebensfremd*). The complex motor task (the office board with instruments; power lifting), he regarded as *lebenswahr*, akin to real life. For Goldstein the question of *ecological validity* was already an important issue. However, he argued that both kinds of tests are important in the assessment phase.

The Russian neuropsychologist, Alexander Luria (see this book, last chapter, p. 220), developed a completely different psychological theoretical framework. After the great revolution of 1917, Russian communist authorities began to look differently at all kinds of things associated with Western bourgeoisie. And this also applied to views on psychology. Individual differences were, according to the new political views, the result of socio-cultural differences in developmental conditions. Capacities are learned, they are not inborn or inherited. They also opposed to the use of psychological tests and quantifying behavioral observations.

Luria treated large numbers of soldiers with brain damage in World War II. He developed a comprehensive test battery which was based on his personal view of the functioning of the brain [18]. He distinguished 3 fundamental units: attention (brainstem), perception (posterior part of the brain), and organization and planning of behavior (anterior part of the brain). For each of the sensory modalities he believed there were 3 levels of processing: primary (picture), secondary (interpretation), and tertiary level (cross-modal integration). He considered it to be a flexible system: in all forms of behavior, all units played a role and multiple subsystems could be deployed to perform a task, depending on which strategy a person followed.

He claimed that each of his many tests examined a specific part of the brain. The empirical basis of that claim was lacking. More important than how well a patient performed on a test was the observation how the patient performed a task. Luria recognized the great plasticity of the functional system: many roads lead to Rome, and if a particular route is blocked, another strategy can be used. Scores are therefore less important than a good observation [18].

In the 1970s, Luria and his work were well-known in the West, even popular. This resulted in a different way of neuropsychological assessment in some Western countries. Luria's tests were the basis for the Luria – Nebraska Neuropsychological Test battery with Anne-Lise Christensen and Charles Golden as major advocates (see Golden, Freshwater and Vayalakkara [19]). The test had a large number of subtests (269 in Form I and 279 in the Form II), but these could be used flexibly.

The Psychometric Approach

The use of objective scores and statistics has increased significantly in the course of the 20th century. It has even become an independent field of research: psychometrics. In many historical accounts of psychological tests, the development of *intelligence tests* is seen as the start (for a very detailed description, see Du Bois [20]).

Two Pioneers

The historical account of the intelligence test (for an overview, see Boake [21]) usually starts with the Englishman Francis Galton (1822–1911). He assumed that intelligence is inherited. He believed that there are no innate functions and that all knowledge is ac-

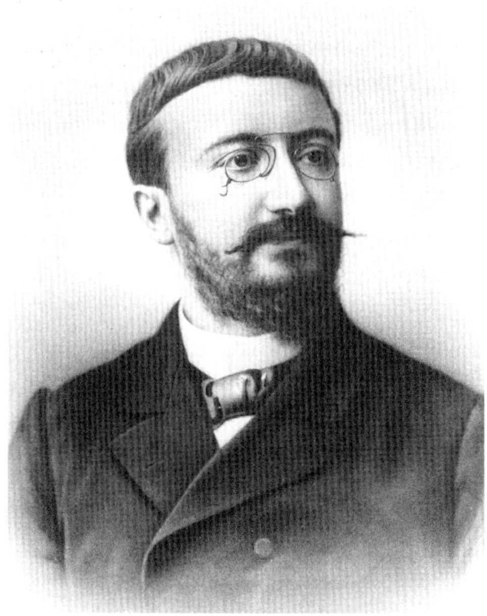

Fig. 4. Alfred Binet (1857–1911), National Library of Science (public domain).

quired through the senses: the dominant associationistic epistemology in England [22]. If someone is very smart, it means he must have a good sense system, and that was the genetic component, according to Galton. Consequently, this basic property can be measured with tests assessing *speed of responding*, such as a reaction time task. Galton's battery contains hardly any cognitive (reasoning, memory) tests. His pupil Charles Spearman (1863–1945) showed that a single factor explains most of the variance in the measurement of intelligence, and he called this factor *g* (from "general").

The second hero in the traditional story of the intelligence test is Alfred Binet (1857–1911; Fig. 4), a French psychiatrist. The French government commissioned him to find a way to better determine which children should be sent from school because they could not function at an appropriate level and would make the work of the teacher difficult. Binet devised, together with his colleague Theodore Simon (1872–1961), a procedure for "screening" (as we would say today) children's *academic skills* [23, 24]. They developed a test with thirty different assignments, which appealed to, amongst others, logical reasoning, searching for rhymes, naming objects, memory, and attention. In order to say something about an individual child, he compared the scores of that child with those of a group of children of the same age, with older and younger children. German psychologist, William Stern (1871–1938), devised a formula in 1912 to express the comparison with older and younger children in a number: the ratio of chronological and mental age; this is the IQ [25].

Binet stressed that any test in itself had little meaning; it did not really matter what tests are used, as long as one uses many different tests, he argued. His test battery was not based on a theory of intelligence, but tapped primarily knowledge and skills important for school.

From Binet to Army Alpha and Beta

The American psychologist, Henry Goddard (1866–1957), introduced Binet's test battery in America. Lewis Terman (1877–1956) adapted the test somewhat, resulting in the Stanford-Binet, published in 1916 [26]. World War I was raging and America prepared itself to attack Germany. A large numbers of men volunteered as soldier. Who was suitable for the army? And who was eligible to become soldier and who was suited for a higher rank? The government established a task force headed by (animal) psychologist Robert Yerkes (pronounced Yer-keez; 1876–1956) to develop a *selection process*. This procedure was not meant to measure intelligence per se. First, the so-called *Army Alpha* was developed, a series of tests, focusing on *knowledge*. It was arranged that the tests could be offered as *group test*. For that purpose, a multiple choice format was used. When converting subtests of the Stanford-Binet for children to tests for adults, it appeared during the selection procedures in the army that many adults were not able to read well enough or had had too little education. The tests were not *valid*! For this reason, a second set of tests was prepared, the *Army Beta*, aiming to screen *skills* or problem solving skills; they were called *performance tests*. These were again designed in the form of group tests. Thus, there were 2 versions (parallel versions, one might say): the Army Alpha and the Army Beta. Another problem Yerkes and his group had to solve was that the ratio of mental age and chronological age was not suitable for adults. Yerkes suggested using *standard scores*: how many people scored higher or lower than a given person, which could take into account social and biological characteristics. Yerkes called this a *point-scale test*.

The Wechsler-Bellevue

David Wechsler (1896–1981), trained as a psychologist, became skilled in the army in evaluating Army Alpha and Army Beta test forms. He received additional training in the field of psychometrics from Charles Spearman and Karl Pearson in London [27]. In 1932, Wechsler became head of the psychology unit of the Bellevue psychiatric hospital in New York, and here he began creating a *better* (as he wrote) intelligence test: the Wechsler-Bellevue, appearing in 1939. He used subtests that were available and that he knew well: components of the Army Alpha and Beta tests, resulting in an intelligence test with a Total IQ, a Verbal IQ, and a Performance IQ.

The Beginning of Standardization of Neuropsychological Tests

The American psychologist, James McKeen Cattell (1860–1944), went for his further education to Wundt's (1832–1920) laboratory in Germany. He thus became familiar with reaction time tasks and was asked by Wundt to investigate the speed of naming words. He subsequently worked for some time with Galton, and then returned to the US. There he introduced the idea of mental testing, not only for experimental research, but also for applied psychological purposes in industry and education. The development of the Color

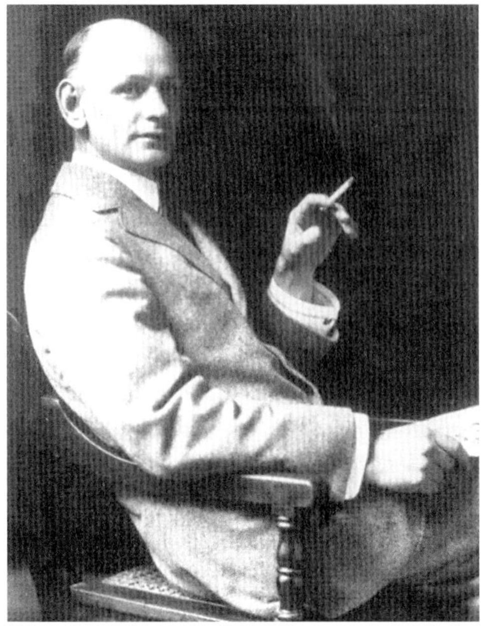

Fig. 5. Shepherd Ivory Franz (1874–1933), around 1920 (public domain).

Word test by John Ridley Stroop (1897–1973) resulted directly from Cattell's and others' laboratory studies on naming latencies for words and objects [29].

The American psychologist, Shepherd Ivory Franz (1874–1933; Fig. 5), wrote his dissertation with Cattell [30]. When Franz in 1907 went to work as a psychologist in the Government Hospital for the Insane in Washington, he designed procedures for diagnostic assessment. He described these in his *Handbook of mental examination methods* from 1912 [31]. The book describes the different steps in the assessment process: first a thorough interview, followed by a series of tests for perception, memory, attention, arithmetic's, speech, language, and movement; then an intelligence test, for example, the Binet-Simon or the Army test; and finally the test for Emotional instability of Woodworth, a questionnaire. Franz found it very important to compare the performance of a patient with standardized data.

One of Franz's most famous students was Karl Lashley (1890–1958), known among neuropsychologists for his animal studies on the localization of memory. Lashley himself has not played a major role in clinical neuropsychology, but some of his students did, such as Donald Hebb (1904–1985) and André Rey (1905–1965), who created the Auditory Verbal learning Test and the Rey Complex Figure Test [32].

In 1935, the psychologist Ward Halstead (1908–1968; Fig. 6) was appointed to the Medical Faculty of the University of Chicago [33]. He examined the biological basis of intelligence in patients with brain injury [34]. He developed a fairly extensive test battery. The Category Test, a concept learning test, is probably the best known of these. In neurosurgical patients, patients with acquired brain disorders, and also in healthy controls, data were collected and analyzed with the newly-designed (by Louis Thurstone [1887–1956]) factor

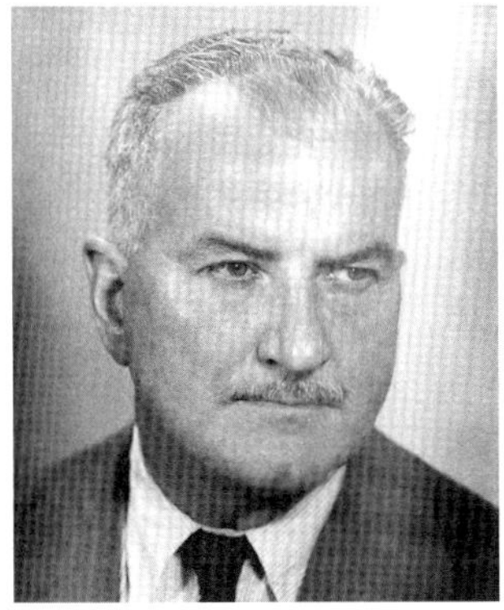

Fig. 6. Ward Halstead (1908–1968). The Drs. Nicholas and Dorothy Cummings Center for the History of Psychology, The University of Akron, with kind permission.

analysis. Ward found 4 factors: Factor A represented abstraction capacity, P stands for Power, C for central integration capacity, and D for differentiated capacities. His pupil Ralph Reitan (1922–2014) contributed to this battery by constructing the Halstead-Reitan Neuropsychological Battery, which counts eleven subtests. Reitan also popularized the Trail Making Test, which was not part of the battery, but was taken regularly [35]. Originally it was claimed that it "measured" "organicity," then "divided attention," and currently it is used for assessing executive functioning [36]. Reitan was also a great advocate of the idea of a *fixed battery*: always using the same battery allowed for the use of psychometric data for interpretation.

Aphasia Test Battery

A special case within the domain of neuropsychological assessment forms the territory of aphasia, usually dominated in the clinic by speech pathologists. Henry Charlton Bastian (1837–1915; Fig. 7) developed a language model with language centers for the various modalities, several years before Wernicke. Recently, Lorch showed that Bastian perhaps theoretically might be considered a misfit in London (he localized functions in the cortex, while in England most neurologists did not believe in localization of function, echoing John Hughlings Jackson's (1835–1911) opinion [37]. However, neurologists there have learned using Bastian's comprehensive test battery to examine aphasia patients. The battery examined various aspects of language behavior and forms of aphasia. It was based on Bastian's language model (for word form centers in the 4 modalities: auditory, visual (reading), motor (articulation), and kinetic (writing).

In America some test batteries were developed for the assessment of aphasia patients [4]. For example, there is one designed by the neurologist Theodore Weisenburg (1876–1934) and the psychologist Katharine McBride (1904–1976) in 1935 (based on Wernicke's sensory-motor theory of language behavior) [38]. Another battery was developed by the American neurologist Joseph Wepman (1907–?) and language pathologist Hildred Schuell (1907–1970): the Language Modalities Test for Aphasia from 1961 [39].

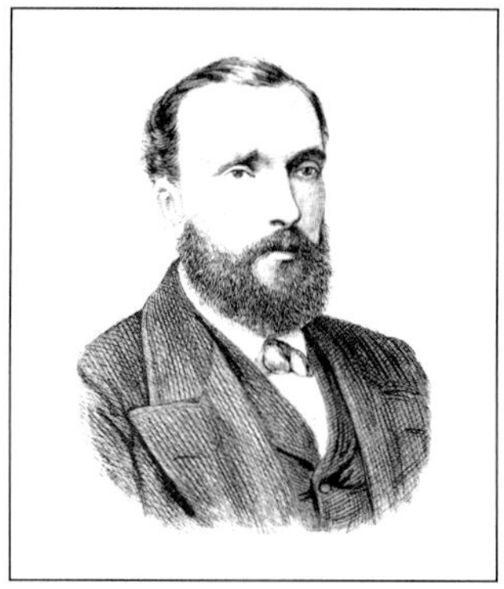

Fig. 7. Henry Charlton Bastian (1837–1915). From The Popular Science Monthly, 1875, Vol. 8 (public domain).

These batteries were based on rather simplistic ideas about language processing. Wernicke's sensory-motor theory of word images had already been strongly criticized by the psycholinguist Heymann Steinthal (1823–1899; 1871), as it fails to capture many important components of language processing [40]. With respect to standardization and validation, these batteries were quite deficient, but they were widely used for classifying patients in groups for further investigation. With much confusing consequences!

Epilogue

I have described various historical roots of neuropsychological assessment procedures up to approximately the beginning of modern neuropsychology, around the 1960s. Of course, new tests and new ideas on assessment have been formulated since and these are well-described in the consecutive volumes on neuropsychological assessment, written by Lezak et al. [14] (Lezak et al. [14], 2012). Roots of current assessment procedures can be traced to the 19th and beginning of the 20th century. Examination of a patient always begins with good observation. "Neuropsychologists" increasingly began to use bed-side tests. Many of these tests were designed by neurologists or psychiatrist, using common sense, rather than a formal theoretical framework. The physician presumably could tell what was normal or abnormal, simply by looking at a patient's performance on a given test.

At the beginning of the 20th century, intelligence tests were developed to discriminate between bright and dull children and for young men applying for a position in the American army. This led to the development of more formal procedures for determining scores and the field of psychometrics. Some neuropsychological test batteries also applied statistical procedures and norm scores for the interpretation of test performance. The Halstead-Reitan test battery is an example of this category. Other neuropsychologists, like Goldstein and Luria, did not rely on simple test scores and they primarily pointed to the importance of observations.

Looking back, it is remarkable to see that many tests from the contemporary repertoire derive from procedures developed before or around 1900. Many tests have been used over the years and scores have been interpreted in different theoretical frameworks used over the years. It suggests that procedures were considered valid even though theoretical views changed.

It is important for a present-day clinical neuropsychologist to be aware of the background of their assessment procedures. Insight provides an opportunity to become aware of the possibilities and limitations of a test, and also for doing something about it. A professional cannot and should not blindly trust that a test actually measures what is written on the box.

References

1 Barr WB: Historical development of the neuro-psychological test battery; in Morgan IE, Ricker H (eds): Textbook of Clinical Neuropsychology. New York, Taylor and Francis, 2008, pp 3–17.

2 Sarton G: The edwin smith papyrus. James henry breasted. Isis 1923;5:447–449.

3 Pomata G: The medical case narrative: distant reading of an epistemic genre. Lit Med 2014;32:1–23.

4 Eling P, Whitaker H: History of aphasia: a conceptual analysis; in Finger S, Boller F, Tyler KL (eds): Handbook of Clinical Neurology (Vol 95). Amsterdam, Elsevier, 2009, pp 571–582.

5 Luzzatti C, Whitaker HA: Johannes schenck and johannes jakob wepfer: clinical and anatomical observations in the prehistory of neurolinguistics and neuropsychology. J Neuroling 1996;9:157–164.

6 Bondy M: Psychiatric antecedents of psychological testing (before Binet). J Hist Beh Sci 1974;10:180–194.

7 Guislain J: Leçons Orales sur les Phrénopathies. Gand, L. Hebbelynck, 1852.

8 Wernicke C: Grundriss der Psychiatrie. Leipzig, Thieme, 1900.

9 Snell L: Über Simulation der Geistesstörung. Allg Z Psychiatr 1881;38:257–266.

10 Nies KJ, Sweat JJ: Neuropsychological assessment and malingering: a critical review of past and present strategies. Arch Clin Neurops 1994;9:501–552.

11 Rieger C: Beschreibung der Intelligenzstörung in Folge einer Hirnverletzung nebst einem Entwurf zu einer allgemein anwendbaren Methode der Intelligenzprüfung. Verhandlungen der Physikalisch-Medicinischen Gesellschaft zu Würzburg 1889:1–56; 1890, 1–46.

12 Ebbinghaus H: Über eine neue Methode zur Prüfung geistiger Fähigkeiten und ihre Anwendung bei Schulkindern. Z f. Psych 1897;15:401–459.

13 Ziehen TH. Die Prinzipien und Methoden der Intelligenzprüfung. Berlin, Karger, 1908.

14 Lezak MD, Howieson DB, Bigler ED, Tranel D: Neuropsychological Assessment, ed 5. New York, Oxford University Press, 2012.

15 Whipple GM: Manual of Mental and Physical Tests, A Book of Directions Compiled with Special Reference to the Experimental Study of School Children in the Laboratory or Classroom. Baltimore, Warwick & York, 1910.

16 Eling P: Kurt Goldstein's test battery. Cortex 2015;63: 16–26.

17 Eling P, Derckx K, Maes R: On the historical and conceptual background of the Wisconsin Card Sorting Test. Brain Cogn 2008;67:247–253.

18 Luria AR: Outline for the neuro-psychological examination of a patient 'with local brain lesions. Neurops Rev 1999;9:9–22.

19 Golden Ch, Freshwater S, Vayalakkara J: The Luria-Nebraska ska neuropsychological battery; in Groth-Marnat G (ed): Neuropsychological Assessment in Clinical Practice: A Guide to Test Interpretation and Integration. New York, Wiley, 2000, pp 263–289.

20 Du Bois L: A History of Psychological Testing. Boston, Allyn and Bacon, 1970.

21 Boake C: From the Binet-Simon to the Wechsler-Bellevue: tracing the history of intelligence testing. J Cinl Exp Neurops 2002;24:383–405.

22 Galton F: Hereditary Genius: An Inquiry Into Its Laws and Consequences. London, Macmillan, 1869.

23 Binet A, Simon T: Méthodes Nouvelles pour le Diagnostic du Niveau Intellectuel des Anormaux. L' Année Psychol 1905;11:191–244.

24 Binet A, Simon T: Application des Méthodes Nouvelles au Diagnostic du Niveau Intellectuel chez des Infants Normaux et Anormaux d'Hospice et d'Ecole Primaire. L' Année Psychol 1905;11:246–336.

25 Stern W: Die psychologischen Methoden der Intelligenzprüfung: und deren Anwendung an Schulkindern. Leipzig, Barth, 1912.

26 Terman L: The Measurement of Intelligence. Boston, Houghton Mifflin, 1916.

27 Wechsler D: The psychometric tradition: developing the wechsler adult intelligence scale. Contemp Educ Psych 1981;6:82–85.

28 Sartran R: GI Rossolimo (1860–1928): neurologist and public benefactor. J Hist Neurosc 2007;16:65–73.
29 MacLeod C: John ridley stroop: creator of a landmark cognitive task. Can J Psych 1991;32:521–524.
30 Eling P: Franz: neuropsycholoog *avant la lèttre*. T Neurops 2010;5:35–39.
31 Franz SI: Handbook of Mental Examination Methods. New York, The Journal of Nervous and Mental Disease Publishing Company, 1912.
32 van der Meer J, Eling P: Andre rey and his complex figure test. T Neurops 2008;3:45–51.
33 Reitan RM: Ward Halstead's contributions to neuropsychology and the Halstead-Reitan neuropsychological test battery. J Clin Psych 1994;50:47–70.
34 Halstead WC: Brain and Intelligence A Quantitative Study of the Frontal Lobes. Chicago, University of Chicago Press, 1947.
35 Reitan R: Trail making test results for normal and brain-damaged children. Percept Mot Skills 1971;33: 575–581.
36 Eling P: Op het spoor van de Trail Making Test. T Neurops 2013;8:53–58.
37 Lorch M: Examining language functions: a reassessment of Bastian's contribution to aphasia assessment. Brain 2013;136:2629–2637.
38 Weisenburg TH, McBride KE: Aphasia: a clinical and psychological study. New York, The Commonwealth Fund, 1935.
39 Wepman JM, Jones LV: The Language Modalities Test for Aphasia. The Industrial Relations Center. Chicago, University of Chicago, 1961.
40 Eling P: The psycholinguistic approach to aphasia of Chajim Steinthal. Aphasiology 2006;20:1072–1084.

Paul Eling
Department of Psychology, Donders Institute for Brain, Cognition and Behaviour
PO Box 9104
NL–6500 HE Nijmegen (The Netherlands)
E-Mail p.eling@donders.ru.nl

Bogousslavsky J, Boller F, Iwata M (eds): A History of Neuropsychology.
Front Neurol Neurosci. Basel, Karger, 2019, vol 44, pp 179–191 (DOI: 10.1159/000494962)

Historical Pathway from Description of Cognitive Recovery to Formal Neuropsychological Rehabilitation

Eloi Magnin[a, b] Ilham Ryff[a] Baptiste Brun[c] Pierre Decavel[a, d]
Sebastien Hague[a] Thierry Moulin[a, b]

[a]Department of Neurology, University Hospital of Besançon, Besançon, France; [b]Clinical and Integrative Neuroscience, Research Laboratory 481, Bourgogne Franche-Comté University, Besançon, France; [c]Department of Contemporary Art History, Rennes 2 University, Rennes, France; [d]Laboratory of Clinical Functional Exploration of Movement, University Hospital of Besançon, Besançon, France

Abstract

Neuropsychological rehabilitation is one of the subspecialties of neuropsychology, along with neuropsychological assessment, cognitive process descriptions, and anatomo-functional correlation, but it is still frequently underrecognized, even from a historical point of view. In this chronological review, we propose following some of the historical descriptions of cognitive recovery, and the suggested procedures and therapies to improve this recovery from mythological periods and the antiquity to recent contemporary periods and the birth of formal neuropsychological rehabilitation in neurological and psychiatric conditions.

Introduction

Definition

Neuropsychology, a term that was used for the first time by Sir William Osler in 1913 [1], is a discipline that studies cognitive mechanisms, behaviors, and their relation to brain structure.

Cognitive or neuropsychological rehabilitation, an art and a science [2], is a therapeutic program including both restorative and compensatory components to help cognitively impaired individuals to totally or partially restore normal functioning, or to compensate for cognitive, emotional, psychosocial and behavioral deficits, and improve the quality of life.

The term rehabilitation is the most commonly used term in literature, but other terms, such as remediation, revalidation or reeducation, are also used. In France, the term "re-education" was used for many years to describe this discipline and highlighted the parallel with the learning process of children in the understanding of neuropsychological mechanisms and the rehabilitation procedure, inducing a "re-learning" that will be discussed later. Cognitive rehabilitation is multidisciplinary and includes speech pathology, occupational therapy, special education, physical medicine, neurology, cognitive psychology, cognitive neuroscience, rehabilitation psychology, and neuropsychology [3].

Background and Aims

The history of neuropsychology frequently focuses on detailed semiological case descriptions, interpretation of the potential underlying cognitive mechanisms, and the relationship with anatomical structures [4]. However, the cognitive recovery of these deficits and the potential rehabilitation procedures to improve their recovery were also reported in parallel [5], frequently by the same authors who reported the follow-up of their patients, but these parts of their work were rather less highlighted in the literature.

Therefore, in this review we propose chronologically following some of the historical descriptions of cognitive recovery and the suggested procedures and therapies to improve this recovery from mythological periods, and the antiquity to recent contemporary periods and the birth of neuropsychological rehabilitation. This concept evolved in parallel to the perception of handicap and behavioral disorders over the ages. The purpose of our work is not to prepare an exhaustive list, but rather to present the evolution of concepts and methods in some neurological and psychiatric conditions.

Mythology and Religious Concepts

During older ages, disease and symptoms were frequently considered as curses given by offended gods, goddesses or by puissant sorcerers.

One of the first references to neuropsychological symptoms and recovery was a language disorder associated with a probable facial palsy that might correspond to a stroke reported in a Hittite text in 14th century BC about the Mesopotamian king Mursilis II (1343–1295 BC) [6]. An oracle suggested that as language disorders occurred after thunder, it was a curse of Manuzziya, the Storm god. The first "rehabilitation" procedure proposed by the oracle was to perform 2 rituals after a water-cleansing purification and a night of chastity. The first was a sacrifice by a ritual fire of a "surrogate ox" with all the King's clothes and belongings (weapons, flatware, furniture, horses, and carriages) playing the role of scapegoat to replace Mursulli in the sight of the offended god. The second ritual was also a sacrifice by fire of birds and a lamb as an offering to appease the Storm god.

In Homer's odyssey, written around 7th century BC, neuropsychological symptoms, focusing especially on memory disorders and apathy, are also reported as divine plots against Ulysse in different stages of his return to Ithaka. Lotos fruits given by Lotophage to Ulysse's sailors induced apathy and forgetfulness of their goals, which was healed by "weaning" them off this drug. The episode of Siren's songs is quite similar, but also suggests that a "hypermnesia" about general knowledge might be associated with amnesia of his home and family. Avoidance and renunciation of this "temptation" are the methods proposed in these myths [7].

Similar adventures are reported in Sigurdr's Nordic Saga. The queen Grímhildr gave a philter of oblivion that Sigurdr forget his beloved Valkyrie, Brynhildr, and gets married to Gudrun, Grímhildr's daughter. Participating in the wedding of Brynhildr and Gunnar, Sigudr's best friend, permitted him to recover his memory but it was too late [8]. This saga suggests that revalidation of knowledge, cueing, and emotion might be effective cognitive therapy to cure memory impairment.

In Asian religious and philosophical thought, the state of "Illumination" is sometimes described as a mental state acquired after long training (including meditation), permitting the recovery of the forgotten memories of past lives, usually erased during the process of rebirth, as described by Buddha [9] or Pythagoras [10]. Meditation is actually one of the validated procognitive methods frequently studied by neuroscientists and proposed in different neurological and psychiatric pathological conditions [11].

Religious managements sometimes called "religious therapy" of cognitive and behavioral disorders were focused on redemption, prey, exorcism, charismatic healing, spiritual counsels, fasting, and pilgrimage to seek miracles, magical objects, and amulets [12].

From the First Step of Medical School: Management of Cognitive Disorders to First Neuropsychological Rehabilitation Procedure

Founders of Medicine

Hippocrates (460–370 BC) suggested that the brain was the organ of mind and was influenced by the balance of humors. Hippocrates' humors theory [13] (4th century BC), followed later by Galen (130–210) and Avicienna's (980–1037) theories, suggested cognitive disorders, such as aphasia, were frequently considered as an abnormal phlegm and black bile accumulation in the posterior ventricles, obstructing the flow of the "psychic pneuma" or "animal spirits." The use of bloodletting, hot cups, emetics, purges, and complex alchemic polymedication were performed to correct imbalance of humors [14, 15]. These methods were applied until the 18th century, physical as well as behavioral therapies.

Language Pathfinder

In 1558, Nicolas Massa reported a spectacular immediate language recovery in a soldier presenting with head injury immediately after surgical extraction of part of the bone in the wound [16].

The absence of lingual paralysis in aphasia reported by Johann Schenk von Grafenberg (1530–1598) in 1585 [17] was also important knowledge, even if some physicians still proposed to put plasters on the tongue to cure aphasia until the middle of the 19th century [18].

In 1745, Olof von Dalin (1708–1763) reported the case of a mute and right-hemiparetic patient who, after a trip to a mineral spring known as healing spring 3 years after disease onset, presented with a small improvement of motor skills and the capacity to say "yes." Sign communications were possible. A few times later, he was also able, after external cueing, to sing certain hymns. It foreshadowed the "melodic intonation" speech therapy still currently used in aphasic management [16].

In 1683, Peter Rommel (1643–1708) reported the case of a 52-year-old woman who presented with a severe aphasia (with only a few verbal automatisms) without comprehension disorders associated with right-sided motor deficit. However, she was able to give biblical recitation and prayers fluently [16].

These 2 previous cases illustrate dichotomy between automatic and self-willed language and the potential role of music in recovery, which are some of the speech therapy procedures still used in language rehabilitation today [19]. The healing spring effect that might correspond to actual thermal cure seems to be more anecdotic or might also correspond to a placebo effect.

In 1676, Johann Schmidt (1642–1690) reported the case of a 65-year-old man presenting initially with right-sided paralysis and verbal paraphasias. During the follow-up, the patient recovered from oral language disorders, but had alexia without aphasia. He also reported a second case presenting with alexia, which he totally recovered from after relearning and reading re-training. In his article, Schmidt explains that teaching and guidance were, therefore sometimes useful in these patients [16]. A kind of written language rehabilitation protocol was also probably applied in this case.

In 1690, Johannes Jakob Wepfer (1620–1695) reported the progressive recovery of an aphasic bilingual patient during the first week after disease onset. No mention is given about potential rehabilitation procedures in this case [17].

Pioneer in Behavioral and Cognitive Management

Johann Josef Gassner (1727–1779), an Austrian priest, began to practice his own exorcism procedure after 1760 and became quite renowned. In 1775, Franz Anton Mesmer (1734–1815), an Austrian physician renowned for his "animal magnetism" theory, evaluated Gassner's practice as an "involuntary Mesmerism." Moreover, Mesmer proposed the use of "magnetism" or Mesmerism as a treatment for hysteria [20]. Therefore, some part of Gassner's exorcism procedure and Mesmer's magnetism foreshadowed hypnosis and psychotherapy [21]. Hypnosis is actually one of the cognitive interventions frequently studied by neuroscientists and still proposed in different neurological and psychiatric pathological conditions today [22].

Philippe Pinel (1745–1826), considered as one of the precursors of psychiatry, with the help of Jean-Baptiste Pussin, who is considered as one of the precursors of psychiatric nurse jobs, suggested that insane patients should not be jailed and bound and were potentially curable [23, 24]. In parallel to the study by Vincenzo Chiarugi (1759–1820) in Italy [25], they elaborated on "moral therapy" directly derived from and sometimes associated with "religious" therapy, creating confidence between patient and therapist, keeping the patient away from disabling environmental causes, listening kindly to patient's complaints, reappraisal and blaming of behavioral disorders, considered as one of the first psychotherapy procedures in Salpêtrière Hospital in Paris. This procedure can be considered as feedback therapy to improve the patient's insight into their behavioral disorders. Pinel also proposed marriage as a preventive and curative therapy for hysteria.

Moral therapy introduced art therapy in psychiatric management during the first part of the 19th century, following Pinel's legacy. However, as it might deliver the imagination of patients, some physicians feared negative behavioral side effects. This therapy is frequently considered as an occupational task; however, as reported by William Alexander Francis Browne (1805–1885) [26], a physician of Crichton Royal Institution for Lunatics in Scotland in 1841, it can also permit the channeling of behavioral disorders and delusion, and improve feedback and insight of the patients. Therefore, art therapy should also be considered as a neuropsychological therapy.

Indeed, several historical developments in different countries show a common interest in art practice considered as a healing process and recovery at the very end of the 19th century and throughout the 20th century. Originating from moral treatment, it seems that this trend gave good results. Thus, in France, circa 1896, Dr. Montyel de Marandon developed a workshop in the asylum of Ville-Evrard, dedicated to drawing and painting for his patients who were previously artists in their professional life. They found calmness in reconnecting with their old practice. As Montyel de Marandon wrote in1902: "C'est là un point capital, tout le temps consacré au travail est autant de gagné sur la folie; pendant qu'il s'occupe, le cerveau d'un aliéné est tout entier à son travail, et sur ce point fonctionne normalement: que cela dure et l'on peut espérer que de proche en proche les autres rouages de sa pensée reprendront un fonctionnement normal." [This is a crucial point: the amount of time spent working is time won over insanity; whilst he is busy, the brain of a lunatic is at work in its entirety and functions normally. Whether this lasts, however, one can only hope, and that the other cogs in his brain start turning again as normal.] [27].

Whereas the art critic Marcel Réja (also known as Paul Meunier, 1873–1957, a psychiatrist) published a very famous book untitled "*L'Art chez les fous*" in 1907, art production in asylums and psychiatric institutions raised a deep and long-term interest in the medical community [28]. This attention was ambiguous. First, the documentary value of this kind of artifact made psychiatrists use it for diagnosis. However, in some cases, the perspective changed radically and personalities familiar with the development of psychoanalysis began to observe that troubles could evolve from shifts in art production. Reflections of Dr. Auguste Marie (1865–1934), who collected drawings for his "*Musée de la Folie*" in Villejuif Hospital around 1900, witnessed this phenomenon. Walter Morgenthaler (1882–1965) did the same in the asylum of Waldau, near Bern in Switzerland. He encouraged his patients to draw, challenging them to recover calmness and other aptitudes within that kind of work [27].

Later, in Brazil, Dr. Osorio Cesar (1895–1979) institutionalized drawing as a way to heal his patients in the Hospital of Juqueri in Sao Paolo [29]. Occupational workshops he set up would later have a great influence when these works were exhibited during the First International Congress of Psychiatry in Paris in 1950. This major international event, along with "*L'Exposition internationale d'art psychopathologique*" presented in Sainte Anne's Hospital (Paris) led the way for many psychiatric institutions for decades to come, leading to contemporary art therapy [30].

In Paris, the institute for the deaf and mute was created by de l'Epée [31] (1712–1789), who was one of the first to study sign language. Jean Marc Gaspard Itard (1774–1838) [32], considered as one of the fathers of otology, also worked in this institute on speech abilities of mute subjects and rehabilitation of stuttering.

Itard's work focusing on the integration of these patients directly inspired Edourd Séguin (1812–1880), who created the first private school for intellectually impaired children in 1840 using moral treatment and psychosocial rehabilitation to treat his patients [33]. Among his tools, he used a wooden geometric puzzle as a rehabilitation tool, which was later adapted in the mid-20th century to evaluate Intellectual Quotient [5, 34]. Inspired by Itard and Séguin, Maria Montessori (1870–1952) then applied specific learning programs in children with or without cognitive disorders [35].

Désiré Magloire Bourneville (1840–1909) created a dedicated structure in an alienist department of the hospital of Bicêtre (Paris) from 1879, to take care of deficient children who were segregated before this initiative, because they were formerly considered as incurable. In this structure, the "medicopedagogic treatment," a therapy mixing educative lessons and medical rehabilitation, was proposed to improve their autonomy. Therefore, he is considered as one of the founders of the discipline of rehabilitation [36].

A Specific Focus on Language Disorders and Management

Itard is also known for his work with Victor d'Aveyron in 1801 and 1807, a wild child, who he tried to reeducate and to teach how to speak [37, 38]. Wild children (raised alone in nature), pseudo-wild children (patient presenting probably cognitive, behavioral or sensorial disorders excluded from society), and "artificial experimental" wild children (children "voluntarily" raised without any social communication) were studied both to evaluate the existence of a "primal language" and to study language acquisition, learning strategies and the limits of these children [39].

In 1836, Dax [40] (1770–1837), one of the first to describe left predominance of language in the brain, used leeches on the left temple to improve an acute language disorder in a patient who presented with a second episode of transient aphasic disorder. This is the first therapy to take the localization of the lesion into account in the procedure, and therefore corresponds to the neuropsychological way of thinking [40].

In 1843, Lordat [41–43] (1773–1870), professor of physiology at the University of Montpellier, reported his own experience of aphasia and his recovery over several weeks. It is the first medical autobiographical report of aphasia. He also reported the case of a priest who selectively recovered in his provincial dialect only [41–43].

In 1865, Broca [44] (1824–1880) reported that a relearning of words was possible in aphasic patients; however, it should require a significant effort from both the patient and professionals. Initially, he compared this procedure with children's education of language. He also reported his program of rehabilitation from alexia in this patient, beginning with alphabetic relearning. The patient then worked spontaneously on syllabic reading. He reported that it was impossible for the patient to associate syllabi. Instead, Broca proposed to work on word recognition and reported that his patient preferred to use word form instead of letter or syllabi to identify words. The rehabilitation of this patient was described more than half a century before Ferdinand de Saussure's course and more than one century before Coltheart's dual route model of reading based on the lexical semantic route and the grapheme-to-phoneme conversion route. In this description, Broca also identified that the predominance of this lexical semantic strategy during patient rehabilitation is different from infant learning of reading initially based on the grapheme-to-phoneme conversion. We think that this might correspond to one of the first neuropsychological rehabilitation programs, as well as speech therapy based simultaneously on clinical symptoms, underlying cognitive mechanisms and given by a physician with an anatomical knowledge of language network. The modification of his procedure during the follow-up to adapt it to the patient's results foreshadows the actual personalized "tailored" programs used in cognitive rehabilitation (Box 1).

The Challenging Management of Hysteria (for Review See [45])
Briquet [46] (1796–1881) reported in a treatise many empirical and sometimes aggressive "therapeutic" strategies of hysteria used during the 19th century, such as familial isolement (husband, parents), hydrotherapy, fresh milk, and sometimes even blood-letting. He also described the use of cupping glasses or leeches placed on the perinea, and genital compression. Exciting drugs, enemas, antispasmodic remedies, opiates, lotions, frictions, and cauterizations were also proposed as medical treatments. Electrical current (faradization) was also promoted by Guillaume-Benjamin-Amand Duchenne [47] (1806–1875). Briquet suggested preventive strategies in the improvement of familial and social links (especially marriage, as per Pinel), education including music, good nutrition, and thermal water.

In 1843, James Braid (1795–1860) studied hypnosis with a scientific approach, building a neurophysiological theory [48] which later inspired Jean-Martin Charcot (1825–1893) to try this therapy on his hysteria patients. Charcot also used this method to induce suggestion during the process of diagnosis of hysteria [49]. Bernheim [50] (1840–1919), in Nancy, also used hypnosis to cure hysteria during the same period, but criticized Charcot for his process of diagnosing hysteria, suggesting that he artificially induced hysteric crisis with a method of hypnosis [51]. Richer [51] (1849–1933), a disciple of Charcot, also reported the use of musical therapy, vibrations, metallotherapy, and rest cure [52]. Ovariectomy was very controversial, especially to Charcot, but he occasionally proposed it to hysteric patients in the late 19th century.

Box 1. Paul Broca's point of view about neuropsychological rehabilitation.

Puis, comment sait-on que l'aphémique n'est pas capable d'apprendre à parler avec l'hémisphère droit qui lui reste? A-t-on essayé de faire son éducation? lui a-t-on donné ces leçons de tous les jours, de toutes les heures, de tous les instants à l'aide desquelles on finit à la longue par faire parler un enfant? Pour ma part, je suis convaincu que, sans rendre aux aphémiques la partie de leur intelligence quiapéri avec une partie de leur cerveau, on pourrait, en y mettant assez de persévérance, en les traitant avec l'infatigable constance de la mère qui apprend à parler à son enfant, on pourrait, dis-je, obtenir des résultats considérables. Lorsque j'étais à Bicêtre, j'ai gardé plusieurs mois un aphémique dans mes salles; souvent, à la visite, je lui consacrais quelques minute, et j'avais fini par étendre notablement son vocabulaire. Mais, qu'est-ce qu'une leçon aussi courte? Croyez-vous qu'un enfant ferait bien des progrès si on ne ie faisait parler que quelques moments chaque jour? Et n'allez pas croire que, sous ce rapport, l'éducation d'un adulte soit plus facile que celle d'un enfant; elle est-beaucoupplus difficile au contraire. Il y a des choses qu'on n'apprend jamais bien au delà d'un certain âge. (...); il est probable que l'adulte et l'enfant suivent, pour arriver au but, des procédés différents. L'enfant se borne à imiter, il émet des sons au hasard jusqu'à ce qu'il trouve le son qu'on lui demande, et il recommence avec docilité aussi souvent qu'on le désire. L'adulte n'a pas cette patience; il ne peut faire abstraction de ce qu'il sait ou de ce qu'il croit savoir; il discute le procédé; au lieu d'obéir naïvement, il cherche en lui-même les voies et moyens, et les connaissances qu'il possède déjà, loin de lui venir en aide, l'empêchent au contraire de profiter des leçons pratiques qu'on lui donne. [Then, how do we know that the aphemic is not able to learn to speak with the right hemisphere? Have we tried to educate him? Has he been given these lessons every day, every hour, every moment possible, by which, in the long run, a child ends up being made to talk? For my part, I am convinced that, without giving aphemics back the part of their intelligence that was part of their brain, we could persevere and treat them with the indefatigable consistency of a mother teaching her child to talk, we could, I say, achieve considerable results. When I was at Bicetre, I kept an aphemic on my ward for several months; often, during the visit, I dedicated a few minutes to him and ended up expanding his vocabulary significantly. But what is such a short lesson? Do you think a child would make such progress if we only talked to it for a few moments each day? Do not think that, in this respect, educating an adult is easier than educating a child; quite the opposite is true. There are some things you can never really learn past a certain age. (...) It is probable that the adult and the child will follow different methods to reach their goal. The child limits himself to imitating, he utters sounds at random until he finds the sound he is asked for, and he gently repeats it as often as desired. The adult does not have this patience; he cannot ignore what he knows or thinks he knows; he discusses the process; instead of obeying naively, he seeks in himself the ways and means, the knowledge he already possesses, far from helping him, quite the contrary, this prevents him from benefiting from the practical lessons that are taught to him.]

Paul Broca, le 15 juin 1865 [44]

Sollier [52] (1861–1933), a disciple of Bourneville, then of Charcot, elaborates on an original theory about a "mechanic treatment of psychoneuroses" [53], inducing a peripheric "reactivation" of the central functional deficits which was a precursor of cognitive behavioral therapy. During the beginning of the 20th century, he also suggested psychotherapy for the management of "hysteria" and "first world war psychoneurosis" having seldom used shock therapies, such as "torpillage" electrical treatment, unlike his contemporary colleagues [54]. He also treated Marcel Proust and developed the concepts of reviviscent memories [55] or reminiscences in the therapy of hysteria, a theme largely used by Proust in his literary work. Reminiscence is still used today in dementia rehabilitation [56].

20th Century Genuine Take-Off of Neuropsychological Rehabilitation

The Fathers of the Concept

In 1905, Shepherd Franz (1874–1933), an American psychologist, presented a program of speech therapy after working on a brain-injured cat model of rehabilitation, following a habit learning approach with multiple trials, including color naming, number naming and rehearsing, poem, and prayer recitation. He suggested that his program induced new functioning instead of revalidating former pathways in the brain, suggesting compensatory mechanisms in which the right hemisphere may be involved [57].

Janet [57] (1847–1959), who worked with Charcot in Salpetrière Hospital in Paris, introduced progressive exposition to anxiogen stimulus and a method of disengagement of rumination as therapy for depressive patients [58]. These methods foreshadowed the cognitive and behavioral therapy.

In 1913, Watson [58] (1878–1958), followed by Skinner [59] (1904–1990) in the 1930s [60], 2 American psychologists, developed the behaviorism model that was applied in education and rehabilitation processes and opened the field for many current behavioral methods, such as Applied Behavioral Analysis for autist management developed in the 1960s [61].

(1) First World War: Setting-Up of a Rehabilitation Structure for Brain-Injured Patients and the First Formal Cognitive Rehabilitation Programs

Formal neuropsychological rehabilitation, with dedicated centers and a pluridisciplinary approach, really started at the beginning of the 20th century, particularly during the First World War, to help brain-injured soldiers. Germany and Austria were the most advanced in this domain with the creation of dedicated medico-social structures. Poppelreuter [62] and Goldstein [63] were the most renowned authors and directors of these structures. Goldstein mostly worked on oral and written language therapy with elaboration of compensatory strategies (e.g., to mimic the blowing of tobacco smoke to relearn some phonemes). He also highlights the importance of valuating the clinical aspect of the patient, as "real life" ecological future socio-professional needs to personalize in the rehabilitation and focus on useful objectives [62, 64]. His work has also helped to develop behavioral methods for shaping desired behaviors. Poppelreuter [62], a highly critiqued figure for having later followed Nazi ideology, suggested that initial learning of a skill should be quite slow and accurate, then progressively speed-up during training [65, 66]. This foreshadowed Milner's procedural memory theory, which came about 4 decades later [67].

(2) Second World War: Rehabilitation of Cognitive Functions Other than Language and the First Scientific Evaluation of Effects of Cognitive Rehabilitation Programs

In the 1920s, Lev Semenovich Vygotsky (1896–1934), a Russian psychologist, proposed a cognitive rehabilitation of Parkinsonian patients using "cognitive prosthesis" as a cue to initiate movement, suggesting the possibility of the restructuring and reorganization of mental processes [68].

The Second World War was also a period of development for the neuropsychological rehabilitation of brain injured patients. Contrary to the rest of the world, who were mainly focused on language, Alexander Luria (1902–1977), a Russian psychologist and neurologist and disciple of Vygotsky, widens the vision of neuropsychological rehabilitation beyond language disorders to other cognitive functions, particularly executive ones [69, 70]. Therefore, he inspired future rehabilitation programs which include executive functions, even in reading rehabilitation such as PASS Reading Enhancement Program [71].

In Edinburgh, Edna Butfield and Oliver Zangwill tried to develop experimental studies to scientifically evaluate the efficacy of a language rehabilitation inspired by Goldstein's programs and vocational outcome. Zangwill [72] proposed 3 principles of rehabilitation strategies that are still considered in contemporary neuropsychological rehabilitation programs today: direct retraining, compensation, and substitution.

(3) Post-World-War Era: Improvement of Neuropsychological Rehabilitation Programs and Tools along with Neurosciences' Take-Off

After both World Wars, the era of motor vehicles also induced a brain-injury epidemic in parallel with the advanced medical technologies that increased survival rates for persons with brain injuries. Therefore, it justified the pursuit of neuropsychological rehabilitation development.

During the 1970s and 1980s, the field of cognitive rehabilitation grew rapidly and evolved, stimulated by advances in cognitive psychology and neurosciences. Memory disorders and neglect were more accurately described and therefore a new focus on the rehabilitation of these disorders was initiated, especially in the US. In New York, Leonard Diller's team developed a program with progressive difficulty, using verbal and visual cues to direct attention towards the neglected field or body part [73]. These programs are still widely used by neurorehabilitation therapists.

Another example of how wartime casualties have induced the need for neuropsychological rehabilitation programs is that of Yehuda Ben-Yishay. After the Yom Kippur War in Israel in 1973, he recognized the importance of the interpersonal and social needs of patients to re-enter their social environment [74, 75]. The program included small groups of veterans, patients who performed cognitive exercises, psychotherapy and therapeutic community activities following Goldstein's theory of "therapeutic environment." One of the objectives of the therapeutic activities was to increase the patients' awareness of injury-related impairments and to define and accept realistic outcomes, particularly vocational goals. It foreshadowed the "holistic" approach of rehabilitation programs, which is currently one of the most efficient in TBI management [76]. Following Ben-Yishay's theory, in 1986 Muriel Lezak worked on the emotional needs and responses of brain-injured patients and their families, highlighting the importance of this dimension in neuropsychological rehabilitation [77]. A holistic approach includes patient characteristics involving physical, physiological, cognitive and emotional-personal components, interaction between the patient and therapists, family, friends, and society in general.

One of the first computer programs of cognitive rehabilitation was developed in the 1980s by Rosamond Gianutsos, for remediation of memory and visual disorders by using mass practice as retraining [78].

Future Directions of Neuropsychological Rehabilitation

The neuropsychological rehabilitation program should be improved and modified in accordance with the better understanding of cognitive process and brain structures [78].

A major effort should be made to evaluate cognitive rehabilitation with evidence-based methodology. The validated methods should then be used preferentially in rehabilitation structures compared to methods which have no proven significant effect.

With the technological boom of the 21st century, the development of advanced technology applications as part of the rehabilitation process should continue, but not overshadow psychosocial issues.

References

1 Bruce D: On the origin of the term "neuropsychology". Neuropsychologia 1985;23:813–814.
2 Parente R, Stapleton M: History and systems of cognitive rehabilitation. NeuroRehabilitation 1997;8:3–11.
3 Koehler R, Wilhelm EE, Shoulson I: Cognitive Rehabilitation Therapy for Traumatic Brain Injury: Evaluating the Evidence. Washington, National Academies Press, 2012.
4 Barr WB, Bielauskas LA: The Oxford Handbook of History of Clinical Neuropsychology. New York, NY, Oxford University Press, 2016.
5 Boake C: Stage in the history of neuropsychological rehabilitation; in Watson BA (ed): Neuropsychological Rehabilitation: Theory and Practice. Lisse, Swets and Zeitlinger B.V., The Netherlands, 2003, pp 11–21.
6 Lebrun R: Aphasie de Mursili II. Hethitica 1985;6:103–137.
7 Bouvier D: La mémoire et la mort dans l'épopée homérique. Revue internationale et pluridisciplinaire de religion grecque antique. Kernos 1999;12:57–71.
8 Boyer R. La Saga de Sigurd ou La Parole Donnée. Paris, Editions du Cerf, 1989.
9 Martin R: Before Buddha Was Buddha: Learning from the Jataka Tales. Somerville, Wisdom Publications, 2018.
10 Cornelli G, McKirahan R: In Search of Pythagoreanism: Pythagoreanism as an Historiographical Category. Berlin, Walter de Gruyter, 2013.
11 Dahl CJ, Lutz A, Davidson RJ: Reconstructing and deconstructing the self: cognitive mechanisms in meditation practice. Trends Cogn Sci 2015;19:515–523.
12 Józsa L: Magical and religious healing in Byzantium. Orvostort Kozl 2010;56:171–185.
13 Contreras Mas A: Libro de la Melancholía by Andrés Velázquez (1585). Part 1. The intellectual origins of the book. Hist Psychiatry 2003;14:25–40.
14 Karenberg A, Hort I: Medieval descriptions and doctrines of stroke: preliminary analysis of select sources. Part II: between Galenism and Aristotelism – Islam theories of apoplexy (800–1200). J Hist Neurosci 1998;7:174–185.
15 Rocca J: Galen and the ventricular system. J Hist Neurosci 1997;6:227–239.
16 Benton AL, Joynt RJ: Early descriptions of aphasia. Arch Neurol 1960;3:205–222.
17 Luzzatti C, Whitaker HA: Johannes Schenck and Johannes Jakob Wepfer: clinical and anatomical observations in the prehistory of neurolinguistics and neuropsychology. J Neurolinguistics 1996;9:157–164.
18 Prins R, Bastiaanse R: History of aphasia. The early history of aphasiology: from the Egyptian surgeons (c. 1700 BC) to Broca (1861). Aphasiology 2006;20:762–791.
19 Lim KB, Kim YK, Lee HJ, Yoo J, Hwang JY, Kim JA, Kim SK: The therapeutic effect of neurologic music therapy and speech language therapy in post-stroke aphasic patients. Ann Rehabil Med 2013;37:556–562.
20 Forrest D: Mesmer. Int J Clin Exp Hypn 2002;50:295–308.
21 Peter B: Gassner's Exorcism – not Mesmer's Magnetism – is the Real Predecessor of Modern Hypnosis. Int J Clin Exp Hypn 2005;53:1–12.
22 Deeley Q. Hypnosis as therapy for functional neurologic disorders. Handb Clin Neurol 2016;139:585–595.
23 Pinel P: Traité Médico-Philosophique sur l'aliénation Mentale ou La manie. Paris, Librairie Bresson, 1800.

24 Pelletier JF, Davidson L: At the very roots of psychiatry as a new medical specialty: the Pinel-Pussin partnership. Sante Ment Que 2015;40:19–33.
25 Grange KM: Pinel or Chiarugi? Med Hist 1963;7:371–380.
26 Browne WAF: Second Annual Report of the Crichton Royal Institution for Lunatics, Dumfries, November 11, 1841.
27 Décimo M: Des fous et des hommes avant l'art brut. Dijon, Les presses du réel, 2018, p 25.
28 Réja M: L'Art chez les fous. Société du Mercure de France, 1907.
29 Cabanas KM: Learning from Madness: Brazilian Modernism and Global Contemporary Art. Chicago, University of Chicago Press, 2018.
30 Volmat R: L'Art Psychopathologique. Paris, PUF, 1956.
31 de l'Epée CM: Institution des Sourds et Muets: par la voie des signes Méthodiques. Paris, Librairie Nyon, 1776.
32 Chalat NI: History of medicine Jean Marc Gaspard Itard 1774–1838. Laryngoscope 1982;92:627–629.
33 Séguin E: Traitement Moral, Hygiène et éducation des Idiots et des Autres Enfants Arriérés. Paris, Librairie Baillière, 1846.
34 Pichot P: French pioneers in the field of mental deficiency. Am J Ment Defic 1948;53:128–137.
35 Cascella M: Maria Montessori (1870–1952): Women's emancipation, pedagogy and extra verbal communication. Rev Med Chil 2015;143:658–662.
36 Gateaux-Mennecier J: L'oeuvre médico-sociale de Bourneville. Hist Sci Med 2003;37:13–30.
37 Itard JM: Mémoire sur les Premiers Développements de Victor de l'Aveyron. Paris, F. Alcan, 1801.
38 Itard JM: Rapport sur les nouveaux développements de Victor de l'Aveyron. Imprimerie imperiale. Paris, F. Alcan, 1807.
39 De Adam de Parme S. Cronica. Scalia (éd.). Bari, Laterza, 1966.
40 Dax M: Lésions de la moitié gauche de l'encéphale coïncidant avec l'oubli des signes de la pensée. Gazette Hebdomadaire de Médecine et de Chirurgie, 1865.
41 Lordat J: Analyse de la parole pour servir à la théorie de divers cas d'Alalie et de Paralalie (de mutisme et d'imperfection du parler) que les Nosologistes ont mal connus. Journal de la Société de médecine pratique de Montpellier 1843;7:333–353.
42 Lordat J: Analyse de la parole pour servir à la théorie de divers cas d'Alalie et de Paralalie (de mutisme et d'imperfection du parler) que les Nosologistes ont mal connus. Journal de la Société de médecine pratique de Montpellier 1843;7:417–433.
43 Lordat J: Analyse de la parole pour servir à la théorie de divers cas d'Alalie et de Paralalie (de mutisme et d'imperfection du parler) que les Nosologistes ont mal connus. Journal de la Société de médecine pratique de Montpellier 1843;8:1–17.
44 Broca P: Sur le siège de la faculté du langage articulé. Bulletin de la Société d'Anthropologie, 15th June 1865;6: 337–393.
45 Broussolle E, Gobert F, Danaila T, Thobois S, Walusinski O, Bogousslavsky J: History of physical and 'moral' treatment of hysteria. Front Neurol Neurosci 2014;35: 181–197.
46 Briquet P: Traité clinique et thérapeutique de l'hystérie. Paris, JB Baillières et Fils, 1859.
47 Duchenne G: De l'électrisation localisée et de son application à la physiologie, à la pathologie et à la thérapeutique. Paris, Baillière, 1855.
48 Braid J: Neurohypnology, or a Rationale of Nervous Sleep, Considered in Relation with Animal Magnetism. London, Churchill, 1843.
49 Charcot JM: Sur les divers états nerveux déterminés par l'hypnotisation chez les hystériques. Comptes-rendus hebdomadaires des séances de l'Académie des Sciences 1882;94:403–405.
50 Bernheim H: De la suggestion dans l'état hypnotique et dans l'état de veille. Paris, Octave Doin, 1884.
51 Richer P: Etudes cliniques sur l'hystéroépilepsie ou Grande Hystérie. Paris, Adrien Delahaye et Emile Lecrosnier, 1881.
52 Sollier P: Genèse et Nature de l'hystérie: Recherches Cliniques et Expérimentales de Psycho-Physiologie, vol 2. Paris, F. Alcan, 1897.
53 Tatu L, Bogousslavsky J, Moulin T, Chopard JL: The "torpillage" neurologists of World War I: electric therapy to send hysterics back to the front. Neurology 2010; 75:279–283.
54 Sollier P: Le problème de la mémoire: essai de psychomécanique. Leçons faites à l'Université nouvelle de Bruxelles, 1898–1899. Paris, F. Alcan, 1900.
55 Bogousslavsky J, Walusinski O: Paul Sollier: the first clinical neuropsychologist; in Bogousslavsky J (ed): Following Charcot: A Forgotten History of Neurology and Psychiatry. Front Neurol Neurosci, Basel, Karger, 2011, vol 29, pp 105–114.
56 Franz SI: The reeducayion of an aphasic. J Philos Psychol Sci Methods 1905;2:589–597.
57 Janet P: L'automatisme Psychologique. Paris, F. Alcan, 1889.
58 Watson JB: Psychology as the behaviorist views it. Psychol Rev 1913;20:158–177.
59 Skinner BF: The Behavior of Organisms. New York, Appleton-Century-Crofts, 1938.
60 Ayllon T, Michael J: The psychiatric nurse as a behavioral engineer. J Exp Anal Behav 1959;2:323–334.
61 Poser U, Kohler JA, Schönle PW: Historical review of neuropsychological rehabilitation in Germany. Neuropsychol Rehabil 1996;6:257–278.
62 Poppelreuter W: Die psychischen Schädigungen durch Kopfschuss im Kriege 1914/17: mit besonderer Berücksichtigung der pathopsychologischen, pädagogischen, gewerblichen und sozialen Beziehungen. Leipzig, Voss, 1917.
63 Goldstein K: Die Behandlung, Fürsorge, und Begutachtung der Hirnverletzten: Zugleich ein Beitrag zur Verwendung psychologischer Methoden in der Klinik. Leipzig, F. C. W. Vogel, 1919.
64 Goldstein K, Marmor J: A case of aphasia with special reference to the problems of repetition and word findings. J Neurol Psychiatry 1938;1:329–341.

65 Hellebrandt FA: The physiology of motor learning; in Singer RN (ed): Readings in Motor Learning. Philadelphia, Lea & Febiger, 1972, pp 397–409.
66 Milner B: Physiologie de l'hippocampe; in Passouant P (ed): Centre National de la Recherche Scientifique. Paris, Editions du CNRS, 1962, pp 257–272.
67 Vygotsky LS: The Collected Works of L.S. Vygotsky, vol 4. The History of the Development of the Higher Mental Function. New York, Plenum Press, 1997.
68 Luriya AR: The Making of Mild: A Personal Account of Soviet Psychology. Cambridge, MA, Harvard University Press, 1979.
69 Luriya AR: The Man with a Shattered World: The History of a Brain Wound. Basic Books. New York, NY, Harvard University Press, 1972.
70 Das JP: PASS Reading Enhancement Program, Sarka Educational Resources. Deal, NJ, 1999.
71 Butfield E, Zangwill OL: Re-education in aphasia; a review of 70 cases. J Neurol Neurosurg Psychiatry 1946;9: 75–79.
72 Zangwill OL: Psychological work at the edinburgh brain injuries unit. Br Med J 1945;2:248–251.
73 Diller L, Ben-Yishay Y, Gerstman LJ, Goodkin R, Gordon W, Weinberg J: Studies in Cognition and Rehabilitation in Hemiplegia. New York, NYU Medical Center, 1974.
74 Ben-Yishay Y, Diller L: Rehabilitation of cognitive and perceptual defects in people with traumatic brain damage. Int J Rehabil Res 1981;4:208–210.
75 Ben-Yishay Y, Diller L: Handbook of holistic neuropsychological rehabilitation: outpatient rehabilitation of traumatic brain injury. New York, Oxford University Press, 2011.
76 Lezak M: Psychological implications of traumatic brain damage for the patient's family. Rehabil Psychol 1986; 31:241–250.
77 Gianutsos R: Training the short- and long-term verbal recall of a postencephalitic amnesic. J Clin Neuropsychol 1981;3:143–153.
78 Brewer-Mixon KK, Munro Cullum C: Historical principles and foundations of neuropsychological rehabilitation; in Noggle CA, Dean RS (eds): Neuropsychological Rehabilitation. New York, Springer Publishing Company, 2013.

Dr. Eloi Magnin, CMRR
Department of Neurology, Besançon University Hospital
Boulevard Fleming
FR–25000 Besançon (France)
E-Mail eloi.magnin@laposte.net

Bogousslavsky J, Boller F, Iwata M (eds): A History of Neuropsychology.
Front Neurol Neurosci. Basel, Karger, 2019, vol 44, pp 192–229 (DOI: 10.1159/000494964)

Shining a Light on Some of the Most Famous 19th and 20th Century's Neuropsychologists

Olivier Walusinski[a] François Boller[b] Victor W. Henderson[c]

[a]Private Practice, Brou, France; [b]Department of Neurology, George Washington University Medical School, Washington, DC, USA; [c]Departments of Health Research and Policy (Epidemiology) and of Neurology and Neurological Sciences, Stanford University, Stanford, CA, USA

Abstract

This chapter pays homage to the masters who made neuropsychology an esteemed and legitimate field in the 19th and 20th centuries. Here we offer a brief biography for each of them and an analysis of their discoveries: Théophile Alajouanine (1890–1980), Henry Charlton Bastian (1837–1915), Arthur L. Benton (1909–2006), Julian de Ajuriaguerra (1911–1993), Ennio De Renzi (1924–2016), Norman Geschwind (1926–1984), Kurt Goldstein (1878–1965), Henry Head (1861–1940), Henry Hécaen (1912–1983), Pierre Janet (1859–1947), François Lhermitte (1921–1998), Jean Lhermitte (1877–1959), Hugo Karl Liepmann (1863–1925), Heinrich Lissauer (1861–1891), Alexander Romanovich Luria (1902–1977), Brenda Milner (1918–), Théodule Ribot (1839–1916), Charles Richet (1850–1935), Paul Sollier (1861–1933), and Carl Wernicke (1848–1905).

Introduction

Neuropsychology, a field at the crossroads between neurology and psychology, is rooted in Egyptian and Greek Antiquity (Imhotep and Eratistrate, respectively). By pondering intelligence, Descartes and Spinoza, the most famous philosophers of the 17th century, conceived a way of thinking about memory and emotion, the foundations of the concepts that contemporary neuroscience endeavors to explore with precision. The advances the discipline has made from the end of the 19th century to the present result from the work of neuroscientists and no longer that of philosophers. Here we present a brief biography of each of the most noteworthy personalities in this young discipline, a discipline that has achieved its most important advances in the 20th century. Each of these biographies identifies key aspects of the training and work of these individuals, who are too often forgotten. They are listed here in alphabetical order.

Théophile Alajouanine (1890–1980)

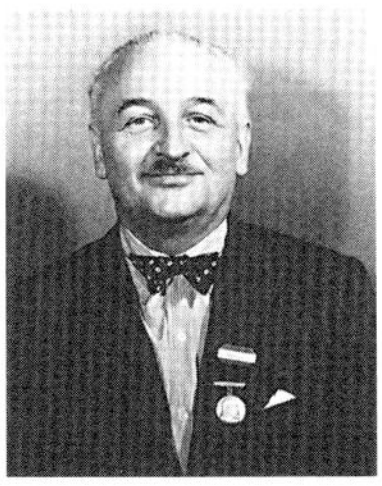

Théophile Alajouanine
Bibliothèque médicale Henri Ey (Paris), with kind permission.

Théophile Alajouanine (1890–1980) may not be universally known to neuropsychologists, yet he deserves to be remembered because he founded a working group which was one of the most active in the world in the years that followed World War II. He contributed to our understanding of several aspects of aphasia and he arguably can be considered one of the fathers of neurolinguistics [1].

Nothing in his family background could have predicted his career. He was born in a small village of Central France, an area known as Bourbonnais, from a relatively humble family and went to a high school in Moulins, the nearest large town. There his brilliant intelligence was noted and he went to Paris where he had to make a hard choice between art, his first passion, and medicine. He performed brilliantly in medical studies, but also befriended many famous artists, prominent among them Valery Larbaud (1881–1957) whom he examined and superbly described, after the cosmopolitan writer, translator of James Joyce's Ulysses, became aphasic. Perhaps because his interest in the arts was well known, he examined other famous artists. This led to a publication in *Brain* [2] in which he described the effect of aphasia on the artistic production of Larbaud, of Maurice Ravel (1875–1937) and of a painter whom he did not name, but whose identity, Paul Elie Gernez (1888–1948), is now well established [3]. In 1914, he was named Interne des Hôpitaux. World War I had just started and he soon was drafted as a physician where he started as an "alienist," but he left it as a neurologist. His first teachers were psychiatrists including Philippe Chaslin (1857–1923) and Jules Séglas (1856–1939). His neurology mentors included Georges Guillain (1876–1961), Pierre Marie (1853–1940) and above all Charles Foix (1882–1927) [1] with whom he described the so called Foix-Alajouanine syndrome in 1926, also known as angiodysgenetic necrotizing myelopathy.

In 1927, he became Professeur Agrégé and when he finally obtained a Chair, it was not in Neurology, but in History of Medicine. It was only in 1947, when Guillain retired, that he was named to what had been Charcot's Chair at the Salpêtrière. Alajouanine's approach to brain and behavior was influenced by Jackson's ideas and he often applied to the analysis of language disorders, the so-called Baillarger-Jackson principle of dissociation between voluntary and automatic or emotional language. He applied this principle in studying such diverse phenomena as dysprosody, agraphia, and stereotypes. He was prompted to study the latter by the famous "Tantan" case described by Paul Broca (1824–1880) and by the case of the writer Valery Larbaud whose only verbal output was the literary sounding "bonsoir, les choses d'ici-bas" (farewell, material things from this earth).

It has been stated that the publication, in 1939, of the book "*Le Syndrome de Désintégration Phonétique*" (SDP), by Alajouanine, André Ombredane (1898–1958) and Marguerite Durand (1904–1962) marks the beginning of modern Neurolinguistics [1]. SDP was meant to characterize the language output of patients with anarthria and Broca's aphasia. Alajouanine and his colleagues studied articulatory phenomena first by transmitting pressure changes to a pen on a rotating cylinder and later with an oscilloscope. They were able to study the phonetic aspects of these articulatory disorders and inferred their physiopathological basis by isolating within the disorder paralytic aspects, dystonic aspects, and apraxic aspects.

Another contribution of Alajouanine was to postulate the existence of 2 language systems. The first is sensory-motor or auditory-phonemic and is responsible for both the production and reception of phonemic units. It is typically impaired in phonemic jargon. The second is a semantic system supposed to control the connection of thoughts and language. Semantic jargon was proposed as a typical effect of disruption of this system. These ideas had the advantage of suggesting a general parallel between language input and output. Modern psycholinguistics abandoned this approach, but some aspects of semantic dementia and the handling of functor words by patients with Broca's aphasia can be explained by principles resembling the postulates of Alajouanine and his group. Many other aspects of language and aphasia, particularly aphasia in children, were developed in a monograph that still provides worthwhile reading [4].

Through the years, Alajouanine attracted many excellent researchers to his laboratory, namely André Ombredane, François Lhermitte (1921–1998), André Roch-Lecours (1936–2005), Olivier Sabouraud (1924–2006), Blanche Ducarne de Ribaucourt (1927–2018), Jean-Louis Signoret (1933–1991), and Luigi Vignolo (1934–2010).

Alajouanine was very attached to his native Bourbonnais. When he retired in 1960, he became a self-described bibliophile. I visited him in his estate in Central France in 1974. Rather than talk about the brain, he preferred showing his beautiful garden and proudly described his rare book collection, many of which he had bound in luxurious leather with his own hands. He lived there, obviously enjoying life, until his death in 1980 at the ripe age of 90.

François Boller

References

1 Lhermitte F, Lecours AR, Signoret JL: Obituary: Théophile Alajouanine (1890–1980). Brain Lang 1981;13:191–196.
2 Alajouanine T: Aphasia and artistic realization. Brain 1948;71:229–241.
3 Boller F: Alajouanine's painter: Paul-Elie Gernez; in Bogousslavsky J, Boller F (eds): Neurological Disorders in Famous Artists. Front Neurol Neurosci. Basel, Karger, 2005, vol 19, pp 92–100.
4 Alajouanine T: L'aphasie et le Langage Pathologique. Paris, Baillière, 1968.

Henry Charlton Bastian (1837–1915)

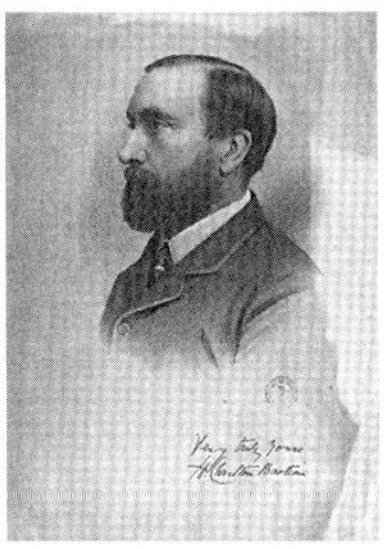

Henry Charlton Bastian
© Bibliothèque de l'Académie nationale de médecine.

Henry Charlton Bastian (1837–1915), born in Cornwall, graduated at the University College of London in 1861, and obtained his medical degree in 1866. He practiced at the National Hospital, Queen Square from 1868 to 1902, eventually becoming a Professor of pathological anatomy at his alma mater. Although he described the anterior spinocerebellar tract in 1867, it became known as Gowers's tract after 1880. In 1878, he was appointed to the Chair of Medicine [1]. From 1884 to 1898, he was an advisor for the Crown in cases of questionable insanity. Bastian had published numerous papers on parasitology. He gained international recognition for his methods of diagnosis and the quality of his teaching in neurology.

Bastian was interested in hysteria, as Charcot was in Paris, but when speaking of the so-called "hysteria major," he noted: "Anything like a complete form is only very rarely met with in this country" [2]. In 1887, his controversial paper on "*the muscular sense, its nature and cortical localization*" was published, in which Bastian contended that "neither on physiological nor on psychological grounds was it needful to postulate the existence of motor centres in the cortex."

In 1869, he described a characteristic speech impairment; this was the first account of word blindness (alexia) and of word deafness, which Carl Wernicke (1848–1905) described 5 years later as sensory aphasia. Since then the disorder has been known as Wernicke's aphasia. As a Lumleian lecturer, Bastian dealt with aphasia and other speech defects. It was his belief that we think with words representing a recollection of sound impressions stored in the auditory brain centers. He also held that aphasia depends either on damage of one or the other of 4 centers in the cortex which are involved in the production of spoken or written language, or on disruption of the neural tracts connecting them. Bastian's emphasis on cell-circuit physiology enabled him to formulate the distinction between punctuate, topographical localization, and distributed localization in a remarkable fashion [3]. Taken together, his lectures on aphasia formed the basis of a classical treatise on the subject: "*A treatise on aphasia and other speech defects,*" 1898.

In 1890, Bastian was the first to demonstrate that after transection of the upper spinal cord, reflexes and muscle tone are abolished in the lower limbs (Bastian's law) [4]. Bastian considered his 1880 book, The Brain as an Organ of Mind, to be his greatest contribution to neuro-philosophy. He presented in this book several prescient ideas, for example that memories activate the same cortical areas as those activated during initial perception, to put it briefly. At the end of his life, Bastian spent time unsuccessfully defending an unorthodox theory of the origins of life [5].

Olivier Walusinski

References

1 Anonymous: Orbituary of Henry Charlton Bastian. Lancet 1915;2:1220–1224.
2 Bastian HC: Various Forms of Hysterical or Functional Paralysis. London, Lewis, 1893.
3 Bastian HC: On the various forms of loss of speech in cerebral disease. Br Foreign Med Chir Rev 1869;43:209–236.
4 Bastian HC: On the symptomatology of total transverse lesions of the spinal cord; with special reference to the condition of the various reflexes. Med Chir Trans 1890;73:151–217.
5 Bastian HC: The Brain as an Organ of Mind. London and New York, Appleton, 1880.

D. Frank Benson (1928–1996)

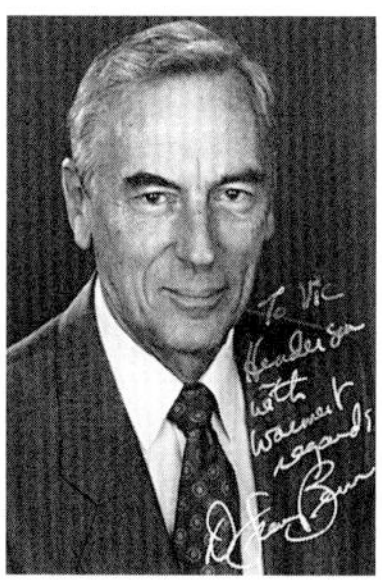

D. Frank Benson
Victor W. Henderson, personal collection.

Through clinical research and mentoring, Frank Benson was instrumental in establishing behavioral neurology as a neurological specialty. Born in Grand Forks, North Dakota, he received his undergraduate degree from the University of North Dakota. After serving 2 years in the United States Army during World War II, he took his M.D. from Northwestern University and completed an internship at Good Samaritan Hospital in Portland, Oregon. Before resuming his education in the neurology program at the Veterans Administration Hospital in San Francisco, California, he was a general practitioner in Sweet Home,

Oregon. After neurology residency, he was in the private practice of neurology in Eugene, Oregon, for 3 years.

In 1965, Benson completed a research fellowship with Norman Geschwind (1926–1984) at the Aphasia Research Center at the Boston Veterans Administration Medical Center. This was the year of Geschwind's landmark article on cortical disconnection syndromes [1], sometimes viewed as the inception of behavioral neurology. Afterwards, Benson remained as the new Section chief and a member of the Boston University neurology faculty. He remarked that he was given few resources but had the freedom to rename his service, which he did in 1972, following a sabbatical at the Institute of Psychiatry, University of London. His new designation – the Neurobehavioral Center – was central to the branding of behavioral neurology as an emerging discipline. In 1979, Benson became the first behavioral neurologist honored with an endowed academic chair, when he moved to the University of California, Los Angeles.

Benson's early, highly-influential work focused on classic disorders of higher cortical function: agnosia, amnesia, acalculia, and – above all – aphasia [2]. He and his collaborators went on to study frontal lobe functions [3] and psychiatric manifestations of neurological disease. In Los Angeles, he focused increasingly on neurobehavioral aspects of Alzheimer's disease and other dementias at a time when dementia was only beginning to be recognized as a highly prevalent, devastating disorder of great importance to neurology.

Benson's preferred methodology was the descriptive case series, often focused on clinical-anatomical associations. He used a large repertoire of bedside techniques to reveal and parse impairments in cognition and behavior. He wrote prolifically and well, publishing nearly 250 articles and chapters, and 9 books. A forte was clinical nosology and the enumeration and tabulation of key clinical findings, distinguishing characteristics, associated features, and differential diagnoses.

Benson was an astute clinician, deeply committed to his patients, and an enthusiastic, nurturing teacher [4]. He had the uncommon ability to see through a morass of distracting symptoms and signs, discern the clinical essence, and then – as often as not – proclaim the case as "absolutely classic" for conduction aphasia [5], for posterior cortical atrophy [6], or for some other neurobehavioral disorder. He attracted a steady stream of postgraduate trainees from neurology and psychiatry, many of whom rose to leadership positions in research and academia. Benson inspired a generation of behavioral neurologists, neuropsychiatrists, neuropsychologists, and scientists with interests in brain-behavior relations and – in doing so – helped secure the foundation of behavioral neurology.

Victor W. Henderson

References

1 Geschwind N: Disconnexion syndromes in animals and man. Brain 1965;88:237–294, 585–644.
2 Benson DF: Aphasia, Alexia, and Agraphia. New York, Churchill Livingstone, 1979.
3 Stuss DT, Benson DF: Neuropsychological studies of the frontal lobes. Psychol Bull 1984:95:3–28.

4 Cummings JL: In memoriam – D. Frank Benson, MD. Arch Neurol 1997;54:98.
5 Benson DF, Sheremata WA, Bouchard R, Segarra JM, Price D, Geschwind N: Conduction aphasia – clinicopathological study. Arch Neurol 1973;339–346.
6 Benson DF, Davis RJ, Snyder BD: Posterior cortical atrophy. Arch Neurol 1988;45:789–793.

Arthur L. Benton (1909–2006)

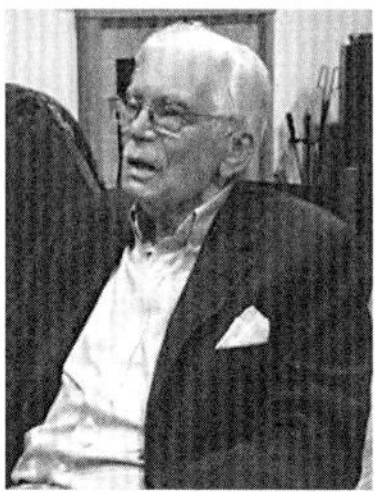

Arthur L. Benton
François Boller collection.

Following World War II, Neuropsychology developed considerably in the US. Similarly to what had happened in Europe, several of the founders of this new field were neurologists such as Derek Denny-Brown (1901–1981), Fred Quadfasel (1902–1981) and, most importantly Norman Geschwind (1926–1984). Among the many PhDs who contributed to this rise, Arthur Lester Benton (1909–2006) stands out because of his considerable interest in and knowledge of the brain-behavior relationships, his introduction of new tests and his rigorous attachment to the methodology. In addition, throughout his life and particularly during his long tenure in Iowa City, he founded a laboratory which trained a large number of students who later became outstanding researchers and clinicians. He also developed close ties with many of the other main contributors to this new field.

A native of New York City, he received his B.A. and his M.A. from Oberlin College, where he studied until 1933. Close to Cleveland, but remote in spirit from the metropolis, Oberlin with its combination of small rural town and cosmopolitan attitude was the perfect place for him to start forming and developing. He went back to New York City and Columbia University for his PhD, which he obtained in 1935. There he could trace his educational lineage to Karl S. Lashley (1890–1958), John B. Watson (1878–1958) and back to Hermann Emminghaus (1845–1904) and Wilhelm M. Wundt (1832–1920) [1]. He was training as a psychologist at the Payne Whitney Psychiatric Clinic of New York Hospital when World War II started and he volunteered for service in the US Navy where he was commissioned as a lieutenant in the medical department. During that time, he worked at the San Diego Naval Hospital with the neurologist Morris Bender (1905–1983) and together they examined a large number of servicemen who had sustained penetrating brain wounds. He was discharged from the Navy in 1946. After a short stay in the Department of Psychology at the University of Louisville, in 1948, he moved to the University of Iowa where Arthur Sachs, one of the founders of neurology in the Midwest offered him a position within his Department of Neurology. There he reached the grade of Director of graduate training in clinical psychology as well as Professor of Psychology and Neurology, retiring in 1978, at which time the Benton Laboratory of Neuropsychology in the Division of Behavioral Neurology was dedicated.

With patients, both children and adults, his approach was to develop appropriate tests to evaluate the presence of specific deficits. He emphasized the need to always compare the performance with that of normal controls of similar educational and demographic levels [2]. His contributions are many, most of them aimed at offering objective assessment of the main symptoms with particular emphasis on memory and visuospatial abilities. We owe to him the Benton Visual Retention Test, the test of Judgment of Line orientation, the test of Facial Recognition [3] and many others. He contributed significantly to the History of Neurology and Neuropsychology, particularly to the history of aphasia before Paul Broca (1824–1880) and early description of prosopagnosia [4]. At Iowa, he supervised no less than 46 doctoral dissertations and 24 master's theses. He was the author of numerous books. He contributed to the foundation of the Research Group on Aphasia of the World Federation of Neurology (Secretary General from 1971 to 1978) and that of the International Neuropsychological Society (President in 1970).

I was fortunate for having a personal interaction with him on many occasions, starting in 1964 when he came to Milano for a 2 months course which led to a book [5]. As pointed out in the article on Ennio De Renzi (1924–2016), the translation of Benton's lectures by De Renzi and Luigi Vignolo (1934–2010) played an important role in spreading the knowledge of neuropsychology among neurologists and psychologists. Benton urged the Milan group to adopt a set of rigorous experimental procedures, which was further elaborated and refined in subsequent years. He had sufficient knowledge of French, Italian, and German to discover hitherto obscure early descriptions of many disorders. Together with his wife Rita, a noted musicologist, he spent considerable time at the Bibliothèque Nationale in Paris and in other great places of learning.

The citation that accompanied the award of the American Psychological Association Gold Medal for Life achievement well summarizes his work "... lifetime contributions that include pioneering clinical studies and brain-behavior relations." One must add that thanks to his warm and endearing personality, he developed close working and personal ties with many other neuropsychologists. They included Ennio De Renzi (1924–2016) and other members of the Milan Group. Norman Geschwind (1926–1984), MacDonald Critchey (1900–1997), Klaus Poeck (1926–2006), Henry Hécaen (1912–1983), the Japanese aphasiologist Sumiko Sasanuma and many others. A grossly incomplete list of people associated with his Laboratory includes Helena Chui, Hanna Damasio. Antonio Damasio who later chaired the Department of Neurology. Paul Eslinger Kerry Hamsher, Julia Hannay, Robert Joynt, Harvey Levin, Manfred Meier. Otfried Spreen, and last but not least his daughter Abigail Sivan. His former student Daniel Tranel currently directs his Laboratory which is now part of an Interdisciplinary Graduate program in Neuroscience.

François Boller

References

1 Joynt RJ: Arthur Lester Benton (1909–2006). Neurology 2007;68:1454.
2 Sivan AB, Levin HS, Hannay J: Arthur L. Benton, Ph.D.: pioneer, colleague, mentor and friend. J Int Neuropsychol Soc 2007;13:559–560.
3 Benton AL: Facial recognition. Cortex 1990;26:491–499.
4 Benton AL: Exploring the History of Neuropsychology. New York, NY, Oxford University Press, 2000.
5 Benton AL: Problemi di Neuropsicologia. Firenze, G. Barbera, 1966.

Julian de Ajuriaguerra (1911–1993)

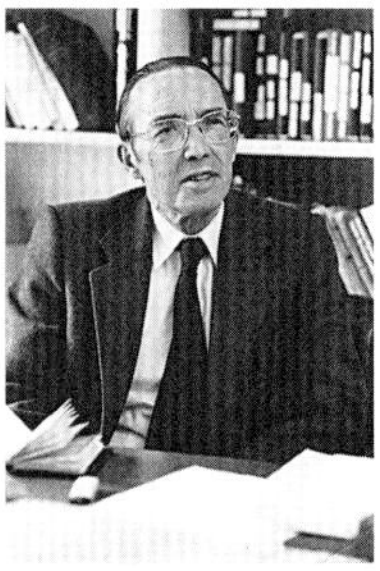

Julian de Ajuriaguerra
© Famille Ajuriaguerra and Bibliothèque médicale Henri Ey. CH Sainte-Anne (Paris), with kind permission.

Julian de Ajuriaguerra (1911–1993) was a French neuropsychiatrist of Spanish Basque origin. He left his native city of Bilbao to study medicine in Paris and become a psychiatrist. After working in Paris psychiatric hospitals as an interne (house officership) from 1933 to 1936, he defended his thesis in 1937, entitled "*La douleur centrale*" (central nervous system pain) [1]. After fighting with the Republicans during the Spanish Civil War, Ajuriaguerra took part in the French Resistance while working in Paris at Hôpital Sainte-Anne between1942 and 1944. In 1946, he became an assistant neurology professor with foreign status, obtaining French nationality in 1950. At that point, he was able to become a practicing physician and thus defended a doctoral thesis entitled "*Aspects des troubles mentaux au cours des tumeurs mésodiencéphaliques*" (mental disorders during mesodiencephalic tumors). As he did not have the possibility to become a full professor in France, he accepted a position at the Geneva medical school in 1959, where he held the Chair of Psychiatry and directed the cantonal university clinic. Finally, in 1975, he was appointed to the Developmental Neuropsychiatry Chair at the College de France in Paris [1].

Continuing the work of his master Jean Lhermitte (1877–1959), Ajuriaguerra focused on aphasia and rejected strict brain mapping based on various deficits, arguing instead in favor of diffuse and evolutive processes. His research on pain led him to identify pseudo-thalamic pain originating in the parietal lobes.

With Ludovic Marchand (1873–1976), in 1948 he published "*Epilepsies, leurs formes cliniques et leurs traitements*" (epilepsy, clinical forms and treatment) in which his aim was to study psychic auras, paroxysmic mental disturbances, and psychomotor automatisms, both in terms of the cerebral substrate and the localization value of these symptoms.

With André Thomas (1867–1963), Ajuriaguerra worked on developmental neurology and neuropsychiatric ontogenesis in children. They identified the evolutive chronology of reflexes present at birth. His 1948 book "*L'axe corporel*" *Musculature et innervation* (corporal axis, musculature and innervation) laid the ground for his 1949 "*Etude sémiologique du tonus musculaire*" (semiological study of muscle tone), which introduced concepts of muscle examination such as consistency, extensibility, and passivity, which until then had not been isolated [2]. His partnership with Henry Hécaen (1912–1983) led him to study left-handedness (manual prevalence and cerebral dominance), writing, and "integration and disintegration of somatognosis" during hemispatial neglect and corporal hallucinations.

With Jean Piaget (1896–1980), Ajuriaguerra explored the relationships between muscle tone, corporal expression, and emotional experience as well as concepts of non-verbal communication. His psychogeriatric writings highlight the constant order of psycho-behavioral disorganization during dementia, in contrast to the hierarchical order of development. Finally, his "*Manuel de psychiatrie de l'enfance*" is still a reference in the history of child psychiatry, revealing the influence of evolutionist and ethological thinking [3, 4].

Olivier Walusinski

References

1 Aguirre Oar JM, Guimon Ugatechea J: Vie et oeuvre de Julian de Ajuriaguerra. Paris, Masson, 1996.
2 Bergeron M: Julian de Ajuriaguerra (1911–1993). Bulletin de psychologie 1993;46:637–638.
3 Tissot R: Hommage à Julian de Ajuriaguerra. Rev Med Suisse Romande 1993;113:499–500.
4 Diatkine R, Vincent M: Hommage à Julian de Ajuriaguerra. Psychiatr Enfant 1994;37:5–12.

Ennio De Renzi (1924–2016)

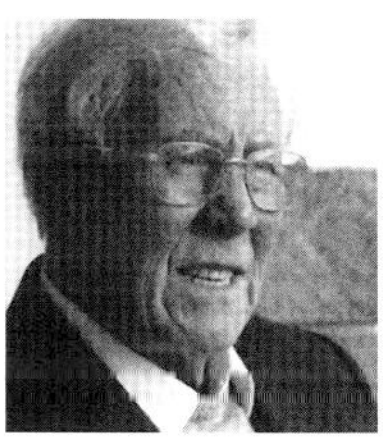

Ennio De Renzi
François Boller collection.

There are prominent early examples of Italian clinicians and researchers who dedicated their work to human neuropsychology. These precursors, active between the end of the 19th and the beginning of the 20th century include Leonardo Bianchi (1848–1927) and Giovanni Mingazzini (1859–1929). However, the systematic development of neuropsychology in Italy started in the early 1960s in Milan with the neurologist Ennio De Renzi (1924–2016). De Renzi was born in Cremona in 1924. In a recent autobiographical paper [1], he elegantly summarized the political climate of Italy during his youth, engulfed in a "repressive, untruthful and boring" fascist dictatorship which inexorably led Italy into the catastrophe of World War II. He also describes leaving the Faculty of Law to study Medicine at the University of Pavia where he was admitted to the prestigious Ghislieri College. He obtained his MD in 1950, and completed his specialization in Neurology and Psychiatry in 1953 at the Institute Casimiro Mondino, then directed by Carlo Berlucchi (1897–1992).

His first interest was psychiatry, specifically, projective tests such as the Rorschach ink block test [2]. However, he soon became frustrated by the difficulty of obtaining reliable and reproducible results from such tests, and, towards the end of the 50s, he focused on behavioral disorders associated with cerebral lesions, with a particular interest in aphasia.

Meanwhile, he had moved from Pavia first to Modena, and then to the Clinica delle Malattie Nervose e Mentali (Clinic of Nervous and Mental Diseases) of the University of Milan, where he found a suitable environment for his research. There he was able to study a large number of patients with histories of stroke and brain tumors. He informally founded the "Milan group," the first nucleus of the Italian neuropsychological school. Among the members of the group, first and foremost was Luigi A. Vignolo (1934–2010), who had been trained in Paris before returning to Italy, and Anna Basso, who also received training in Paris, and who established and directed the first Service for the Rehabilitation of Aphasia, as well as a School for Speech Language Pathologists. They were soon joined by others including Hans Spinnler and Pietro ("Pierino") Faglioni. I was privileged to join the group at that early stage, and to be part of De Renzi's daily patients' rounds. I distinctly remember his clinical acumen, his vast knowledge, his empathy towards the patients and his sense of humor. He conducted rounds in a relaxed yet very demanding style, writing, sometimes to our dismay incisive comments in a fountain pen on our painfully prepared clinical reports.

These early years saw several landmarks which contributed to establishing the position of De Renzi and the Milan group on the international scene. These included an article on the Token Test in *Brain* [3] which can be considered the first modern Italian neuropsychological study to be published in an international journal.

Together with the group he participated in the International Neuropsychological Symposium in 1964, beginning a period of work and personal friendships with neurologists and psychologists from various European countries as well as the US and Canada. He founded the journal *Cortex* which he led as Editor-in-Chief for over 25 years. In 1964, Arthur Benton (1909–2006) taught a 2-month course in Milano. The translation of Benton's lectures by De Renzi and Vignolo was the first textbook on neuropsychology published in Italy, and played an important role in spreading this culture among neurologists and psychologists [4].

From the beginning, De Renzi established a standard of experimental methodology in the group. The approach was primarily based on quantitative assessment of the cognitive ability of interest in left- and right-brain-damaged patients, and in neurologically unimpaired participants (controls), by means of ad hoc devised and standard tests, followed by statistical comparison of the patients' and controls' performances, taking into account, and partialling out the influence of sex, age, and education. Faglioni was the principal developer of these advanced statistical methods.

The group focused mainly on hemispheric differences in higher-order mental processes. Two sets of results may be mentioned: the greater and more frequent impairment of spatial abilities consequent to right than to left hemispheric damage; different patterns of impairment after unilateral hemispheric damage in stimulus recognition: the right hemisphere proved to be more involved in the perceptual discrimination of the stimulus' qualities, the left one in its identification ("recognition," with retrieval of its semantic associations). This hemispheric asymmetry held for visual material, but also involved color processing and auditory stimuli.

In subsequent years, De Renzi became Chairman of Neurology at the University of Modena and continued to be a prominent and productive researcher as well as a superb teacher. His book on *Disorders of Space Exploration and Cognition* [5] is a classic. The list of persons whose professional lives and thinking were influenced by him is too long for this Editorial. Many of them went on to productive careers of their own. To mention only a few, Paolo Nichelli is the current Chair of the Department of Neurology in Modena, Giuseppe Vallar is Head of the Department of Psychology in Milano Bicocca, and Sergio Della Sala is the current Editor-in-Chief of Cortex.

Following his retirement in 2000, Ennio ostensibly focused his interest on other areas, becoming an assiduous visitor to the wonderful Modena Public Library where he could be found just about every afternoon. However, he also enjoyed keeping in touch with his former pupils. A touching contribution of his came on the occasion of a symposium entitled "*Modern Italian Neuropsychology: origins, developments and future perspectives*" organized by Giuseppe Vallar and Guido Gainotti and held in Como in May 2013. Ennio made the keynote introduction and participated actively in the entire symposium. He also thoughtfully reviewed an article summarizing the history of Neuropsychology in Italy [6]. We are grateful to him also for these last contributions to Neuropsychology.

François Boller

References

1 De Renzi E: Ennio De Renzi; In Squire L (ed): The History of Neuroscience in Autobiography. Amsterdam, Elsevier, 2006.

2 De Renzi E, Isotti M, Saraval A: Il test di Rorschach nell'Italiano adulto normale. Arch Psicol Neurol Psichiatria 1957;18:279–321.

3 De Renzi E, Vignolo LA: The token test; a sensitive test to detect receptive disturbances in aphasia. Brain 1962;85:665–678.

4 Benton AL: Problemi di Neuropsicologia. Florence, Universitaria Barbera, 1966.

5 De Renzi E: Disorders of Space Exploration and Cognition. New York, John Wiley, 1982.

6 Vallar G, Boller F, Grossi D, Gainotti G. Italian neuropsychology in the second half of the twentieth century. Neurol Sci 2015;36:361–370.

Norman Geschwind (1926–1984)

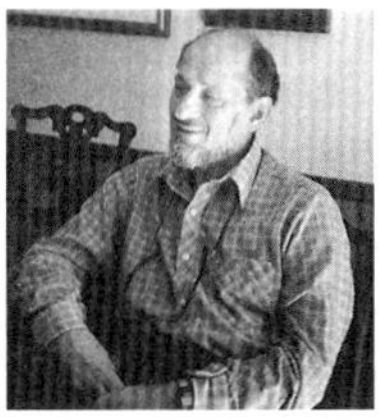

Norman Geschwind
Antonio Damasio, with kind permission.

Many people contributed to the rise of interest in brain-behavior relations in the US after World War II, but Norman Geschwind (1926–1984) unquestionably played a major role. He shaped modern neurology, particularly through his decisive role in the development of Behavioral Neurology and Neuropsychology. These disciplines barely existed in the United States when he arrived on the scene, but, thanks in great part to him, they are now prominent, as attested to by the many Societies and by more than 35 Journals currently dedicated to them. The Geschwind family left Poland for Brooklyn NY in the 19th century. His father, Morris, was religiously skeptical, but the family enrolled Norman in a Jewish elementary school. Although young Norman disliked the Yeshiva education, it provided him with a key element for his future professional life by encouraging him to use his own judgment in interpreting texts rather than relying on what other people said. Just like Henri Hécaen (1912–1983), Ennio De Renzi (1924–2016) and others, he first intended to become a psychiatrist but shifted his interest to neurology, influenced by teachers such as Marcus Singer (1926–2016). At that time, he began to develop an interest in language disorders and epilepsy. He graduated from medical school in 1951 and continued his studies at London's National Hospital, where he studied with Sir Charles Symonds (1890–1978) who also influenced Geschwind's development.

In 1955, Geschwind became the chief resident in the Neurology Department at Boston City Hospital, then directed by Derek Denny-Brown (1901–1981). Following a 2-year fellowship at MIT, Geschwind joined the Neurology Department of the Boston Veterans Administration Hospital in 1958, where he met Alfred (Fred) Quadfasel (1902–1981), a pupil of Karl Bonhoeffer (1868–1948), who was in turn a pupil of Karl Wernicke (1848–1905). Quadfasel played a major role in shaping Geschwind's future development by encouraging him to study aphasia, and also to read classic texts of neurology from the 19th and early 20th century, exposing him to classic localizationist theory. Because of his knowledge of French and German, Geschwind could read these texts in their original language relatively easily. He convinced himself that, contrary to what had been stated by "distinguished neurologists" like Pierre Marie (1853–1940) or Henry Head (1861–1940), the writings by Wernicke, Jules Dejerine (1849–1917), Henry Charlton Bastian (1837–1915) and others were not "the chaotic confabulations of a group of tedious imperceptive 19th century scholars," but rather the healthy disagreements of a lively science [1].

Geschwind became the Chief of Neurology at the Boston VA Hospital and Chair of the Department of Neurology at Boston University in 1966. In 1969, he returned to Harvard Medical School's James Jackson Putnam Professor of Neurology and Director of the Harvard Neurological Unit at Boston City Hospital. In 1975, the Unit moved to Beth Israel where he remained as Chief until the time of his death.

Geschwind created 2 major beehives of research which remain highly active to this day. At the VA, together with Edith Kaplan (1924–2009), he established the Boston University Aphasia Research Center in 1966. The Aphasia Research Center would go on to become a pioneer in interdisciplinary aphasia research, including luminaries like Harold Goodglass (1920–2002) and D. Frank Benson (1928–1996). He kept his ties with the VA after he moved across town.

Geschwind's best known and most often quoted paper is his "*Disconnexion syndrome*" paper published in 1995 [2, 3]. What led to that paper is undoubtedly his reading of papers by Wernicke, Ludwig Lichtheim (1845–1928), Hugo Karl Liepmann (1863–1925), Dejerine and others emphasizing the importance of interruptions of cortical connections. On top of this came the clinical observation by Edith Kaplan (1924–2009) of a patient, the famous Mr. K who could perform praxic (symbolic) movements with his right hand but not with his left hand, even though that hand had no primary motor or sensory deficit. The patient's left hand did not seem to know what his right hand was doing. Geschwind proposed that the patient was displaying a classic disconnection syndrome, one the first documented in humans. In his 1995 paper, Geschwind defined a disconnexion lesion as "a large lesion either of association areas or of the white matter leading from that association area." The paper discusses in a novel fashion such syndromes as conduction aphasia, agnosia, and various forms of apraxia. In the 1980s, the neuroscience world tended to move away from the connectionist views but current imaging techniques have largely contributed to their revival [4].

Geschwind's work on aphasia was also quite significant. Until Geschwind's time, the standard neurological examination paid relatively little attention to language. He emphasized the importance of testing various aspects of language such as fluency, naming, repetition, comprehension, and reading and writing. This was the prelude to a better understanding of specific syndromes like conduction aphasia or pure alexia. Through the work of his colleagues, this led to such classic works such as the Boston Diagnostic Aphasia Examination of Harold Goodglass (1920–2002) and Kaplan, first published in 1972 and still widely used.

His many other achievements include his demonstration of major anatomical asymmetries in the brain, particularly at the level of the planum temporal [5]. He contributed to the understanding of epilepsy and its accompanying behavioral disorders such as hypergraphia. The list of fields where he performed and often pioneered research includes traumatic amnesia, disorders of attention, and the neurology of emotions. Not too long before his death, he went in a completely different and novel direction: showing that left-handed individuals have a higher incidence of autoimmune disorders.

Two crucial inter-related elements are extremely important in understanding Geschwind, the man and the physician. His warm and generous personality and his extraordinary clinical ability. He did not hesitate to offer hospitality in his own house to some of the newly arriving visitors and residents. His clinical ability, acumen, and kindness were on full display when examining patients, with truly amazing results. Through a mixture of deep knowledge and intuition, he was always able to demonstrate "live" clinical elements and signs that illustrated his lectures and rounds.

Geschwind's legacy is illustrated in a striking fashion by the number of persons he trained or otherwise influenced not only in North America, but throughout the world [6]. I will particularly mention 4 "schools" which to this day continue his work: that of Alberto Galaburda in Boston, MA, Kenneth Heilman in Gainesville, FL, M-Marsel Mesulam in Chicago, IL, USA, and Andrew Kertesz in London, Canada.

François Boller

References

1 Geschwind N: The paradoxical position of kurt goldstein in the history of aphasia. Cortex 1964;1:214–224.
2 Geschwind N: Disconnexion syndromes in animals and man. I. Brain1965;88:237–294.
3 Geschwind N: Disconnexion syndromes in animals and man. II. Brain 1965;88:585–644.
4 Mesulam MM: Fifty years of disconnexion syndromes and the Geschwind legacy. Brain 2015;138:2791–2799.
5 Geschwind N, Levitsky W: Human brain: left-right asymmetries in temporal speech region. Science 1968;161: 186–187.
6 Boller F: International figure; in Schacter S, Devinsky O (eds): Behavioral Neurology and the Legacy of Norman Geschwind. New York, NY, Lippinicott Raven Publishers, 1997.

Kurt Goldstein (1878–1965)

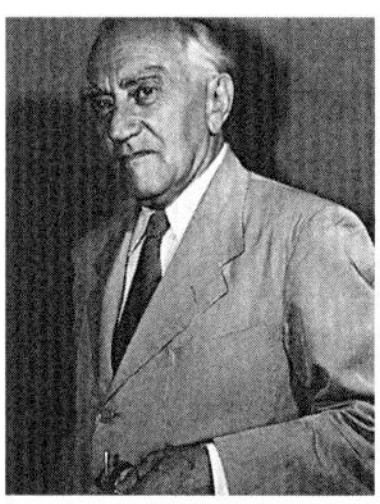

Kurt Goldstein
US National Library of Medicine, public domain.

Kurt Goldstein (1878–1965), born in Kattowicz (Poland), studied philosophy and literature at the universities of Breslau and Heidelberg. He went on to obtain his doctoral degree in medicine in 1903. Studying under Carl Wernicke (1848–1905), he became interested in aphasia. He then worked as a post-doctoral assistant at the Frankfurt neurological institute, where he studied comparative neurology in the neuropathological laboratory of Ludwig Edinger (1855–1918). In 1906, he moved to Königsberg, where he worked as a psychiatrist and neurologist. He also became acquainted with the Würzburg school of experimental psychology, which emphasized "imageless thought." In 1914, based on his clinical work, Goldstein established the Institute for Research into the Consequences of Brain Injuries where he collaborated with Adhémar Gelb (1887–1936). He was appointed to the Frankfurt neurology chair in 1923, succeeding Edinger. In 1930, he left Frankfurt for Berlin, where he was a professor at the university in the neurology and psychiatry department; he also directed a large neuropsychiatric clinic. He developed a close friendship with his cousin Ernst Cassirer, the neo-Kantian philosopher. When Hitler was appointed chancellor in 1933, Goldstein, who was Jewish, was arrested and imprisoned in a basement. After a stay in Amsterdam, he moved to New York City in 1935 where he started a new career at Columbia University and the Montefiori Hospital [1].

Goldstein worked to further understanding of trauma in soldiers returning from duty in World War I. He was particularly interested in soldiers with acute frontal lobe injuries. He developed the finding of Eduard Hitzig (1838–1907) that monkeys with frontal lesions were especially blunted in the domain of abstract thought. In addition, Goldstein was influenced by John Hughlings Jackson (1835–1911) and his concepts of negative symptoms related to local damage and positive symptoms caused by modifications of surrounding areas [2]. After studying the effects of brain damage in soldiers, he argued that the loss of abstract thinking was the key feature of frontal lobe damage [3]. He believed these defects to underlie maladaptive emotional responses and memory loss. Goldstein developed a number of tests for measuring abstract thought and concrete behaviors, notably using fables and proverbs. The so-called Goldstein test battery was also used for neuropsychological rehabilitation [4]. His continued work led him to postulate that memory involved engram patterns spread throughout the cortex, "each of which involved a central figure and a peripheral ground." Goldstein went on to develop a theory that the brain, following traumatic experiences, is in a constant state of active shock and that "slight catastrophic reactions" occur as the individual attempts to come to terms with the world [5].

Goldstein was one of the major proponents of the holistic movement, notably for aphasiology, at the beginning of the 20th century. His holistic views of brain activity were influenced by Naturphilosophie, a current in the philosophical tradition of German idealism. According to Naturphilosophie, both normal and abnormal behaviors are the result of the antagonism between the brain and the environment; thus, both normal and abnormal states of mind are an expression of adaptation. Symptoms of illness are not secondary effects, but a sign of positive development towards a new state, indicative of the organism's struggle to re-establish equilibrium [6]. In this way, Goldstein can be seen as a philosophical scientist.

Olivier Walusinski

References

1 Teuber HL: Kurt Goldstein's role in the development of neuropsychology. Neuropsychologia 1966;4:299–310.
2 Goldstein G: Contributions of Kurt Goldstein to neuropsychology. Clin Neuropsychol 1990;4:3–17.
3 Goldstein K, Scheerer M: Abstract and concrete behavior: an experimental study with special tests. Psychol Monogr 1941;53:1–151.
4 Eling P: Kurt Goldstein's test battery. Cortex 2015;63:16–26.
5 Goldstein K: After Effects of Brain Injuries in War: Their Evaluation and Treatment. New York, NY, Grune & Stratton, 1942.
6 Goldstein K: Language and Language Disturbances: Aphasic Symptom Complexes and Their Significance for Medicine and Theory of Language. New York, NY, Grune & Stratton, 1948.

Sir Henry Head (1861–1940)

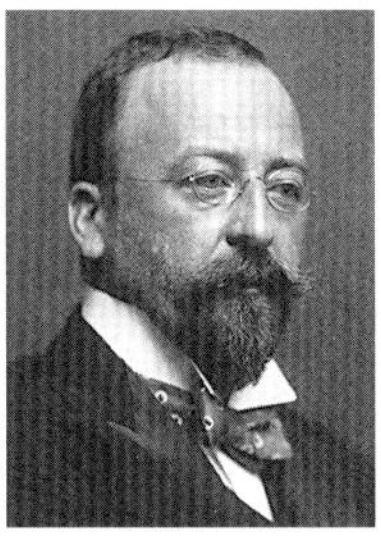

Henry Head
Photo by G.C. Beresford, public domain.

After learning physiology at Cambridge, Henry Head (1861–1940) studied for 2 years in the laboratory of University of Halle in Germany, then worked in Prague in the laboratory of Ewald Hering (1834–1918) on the physiology of respiration. His first paper was on the action potential of nerves. In 1889, he published a masterly treatise on the respiratory effects of the vagus nerve. He is credited with having been the first to use endotracheal intubation for his experiments, now a common technique in anesthesiology. After his house officership at University College Hospital in London, he took his MD at Cambridge in 1892. In 1896, he was appointed to the London Hospital. From 1905 to 1921, he was editor of the journal *Brain* [1].

His thesis "*on disturbances of sensation with special reference to the pain of visceral disease*" was later expanded and published in *Brain* in 1893 [2]. In 1903, with William Rivers's assistance (1864–1922), he was his own subject in an experiment on the transection of cutaneous nerves, the results of which he used to develop theories of 2 separate sensory systems, protopathic and epicritic [3]. Head then investigated pain caused by herpes zoster and thus explained the anatomic distribution of cutaneous disturbances as selective by dermatomes. Following his study on dermatomes, Head's investigations were devoted almost wholly to the sensory system and to refining the clinical method of sensory examination. Collaborating with an Australian neurologist, Alfred Walter Campbell (1868–1937), he was able to chart the cutaneous distribution of different fibers originating from the cells of each ganglion and reaching the corresponding segment of the spinal cord [4]. Head studied the physiological basis for sensation, that is, the manner in which afferent impulses subserving sensation are integrated and conducted to the forebrain, and the specific brain areas that process these afferent impulses. Based on all of his researches, Head can be considered to have provided the first rational explanation of the nature of sensory dissociation.

In 2 other fields, Head's contributions were also outstanding: he shed new light on spinal reflex functions, notably on the nature of the stimulus. His collaboration with Gordon Holmes (1876–1965) led to the first accurate account of the functions of the optic thalamus and its relation to the cerebral cortex. Head and Holmes then defined 2 distinct types of body representation that can be impaired, the body schema and the body image. In their view, the brain constantly updates the status of the body shape and posture as an ongoing, mainly unconscious integration of successive proprioceptive signals (body schema), somehow distinct from a more conscious representation of the body, or body image [5].

Head retired from the hospital in 1919, following the onset of Parkinson's symptoms. He dedicated the end of his career to 2 large volumes under the title Aphasia and Kindred Disorders of Speech (1926). He investigated the psychical processes and the physiological integrations necessary for the comprehension and expression of ideas as language. Thus, he described "semantic aphasia" which provided a link between the linguistic and the intellectual aspects of speech, based on the concepts developed by the French neurologist Pierre Marie (1853–1940). Suffering the effects of his disease, his study was in part concerned with the loss of his own faculties of speech [6, 7].

Olivier Walusinski

References

1 Fremantle F, Stevenson FH: Obituary henry head. Lancet 1940;236:534.
2 Head H: On disturbances of sensation with especial reference to the pain of visceral disease. Brain 1893;16:1–133.
3 Rivers WHR, Head H: A human experiment in nerve division. Brain 1908;31:324–450.
4 Head H, Campbell AW: The pathology of herpes zoster and its bearing on sensory location. Brain 1900;23:353–523.
5 Head H, Holmes HG: Sensory disturbances from cerebral lesions. Brain 1911–1912;34:102–254.
6 Head H: Aphasia and Kindred Disorders of Speech. Cambridge, Cambridge University Press, 1926.
7 Brain R: Henry Head: The Man and His Ideas. Brain 1961;84:561–566.

Henry Hécaen (1912–1983)

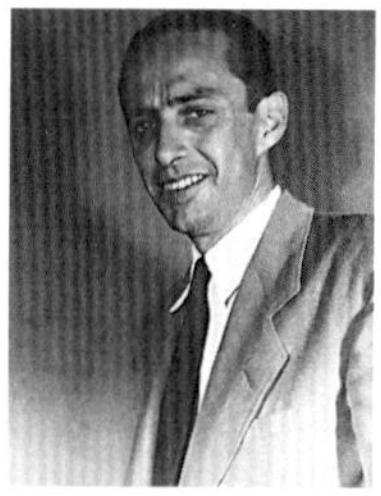

Henri Hécaen
US National Library of Medicine, public domain.

Most persons associate Neurology and Neuropsychology in France with la Salpêtrière, the famous Paris hospital. It is true that major personalities in those disciplines have worked at that Institution. However, some crucial personalities have operated in France without any tie with la Salpêtrière. This is the case for Henry Hécaen (1912–1983) who was based at Sainte-Anne Hospital (now Centre Hospitalier Sainte-Anne) for most of his professional career. Hécaen was born in 1912 in the city of Brest in Brittany. After graduating from medical school in Bordeaux, he started his professional career as a Navy officer, but soon realized that he was not fit for spending his life on boats. He moved to Paris where he selected Sainte-Anne as his place of training to become a psychiatrist. There he met Julian de Ajuriaguerra (1911–1993) and, for a while, their careers developed in parallel. Both men were trained in Psychiatry by Henri Ey (1900–1977), and in Neurology by Jean Lhermitte (1877–1959) who later wrote an affectionate introduction to their book, the 1949 edition of "*Le Cortex Cérébral*," arguably the first textbook of neuropsychology ever written in any language.

This tall, elegant man was quite striking in his appearance and in his demeanor. He was reserved and yet very generous. He and his wife Renée enjoyed receiving friends at their apartment in the Faubourg Saint Germain. Because of the depth of his knowledge and his human warmth, he had an extraordinary ability to communicate in private or in small gatherings. By contrast, his capacity as a public speaker was poor. This was true not only in English (he could or would never overcome his horrendous French accent), but also in French. It has been written that this was because his mind was so quick and acute that when listening to him or reading him, one had "to understand what he had not yet expressed." Nevertheless, in spite of these difficulties, listeners and readers kept listening and reading, "obviously aware that he had great knowledge to share" [1]. After a while, he decided that he was not happy as a psychiatrist and opted for neurology, perhaps because "the ways and means of psychiatry were unsatisfactory to his Cartesian mind" [1].

In 1952, he spent several months at McGill Montreal Neurological Institute where he worked with Wilder G. Penfield (1891–1976) and Brenda Milner (1918–). One paper written after his return to Paris propelled him on the international scene. This paper "*The syndrome of apractognosia due to lesions of the minor cerebral hemisphere*" [2] was based on material he had gathered at the Montreal Neurological Institute. It opened the eyes of the scientific community on the role of the right hemisphere, a portion of the brain often considered until that time without specific functions. In 1968, he moved to the newly constructed Centre Paul

Broca. Over the years, Hécaen and his group grew steadily in size and influence and his INSERM Unit 111 became known all over the world as one of the leading laboratories in the field. Hécaen did not invent the term "neuropsychology" which had been used by William Osler (1849–1919), Kurt Goldstein (1878–1965), Karl S. Lashley (1890–1958), and Donald O. Hebb (1904–1985). However, he was the first to use it in its present meaning when, in 1962, he founded the Groupe de Neuropsychologie et Neurolinguistique.

He was a prolific writer, having written over 300 articles and books [3]. He was among the first in Europe to carry out carefully planned group studies. His research touched practically all aspects of the discipline, with major emphasis on hemispheric cerebral dominance and aphasia. His papers on conduction aphasia, particularly the 1964 article written with 2 linguists (Jean Dubois [1920–2015] and Pierre Marcie) included one of the first neurolinguistic analyses of the disorder [4]. Among the other deficits he investigated, one should mention agraphia, dressing apraxia, and visual agnosia. An article dealing with acalculia provides an example of Hécaen's peculiar style. The paper is in French, includes very little methodology and no references. Yet the conclusions of the paper are cogent. Acalculia is found in patients with predominant alexia or agraphia, with spatial disorders and with an actual disorder of the processing of arithmetic operations which he called anarithmetia. This distinction is valid and the paper is still considered a milestone in the field [5].

Other lasting contributions of Hécaen include the foundation, in collaboration with Oliver Zangwill (1913–1987) and Hans Hof, of the International Neuropsychological Symposium, which met first in 1951 [6]. Another milestone is the foundation of Neuropsychologia in 1963 which he edited until 1981 [6]. In that year he officially retired, but remained Director of the Unit until his death in 1983.

In 1965, he was named Directeur d'Etudes at the Ecole Pratique des Hautes Etudes (now Ecole des Hautes Etudes en Sciences Sociales). As stated by François Lhermitte (1921–1998) et al. [1] "given the rigidity of the French medical pyramid and considering his academic background, the royal roads of the Salpêtrière and of Bicêtre were closed to him" and he was never officially named Professor, because the positions he could have aspired to were occupied by someone else. This was perhaps a blessing in disguise because without being preoccupied with the arcane aspects of academic life, he was free to pursue his own interest and fully develop his potential.

François Boller

References

1 Lhermitte F, Lecours AR, Poncet M, Marcie P, Whitaker H: In memoriam Henry Hécaen (1912–1983). Brain Cogn 1985;4:133–139.

2 Hécaen H, Penfield W, Bertrand C, Malmo R: The syndrome of apractognosia due to lesions of the minor cerebral hemisphere. AMA Arch Neurol Psychiatry 1956;75:400–434.

3 Galtier A. Publications de Henry Hécaen. Neuropsychologia 1984;22:647–659.

4 Dubois J, Hécaen H, Angelergues R, Maufras du Chatelier A, Marcie P: Etude neurolinguistique de l'aphasie de onduction. Neuropsychologia 1964;2:9–44.

5 Hécaen H, Angelergue R, Houllier S: Les variétés cliniques des acalculies. Approche statistique du problème. Rev Neurol (Paris)1961;105:85–103.
6 Boller F: History of the international neuropsychological symposium: a reflection of the evolution of a discipline. Neuropsychologia 1999;37:17–26.

Pierre Janet (1859–1947)

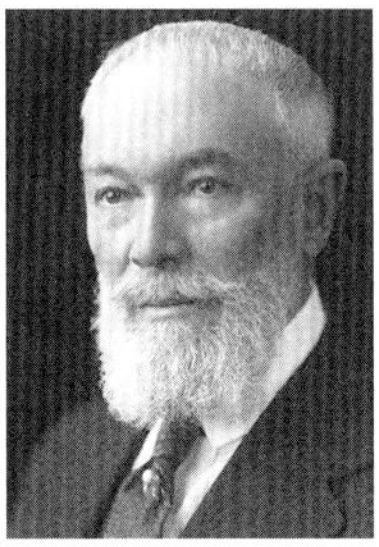

Pierre Janet
BIU santé Paris, public domain.

Pierre Janet (1859–1947) was born in Paris and was the nephew of philosopher Paul Janet (1823–1899). In 1878, at the Ecole Normale Supérieure, he began preparing for the competitive exam to become a philosophy teacher, along with Henri Bergson (1859–1941) and Emile Durkheim (1858–1917). After passing the exam in 1882, he moved to Le Havre in northwest France where he taught for 7 years. One of his students was the son of a hospital alienist, Joseph Gibert (1829–1899). Janet became friends with Gibert and began spending time at the hospital. For his humanities thesis, defended in 1889, he included observations of Léonie Leboulanger, "clairvoyant and magnetizer," which he had prepared in 1885 and 1886. His thesis was entitled *Automatisme psychologique. Essai de psychologie experimentale sur les formes inférieures de l'activité humaine* (Psychological automatism. Essay on the experimental psychology of the inferior forms of human activity). Janet focused on diseases of personality, especially multiple personalities, and tried to reconcile the phenomena of consciousness with the notion of a subconsciousness. Janet met Charcot in Le Havre in 1885. Accompanied by the future Nobel-prize winner Charles Richet (1850–1935), Charcot had come to examine Léonie. In 1890, Charcot created a "psychology laboratory" for Janet at La Salpêtrière where he could investigate scientific philosophy and medicine. Janet remained director of the laboratory until 1910. He defended his doctoral thesis in medicine on July 29, 1893. It was the last defense presided over by Charcot, who died on August 16, 1893. Janet practiced as a clinical psychotherapist at Le Havre and at La Salpêtrière, defending a theory of psychic trauma as the cause of hysteria. In 1897, he was appointed to the Experimental Psychology Chair at La Sorbonne and occupied the Experimental and Comparative Psychology Chair from 1902 to 1934. He founded the Société de Psychologie in 1901 and the *Journal de psychologie normale et pathologique* in 1904 [1, 2].

Janet was the first to assert that a connection existed between past events experienced by a subject and his or her current trauma. To describe the behaviors involved, he coined the words "dissociation" and "subconscious" and later described the phenomenon of transference between patient and therapist [3].

Janet's work covered all fields of psychology: cognitive psychology, social psychology, and dynamic psychology. He attempted to model the relationships between emotions and actions, focusing on secondary regulatory actions (reduction/amplification) that enable adjusting behavior according to the relevance of the context. His model provided the basis for explaining pathological deviations and inappropriate responses to an initial stimulation. Janet's work dealt with fields of consciousness (perception/action), distraction/concentration, emotional responsiveness, will and belief, and judgment (adherence to/rejection of rules) [4, 5].

Olivier Walusinski

References

1 Pichon-Janet H: Pierre Janet, quelques notes sur sa vie. L'Évolution Psychiatrique 1950;15;345–355.
2 Piaget J: Nécrologie: Pierre Janet, 1859–1947. Archives de Psychologie 1948;32:235–237.
3 Leblanc A: The origins of the concept of dissociation: Paul Janet, his Nephew Pierre, and the problem of post-hypnotic suggestion. Hist Sci 2001;39:57–69.
4 Valsiner J, Van Der Veer R: The Social Mind: Construction of the Idea. Cambridge, Cambridge University Press, 2000.
5 Carroy J, Plas R: How Pierre Janet used pathological psychology to save the philosophical self. J Hist Behav Sci 2000;36:231–240.

François Lhermitte (1921–1998)

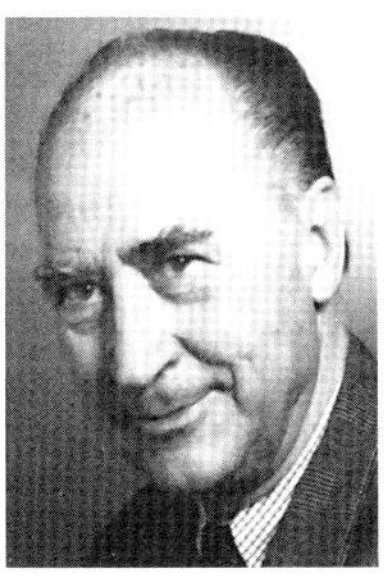

François Lhermitte
ICM La Salpêtrière (Paris), with kind permission.

There are dynasties of musicians (Bach), of mathematicians (Bernouillie), and of writers (Dumas). To the list of these illustrious families, we can add the dynasty of neurologists since in some instances neurology is practiced by the children of famous neurologists. One such family is the Lhermittes. Here we deal with the son of Jean Lhermitte (1877–1959), François Lhermitte (1921–1998) who made advances in several fields, particularly in an area outside the "classical" area of neuropsychology; one that deals with the relationship between individuals and the outside world. François Lhermitte's youth and early adulthood saw a mixture of achievements in patriotism and clinical medicine. He entered Medical School in Paris in 1940, a time when France was being invaded by Germany. He was active in the Resistance, for which he earned the Medal of the Resistance and the Legion of Honor for military reasons. After the war, he became the "enfant prodige" of French Neurology. His doctoral thesis was written when he was only 28 under the direction of Théophile Alajouanine (1890–1980). It is entitled "*Les Leucoencéphalites*" and it remains a landmark for research in multiple sclerosis. Another area of interest was cerebrovascular disease.

However, his creativity found its main fulfilment in neuropsychology. Alajouanine, who had founded the first Center for study and rehabilitation of language disorders in France, entrusted its direction to François Lhermitte in 1954. It became an important Laboratory funded by INSERM for many years. His first neuropsychological studies, following the work of Alajouanine, were devoted to aphasia. He co-edited a book on aphasia with André Roch-Lecours (1936–2005) from Canada. It has been translated into English [1].

Many other eminent neuropsychologists undertook their training in Lhermitte's Center, including Anna Basso and Luigi Vignolo (1934–2010) from Italy, Xavier Seron from Belgium, René Tissot from Switzerland, and Michel Poncet from Marseille. Other prominent cognitive neuropsychologists came from his laboratory: Jean-Louis Signoret (1933–1991), Marie-France Beauvois, Jacqueline Derouesné, and Bernard Pillon among others.

His first study on the neuropsychology of the frontal lobes was published in 1972 with Derouesné and Signoret [2]. This study was inspired by the work of Luria and provided vivid examples of abnormal behaviors in patients with frontal lobe lesions. Lhermitte later described 2 new clinical syndromes [3]. In *utilization behavior*, patients spontaneously grab objects put in front of them, starting appropriate behavior associated with it, but at an inappropriate time. In *imitation behavior*, patients imitate gestures performed by the examiner, although they were not instructed to do so. This may involve fairly conventional gestures such as praying, but also some highly unconventional ones. For Lhermitte, utilization and imitation behaviors were manifestations of a common basic disorder, an imbalance between dependence and independence from external stimuli. Utilization and imitation behaviors have contributed greatly to our clinical understanding of the frontal lobes. But, in our opinion, the major contribution of François Lhermitte to neuropsychology was his description of the "*Environmental dependency syndrome*" [4], a phenomenon where the affected individuals lose much of their autonomy and rely on environmental cues to accomplish goals or tasks, assuming a different, changing social role. This can occur in complex social situations such as a visit to a medical office, a walk in the garden or a gambling room. It was a striking introduction to an "ecological" neuropsychological approach to everyday life and social interactions. For the first time, neuropsychology went from laboratory studies to quasi-experimental studies in everyday life. Incidentally, thanks to Woody Allen and his 1983 movie, the phenomenon is also known as Zelig syndrome [5].

What were the relations between Lhermitte and other neuropsychologists? He was among those who inspired Ennio De Renzi and Luigi Vignolo to go ahead and form what was to become the Milan group [6]. Lhermitte was one of the founding associate Editors of *Cortex* and remained on the Editorial Board of that Journal for many years. The encounter between Lhermitte and the Italians occurred in 1960 at a Paris meeting organized jointly by him and by Hécaen. In subsequent years, it must be said that Henry Hécaen (1912–1983) and Lhermitte often pretended to ignore each other. However, at Henry Hécaen's funeral, François Lhermitte pronounced a moving and very laudatory eulogy, part of which was published in 1985 [7].

A striking facet of François Lhermitte was his clinical skill as a neurologist. When he was shown a patient, his first words were: "Don't tell me anything." He would take the history, propose one or several diagnostic hypotheses, and then examine the patient. In so doing, one sometimes wondered if he wasn't somehow persuading patients to behave or respond in a certain fashion, as if making up the clinical signs to prove his hypothesis. Actually, in most cases, he just showed an extraordinary intuition of what the patient might show or do. Unlike the laconic output of other clinicians such as Alajouanine, François Lhermitte thought aloud, jumping from one hypothesis to another. Inexperienced or inattentive neurologists might have trouble following his mind, but for others, the exercise was very stimulating.

François Lhermitte's talent was widely recognized by the French scientific community. Few people in modern times have been members of both the Académie de Médecine and the Académie des Sciences. All this fame did not quell his brilliant mind and his intellectual curiosity. Until his final years, he lived by the motto he had pronounced at the closing of his own inaugural lecture: "we grow weary of everything, but of learning."

François Boller

References

1 Roch Lecours A, Lhermitte F, Bryans B: Aphasiology. London, Baillière Tindall, 1983.
2 Lhermitte F, Derouesné J, Signoret JL: Analyse neuropsychologique du syndrome frontal. Rev Neurol (Paris) 1972;127:415–440.
3 Lhermitte F, Pillon B, Serdaru M: Human autonomy and the frontal lobes. Part I: imitation and utilization behavior: a neuropsychological study of 75 patients. Ann Neurol 1986;19:326–334.
4 Lhermitte F: Human autonomy and the frontal lobes. Part II: patient behavior in complex and social situations: the "environmental dependency syndrome." Ann Neurol 1986;19:335–343.
5 Conchiglia G, Della Rocca G, Grossi D: On a peculiar environmental dependency syndrome in a case with fronto-temporal damage: Zelig-like syndrome. Neurocase 2007;13:1–5.
6 Boller F, Vallar G, Gainotti G, Grossi D: History of Italian Neuropsychology; in Barr W (ed): History of Neuropsychology. New York, NY, Oxford University Press, 2018.
7 Lhermitte F, Lecours AR, Poncet M, Marcie P, Whitaker H: In memoriam Henry Hécaen (1912–1983). Brain Cogn 1985;4:133–139.

Jean Lhermitte (1877–1959)

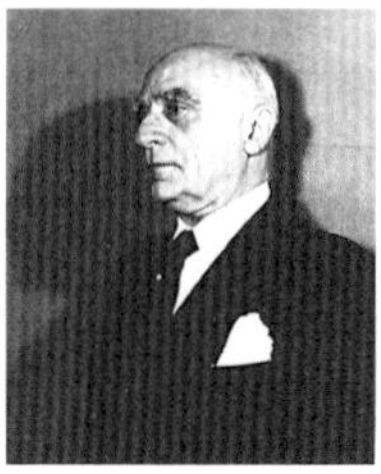

Jean Lhermitte
BIUsanté Paris, public domain.

Jean Lhermitte (1877–1959) highly deserves to be included in this book on *History of Neuropsychology* because he had a definite formative influence on many persons who have occupied the field of neuropsychology in France in more recent years. Jean Lhermitte was born on January 30, 1877 in Mont Saint-Père on the Marne River. He came from a family of artists, in particular his father Léon Lhermitte (1844–1925) was a renowned painter, friend of such artists as Rodin and Van Gogh. Léon Lhermitte's production can be seen in Chateau Thierry and at the Orsay Museum in Paris. His brother was an art photographer.

After High School in Meaux, Jean Lhermitte attended Medical School in Paris and became "interne des hôpitaux" in 1900. His teachers included Gustave Roussy (1874–1948), Fulgence Raymond (1844–1910), and Pierre Marie (1853–1940). His career was interrupted by the Great War. He was a field military doctor for 2 years and later a medical officer in a Neurology Center in Bourges under the direction of Henri Claude who was later to get the direction of Sainte-Anne Hospital in Paris.

His career was atypical. He did not have a formal University title until his retirement in 1947 when he was named Honorary Professor. He remained for most of his professional life Head of the Neuropathology Laboratory (an appointment he had received from Pierre Marie), which was located in rue de l'Ecole de Médecine. In 1919, he became "Chef de Service" at a relatively peripheral institution, the Paul Brousse Hospital in Villejuif.

At that time, it was customary for Neurologists to practice more than one discipline [1], but few persons were as versatile as Jean Lhermitte. He was actively involved in practice, research, and teaching of neuropathology including histology. As early as 1914, he co-authored with Gustave Roussy a classical treatise of neuropathology [2]. With Pierre Marie, he wrote an early description of the pathology of Huntington's disease.

He was a prominent neurologist and is known all over the world for having described a characteristic phenomenon, "Lhermitte's sign." Flexing of the neck produces electric shock-like sensations that extend down the spine and shoot into the limbs. He described it in a patient with multiple sclerosis [3, 4], but it is not pathognomonic as it is known to be caused also by trauma to the cervical portion of the spinal cord, cervical cord tumors, cervical spondylosis, or even vitamin B12 deficiency.

He called himself a Neuropsychiatrist, but when reading the topics he covered under that label, one sees that he was clearly interested in brain and behavior relationships. In other words, his interest was "la discipline qui traite des fonctions mentales supérieures dans leurs rapports avec les structures cérébrales," which is as close as can be to our current definition of Neuropsychology. He wrote extensively on many subjects ranging from phantom limbs to disorders of consciousness and constructional apraxia.

He is perhaps best known to neuropsychologists for his interest in hallucinations. He was one of the first to propose a classification according to whether the patients have no insight or if they realize that the hallucinations do not correspond to reality, a phenomenon he called hallucinosis. He described the syndrome known as peduncular hallucinosis [5] whereas hallucinations are formed, colored, visual images of people, animals, plants, scenes or geometric patterns. They have been reported in vascular and infective lesions of the thalamus, the pars reticulata of substantia nigra, midbrain, pons and basal diencephalon as well as by compression of midbrain. He pointed out that these patients can also have auditory hallucinations and the syndrome of "auditory hallucinosis" as well as its neuropathological basis have been confirmed [6]. He also described a case of Alzheimer disease in a blind man who had vivid visual hallucinations. Yet the patient had defective imaging, for instance, he could not call to mind the visual image of colors [7]. One could argue that there are similarities with the so-called Charles Bonnet syndrome [8].

His biographers are unanimous in recognizing his extraordinary gift for teaching. His captivating eloquence as well as his charm inspired many students to later become involved in the field of neurology, as exemplified by the Peruvian Oscar Trelles (1904–1990). Both Henry Hécaen (1912–1983) and Julian de Ajuriaguerra (1911–1993) were among the persons who discovered neuropsychology thanks to him. They wrote some of their early papers with him [9, 10] and never lost an occasion of referring to him as their Maître.

In concluding his obituary, Trelles wrote that because of his almost unlimited knowledge, Jean Lhermitte was the last of the "Seigneurs de la Neurologie." Fortunately, his memory lives forever through his own work and that of his pupils [11].

François Boller

References

1 Boller F, Duyckaerts F: 1914 to 1917: the Great War years. Arch Neurol 1999;56:882–885.
2 Roussy G, Lhermitte J: Techniques Anatomo-Pathologiques du Système Nerveux, Anatomie Macroscopique et Histologique. Paris, Masson, 1914.
3 Lhermitte J, Bollack J, Nicolas M: Les douleurs à type décharge électrique consécutives à la flexion céphalique dans la sclérose en plaques. Un cas de la sclérose multiple. Rev Neurol (Paris) 1924;39:56 62.
4 Lhermitte J: Multiple sclerosis. Arch Neurol Psychiatry. 1929;22:5–8.
5 Lhermitte J: Syndrome de la calotte du pédoncule cérébral. Les troubles psychosensoriels dans les lésions du mésocéphale. Rev Neurol (Paris) 1922;38:1359–1365.
6 Cascino GD, Adams RD: Brainstem auditory hallucinosis. Neurology 1986;36:1042–1047.
7 Lhermitte J, Nicolas M: Sur la maladie d'Alzheimer, une observation clinique. Ann Med Psychol 1923;92:435–448.
8 Boller F, Birnbaum DS, Caputi N: Charles Bonnet syndrome and other hallucinatory phenomena; in Bogousslavsky J (ed): Neurologic-Psychiatric Syndromes in Focus – Part I. From Neurology to Psychiatry. Front Neurol Neurosci. Basel, Karger, 2018, vol 41, pp 117–124.
9 Lhermitte J, de Ajuriaguerra J: "Asymbolie tactile et hallucinations du toucher. Etude anatomo-clinique." Rev Neurol (Paris) 1938,70.492–495.
10 Lhermitte J, Hécaen H: Sur les troubles de la psycho-motilité chez le vieillard. Ann Med Psychol 1942;11:62–70.
11 Hécaen H, Dubois J: La Naissance de la Neuropsychologie du Langage. Paris, Flammarion, 1969.

Hugo Karl Liepmann (1863–1925)

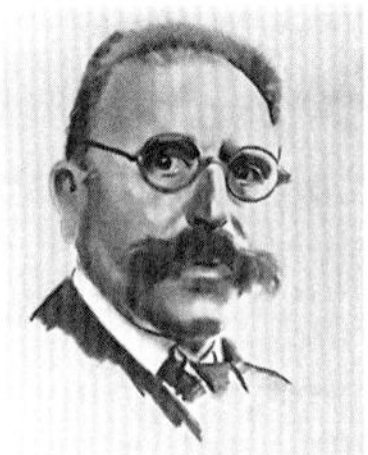

Hugo Karl Liepmann
From Monatsschrift für Psychiatrie und Neurologie 1923, vol. 54.
Redrawn by Herman Van Cott (1901–1978).

Hugo Karl Liepmann (1863–1925) was a neuropsychiatrist born in Berlin. After studying chemistry and defending a doctoral thesis in philosophy, he pursued medical studies, becoming in 1895 assistant to Carl Wernicke (1848–1905) in Breslau. From 1899 onward, he practiced psychiatry in Berlin, treating several patients with general paralysis [1]. Observing the motor difficulties of one of his patients, referred to as "the imperial counsellor," in 1900 he described dissociation in the execution of movements upon command and approximative execution with interference on one side of the body by inappropriate activity on the other side. The patient was not able to handle everyday objects or dress himself, but his movements improved when he was given commands. The patient presented neither paralysis nor motor incoordination but rather a disturbance of planning functions [2]. Liepmann called this symptom "apraxia," a term first used by the German linguist Heymann Steinhal (1823–1899) in 1871 [3]. The pathophysiological explanation proposed by Liepmann was damage to the fiber tracts linking frontal regions involved in movement to the parietal lobe, rather than a localized cortical lesion. For Liepmann, a disconnection occurred between the memory of coordinated goal-oriented or functional movement ("kinetic-kinaesthesic images") and the cortical regions controlling movement and movement perception ("movement formula"): "If one speaks of a movement image, one should be aware that the kinaesthesis part of the word 'image' does not apply in a strict sense; it serves only to summarize the entirety of the permanent material traces of previous centripetal stimuli. It designates not a psychological idea but a physiological one." Liepmann highlighted the distinction between procedural learning (automated movements) and conscious representation of actions. In 1905, Liepmann added the notion of apraxia, of which he distinguished 3 varieties: ideational, ideomotor, and kinetic. Ideational apraxia or "object blindness" renders patients incapable of making appropriate use of familiar objects upon command, even though they can name the object and describe how to use it. Ideomotor apraxia is the inability to follow verbal commands or imitate actions even though the patient performs the gesture spontaneously or as an emotional response. Kinetic apraxia refers to clumsiness in performing a skilled act that is not due to paralysis, muscle weakness, or sensory loss [4]. In 1899, one year before Liepmann's publication, the Belgian physician David de Buck used the term "parakinesis" to describe this type of motor disturbance and its pathophysiology: "The patient can conceive of actions, but cannot call to mind the corresponding kinetic images. There is disconnection between movement centres and ideational areas" [5].

Olivier Walusinski

References

1 Goldenberg G: Apraxia and beyond: life and work of Hugo Liepmann. Cortex 2003;39:509–524.
2 Liepmann H: Das Krankheitsbild der Apraxie (motorische Asymbolie) auf Grund eines Falles von einseitiger Apraxie. Monatschrift für Psychaitrie und Neurologie 1900;8:15–44, 102–132, 182–197.
3 Steinthal H: Einleitung in die Psychologie und Sprachwissenschaft. Berlin, F. Dümmler, 1871.
4 Liepmann HK: Der weitere Krankheitsverlauf bei dem einseitig Apraktischen und der Gehirnbefund auf Grund von Serienschnitten. Monatschrift für Psychatrie und Neurologie 1905;17:289–311, 1906;18:217–243.
5 de Buck D: Les parakinésies. Journal de Neurologie (Société belge de Neurologie) 1899;4:361–374.

Heinrich Lissauer (1861–1891)

During his short life, the German neurologist Heinrich Lissauer (1861–1891), born in Neidenburg (today Nidzica, Poland), described "Lisssauer's tract" and improved on the concept of visual agnosia. Lissauer studied at the universities of Heidelberg, Berlin, and Leipzig. He practiced as a neurologist at the psychiatric hospital in Breslau, serving as assistant to Carl Wernicke. He died while on vacation in Hallstatt (Austria).

"Lisssauer's tract" is a dorsolateral tract of the spinal cord consisting of a longitudinal bundle of poorly myelinated fibers between the apex of the posterior horn and the surface of the spinal marrow. This tract transmits surface sensibility, pain, and temperature sensibility.

Lissauer was not the first to describe impaired visual object recognition. The physiologist Herman Munk (1839–1912) and the ophthalmologist Herman Wilbrand (1851–1935) tried to correlate the defective function they observed with a cortical lesion, in 1878 and 1881, respectively. Lissauer's novel interpretation made his publication a milestone in neuropsychology [1]. He proposed that visual recognition may break down at either an apperceptive or associative level. Lissauer examined an 80-year-old patient 6 weeks after the sudden loss of his capacity to recognize objects even though he could see them. If he could touch and palpate the objects or if he could hear them, he was able to recognize them. Lisssauer developed a model of the recognition process, based on 2 successive stages: first apperception (conscious perception confined to one sensory modality) and then association (perception is linked with previously acquired knowledge and thus understood). According to Lissauer, apperception is dependent on localized cortical activity, while association involves activity of the cortex as a whole. His patient's brain was examined post-mortem and showed impaired conduction in the splenium of the corpus callosum. For Lissauer, "psychic blindness" implied that both hemispheres would be affected simultaneously [2].

In 1883, Désiré Bernard (1853–1887) transcribed a lesson given by his teacher, Jean-Martin Charcot (1825–1893), who presented a case similar to that of Lissauer. Charcot used the expression "amnésie musculaire verbale," attributing pathophysiology to partial amnesia [3].

Olivier Walusinski

References

1 Baumann C: Psychic blindness or visual agnosia: early descriptions of a nervous disorder. J Hist Neurosci 2011; 20:58–64.
2 Goldenberg G: Apraxia, the Cognitive Side of Motor Control. Oxford, Oxford University Press, 2013.
3 Charcot JM, Bernard D: Un cas de suppression brusque et isolée de la vision mentale des signes et des objets (formes, couleurs). Le Progrès Médical 1883;11:568–571.

Alexander Romanovich Luria (1902–1977)

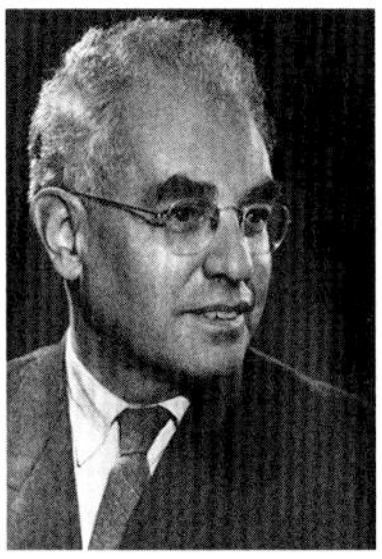

Alexander Romanovich Luria
Photograph by Ria Novosti. Keystone/Sputnik, with kind permission.

Alexander Luria (1902–1977), born in Kazan, moved to Moscow in 1921 where his mother became a dentist and his father a physician. Involved in the fervent cultural atmosphere of the post-revolutionary years, he began to work in psychology in the early 1920s. After a brief foray into the field of psychoanalysis, an approach which Luria soon rejected, the need for sound scientific training led him to medical studies, which he completed in 1936 at the Institute of Tbilisi. After he met Lev S. Vygotsky (1896–1934), his true mentor, in 1924, and then Aleksey N. Leontiev (1903–1979), Luria launched a project to develop a new kind of psychology, rejecting the limitations of physiological psychology based on Russian reflexology [1]. The trio replaced it by an approach which emphasized social and historical aspects of mental functions, that is, they stressed on the importance of personal and social experience in the development of cognitive abilities. Logically, they emphasized the mediatory role of language and writing in the development of higher mental functions.

During the 1930s, Luria made expeditions to Central Asia where he investigated various psychological changes (in perception, problem solving, memory, etc.) that took place in undereducated minorities as a result of cultural development [2, 3].

After the end of World War II, Luria was assigned a permanent position in General Psychology at the central Moscow State University, where he would spend most of his remaining years, becoming the director of the Neuropsychology Department. There, Luria devoted himself to the analysis of cerebral mechanisms underlying mental functions. He was particularly interested in how complex human behavior develops and how recovery takes place following injury or illness. In treating brain-injured soldiers, Luria developed the theory of neuropsychological rehabilitation, identifying uninjured components and supplementing them with external aids to reconstruct activity based on a new functional system. He used the term "syndrome analysis" for differentiation among symptoms according to higher or lower levels of integration in the damaged brain components [2, 3].

Luria can also be called a neuropsychologist in the field of special education for individuals with mental retardation. Using the same approach as for brain injuries, he considered the various brain regions as components of functional systems involved in complex psychological functions. Therefore, damage in a particular brain area should be judged by its role in the functional system and the functional system's role in the individual's future development [4, 5].

Early on, Luria together with Vygotsky described the role of speech in the regulation of behavior. He extended his researches after WWII, studying the functions of human frontal lobes, showing that the frontal lobes play an essential part in higher regulation of the states of activity. Luria contributed to understanding the manifold expressions of frontal lobe syndrome seen clinically by considering the evolutionary origins of these signs. He standardized neuropsychological qualitative assessments which provide a broad-scale evaluation of sensorimotor, linguistic, academic, memorial, and conceptual reasoning ability domains [4, 5].

The prodigious variety of Luria's publications reflects the heterogeneity of his work, which moved from developmental psychology to neuropsychology, from normal child to brain-injured adult, from animal brain to human brain, from theory to rehabilitation, from clinical to experimental researches [4, 5]. According to MacDonald Critchley (1900–1997), "his achievements were a compound of intellectual tirelessness, agility and thought, and unpredictable lateral thinking." [6].

Olivier Walusinski

References

1 Gardner H: The lives of Alexander Luria. Psychol Today 1980;14:84–91.
2 Homskaya ED: Alexander Romanovitch Luria: A Scientific Biography. New York-Boston-Dordrecht-Moscow, Kluwer Academic/Plenim Publishers, 2001.
3 Tupper DE: Alexander Luria's continuing influence on worldwide neuropsychology. Neuropsychol Rev 1999;9: 1–7.
4 Mecacci L: Luria: a unitary view of human brain and mind. Cortex 2005;41:816–822.
5 Homskaya ED: Alexander Romanovich Luria: A Scientific Biography (Plenum Series in Russian Neuropsychology). New York, Kluwer Academic, 2001.
6 Critchley M: In memoriams: A.R. Luria. Brain Lang 1978;5:5–6.

Brenda Milner (1918–)

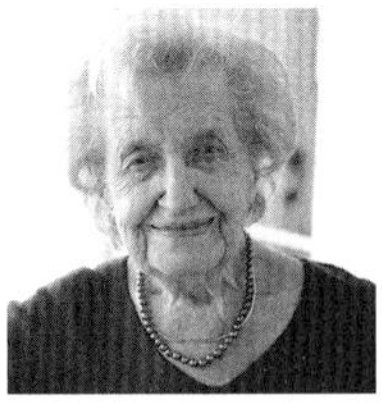

Brenda Milner
©Meera Paleja for Montreal Neurological Institute and Hospital, with kind permission.

Brenda Milner (1918–) is a British-Canadian neuropsychologist who has been an essential key in neuropsychology development since the early days of World War II. After receiving a scholarship in 1936 from Cambridge University, she became, during the war, part of a team interested in distinguishing fighter pilots from bomber pilots in aptitude tests. Brenda married in 1941 Peter Milner, an electrical engineer, and they moved to Canada after the war where he was invited to work with physicists on atomic research. She graduated in experimental psychology in 1949 in Montreal. Working for a PhD in psychophysiology at McGill University, under the direction of Donald Olding Hebb (1904–1985), she had to explore the patient P.B. who had undergone a medial temporal lobectomy and had subsequent memory impairment. Her research garnered the attention of Wilder Penfield (1891–1976) from the Montreal Neurological Institute. Alongside Penfield, she studied the behavior of a young adult epileptic patient treated with elective focal ablation of brain tissue to treat uncontrolled seizures. Milner earned her PhD in experimental psychology in 1952. Milner's thesis was a study on the lateralization of temporal lobe functions. She was one of the first to show that temporal lobe damage can cause emotional and intellectual changes in humans and lower primates [1]. That was the beginning of fruitful researches on the effects of damage to the medial temporal lobe on memory. Brenda Milner described the deficits in the most famous patient in cognitive neuroscience, Henry Molaison (1926–2008), formerly known as patient H.M., who, in an attempt to treat seizures had undergone a bilateral temporal lobectomy. Surgery included removal of major portions of the hippocampus. H.M. suffered severe anterograde amnesia, adding to the evidence that the hippocampus was crucial in the formation of new memories. H.M. also had an inability to recall established memories from a few years immediately before damage while memories from the more remote past and other cognitive abilities, including language, perception, and reasoning were intact [2].

Brenda Milner tried to teach him to reproduce a drawing of a star by looking at it in a mirror. As with a normal subject, H.M.'s performance improved over the 3 days' experiment but the major difference was that he had no memory of all these trials he had been through leading to a total dissociation between his experience and his normal performance. This finding introduced the concept of multiple memory systems within the brain and stimulated an enormous body of research. She also made major contributions to the understanding of the role of the frontal lobes in memory processing, in the area of organizing information, that is, the critical role of the dorsolateral frontal cortex for the temporal organization of memory. She showed that the neural circuits subserving recognition memory are partially separated from those mediating memory for temporal order. She wrote: "interest in human memory processes and their neural substrates has grown steadily over the past 30 years, and the early pioneering work with H.M. certainly provided some of the impetus for this growth" [3].

Brenda Milner was also interested in studying the lateralization of function in the human brain. In 1949, Juhn Atsushi Wada (1924–) described the use of the intracarotid amobarbital procedure (i.e., Wada test) to determine cerebral language dominance. Brenda Milner modified the test to assess hemispheric memory and after that "The Wada test" was used to evaluate the risk of postoperative amnesia, to assess the risk of material-specific memory deficits, to lateralize hemispheric dysfunction, and to predict postoperative seizure outcome [4]. In this manner, she confirmed the existence of bilateral speech representations in about 15–20% of non-right-handed patients.

Theodore B. Rasmusssen (1910–2002) and Brenda Milner were the first to demonstrate convincingly that damage to the brain can lead to dramatic functional reorganization: "lesions in the Broca's area or to the posterior parieto-temporal speech zone in infancy was likely to bring about a functional reorganization of the brain in which the right hemisphere became dominant for language or in which they were bilateral representation, but that, in contrast, left-hemisphere lesions that spared these critical regions rarely affected the lateralization speech." Brenda Milner had found a deficit in memory for new faces after right temporal lobectomy but not after left. All these data are arguments for a greater contribution from the right temporal lobe than the left to memory of visual patterns [5].

During the following years, she also demonstrated that patients with frontal lobe lesions had a heightened susceptibility to interference from the effects of preceding trials, rather than an inability to retain new information over a short time interval. Since the 1990s, neuroimaging work with normal subjects complements rather than replaces the analysis of the behavioral effects of brains lesions. All the works of Brenda Milner point out that her researches had been data-driven rather than theory-driven, authorizing her to discover the memory functions of the medial temporal lobe, hemispheric specialization, and the functions of the frontal lobes [6].

Brenda Milner concludes her autobiography with these words: "as I look over the past 50 years, it seems to me that I have had a lot of luck in being in the right place at the right time, but also enough tenacity of purpose not to be discouraged when the going got rough, as it frequently did in the early days at the Montreal Neurological Institute" [1].

Olivier Walusinski
François Boller

References

1 Milner B: Autobiography in Squire LR. The History of Neuroscience in Autobiography, vol 2. New York, NY, Academic Press, 1998.
2 Scoville WB, Milner B: Loss of recent memory after bilateral hippocampal lesions. J Neurol Neurosurg Psychiatry 1957;20:11–21.
3 Milner B: Memory and the medial temporal regions of the brain; in Pibram KH, Broadbent DE (eds): Biology of Memory. New York, NY, Academic Press, 1970, pp 29–50.
4 Milner B: Amobarbital memory testing: some personal reflections. Brain Cogn 1997;33:14–17.
5 Rasmussen T, Milner B: The role of early left-brain injury in determining lateralization of cerebral speech functions. Ann NY Acad Sci 1977;299:355–369.
6 Milner B, Petrides M: Behavioral effects of frontal-lobe lesions in man. Trends Neurosci 1984;7:403–407.

Théodule Ribot (1839–1916)

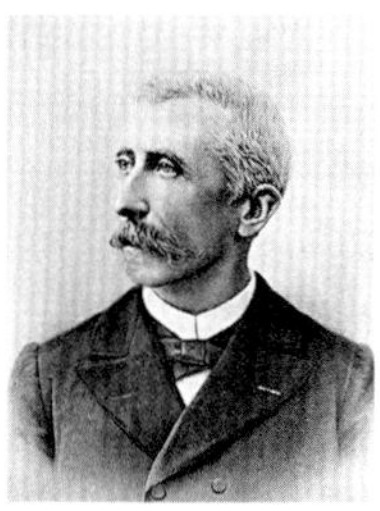

Théodule Ribot, 1898
Wellcome collection, public domain.

Théodule Ribot (1839–1916), who became an associate philosophy professor in 1866, went on to translate *The Principles of Psychology* by Herbert Spencer (1820–1903). Inspired by Spencer, he based his investigation on the mechanisms of thought, affectivity, and will on nervous and psychiatric pathology, fields which progressed rapidly during the last third of the 19th century. Ribot is known as the founder of French scientific psychology, an independent scientific discipline distinct from philosophy. After studying with Jules Baillarger (1809–1890) and Jacques-Joseph Moreau de Tours (1804–1884) at La Salpêtrière, he defended a doctoral thesis in literature in 1873. The subject was heredity – its phenomena, laws, causes, and consequences approached from a psychological perspective. This innovative theme contained the seeds of his later work. Enrolling in 1872 at the medical school, he studied under Claude Bernard (1813–1878), Alfred Vulpian (1826–1887), and Jean-Martin Charcot (1825–1893), regularly attending Charcot's Tuesday dinners. For 3 years, he dissected brains in the histology laboratory of Charles Robin (1821–1885). He did not defend his thesis in medicine. As a close friend of Charcot, he was depicted in the famous painting by André Brouillet (1857–1914), Une leçon clinique à La Salpêtrière [1].

In 1876, he founded La Revue philosophique de la France et de l'étranger and succeeded in bringing together the best minds in science and philosophy. Also in 1876, Ribot presented a report on his research on "the duration of psychic acts, based on current studies," in which he distanced himself from philosophy in favor of scientific experimentation [2].

In 1881, in his successful book on diseases of memory, Ribot combined his method for studying pathology with the theory of evolution and presented his "law of regression of memories," according to which the most recent memories are forgotten first, whereas the oldest memories are forgotten last. Ribot was appointed to the first Chair of Experimental Psychology at the Sorbonne in 1885 and entered the Collège de France in 1888. In addition to memory, Ribot investigated other areas of intellectual and affective function: Les maladies de la volonté (diseases of the will, 1883), Les maladies de la personnalité (diseases of personality, 1885), Essai sur l'imagination créatrice (essay on the creative imagination, 1900), La psychologie de l'attention (psychology of attention, 1889), La psychologie des sentiments (psychology of feelings, 1896), La logique des sentiments (logic of feelings, 1905), and Problèmes de la psychologie affective (problems of affective psychology, 1910). In each study, he used the same methodology, based on pathologies viewed as regressive, from acquisition to dissolution. According to Ribot, pathology made it possible to analyze the disorganization of mental mechanisms in the same way that dissection made it possible to penetrate anatomical parts. His use of the word "sentiment" (feeling) referred to both physical sensitivity (cenesthesia and pain) and moral sensitivity (emotions). He distinguished between the basic forms and described their complex aggregates. In 1914, he investigated "unconscious functions and movements," studying the role of motor images, "procedural" memory, and unconscious activity; this led him to consider the existence of thought without images or words [3].

With Charles Richet (1850–1935), Ribot founded the Société de Psychologie Physiologique in 1885, presided over by Charcot for its first international congress in 1889, during the World's Fair in Paris [4].

Olivier Walusinski

References

1 Sertilanges AD: Notice sur la vie et les travaux de M. Théodule Ribot lue dans la séance du 20 novembre 1920 de l'Académie des sciences morales et politiques. Compte-rendu des séances et travaux de l'Académie des Sciences Morales et Politiques 1921;162:193–220.

2 Ribot TH: La durée des actes psychiques, d'après les travaux actuels. Revue Philosophique de la France et de l'Etranger 1876;1:267–288.

3 Nicolas S, Charvillat A: Introducing psychology as an academic discipline in France: Théodule Ribot and the Collège de France (1888–1901). J Hist Behav Sci 2001;37:143–164.

4 Ribot TH: Congrès International de Psychologie Physiologique. Revue Philosophique de la France et de l'Étranger 1889;28:109–111.

Charles Richet (1850–1935)

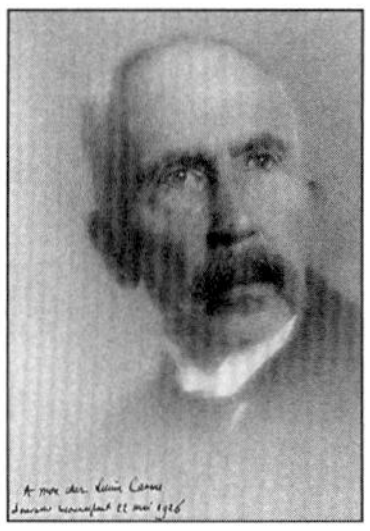

Charles Richet

Charles Richet (1850–1935) is best known for being awarded the Nobel Prize in Physiology or Medicine in 1913 for his work on anaphylaxis. He began his extensive and varied research while only an interne (house officership). His work focused on psycho-physiological phenomena that occur at the limits of ordinary psychic function, coining the term "metapsyche" in 1905. Influenced by the research of Jean-Martin Charcot (1825–1893) on hysteria and hypnosis (Richet used the term "magnetic somnambulism"), Richet tried to materialize mental states, drawing on physiological data and attempting to objectify signs that might elucidate the enigmas of thought [1]. After his thesis in medicine in 1877 "*Recherches expérimentales et cliniques sur la sensibilité*," Richet passed the competitive exam to become an associate professor in 1878, for which his thesis was entitled "*Structure des circonvolutions cérébrales.*" In 1887, he was appointed to the Chair of Physiology. Also in 1887, he published "*Un essai de psychologie générale*," basing his work on studies of the nervous system and proposing explanations of mental activity [2]. In 1890, he founded the journal *Annales de Sciences psychiques.* Although he conducted scientific research on paranormal phenomena, studying seers and ghosts, his scientific integrity leaves no room for doubt, in light of the research he conducted on serotherapy and anaphylaxis. Richet's studies make it clear that he was tricked, but they also reveal the type of interference that may occur between the researcher and what or whom is being investigated. Deeply affected by the horrors of World War I, during which he practiced as a physician, in 1919 he published "*L'homme stupide*" in which he set forth his highly pessimistic view of humanity and argued in defense of pacifism. As was common in his day, Richet expressed opinions that were clearly eugenicist and racist, glorifying the colonization of African and Southeast Asian peoples [3].

Olivier Walusinski

References

1 Mayer A: Notice nécrologique sur M. Charles Richet (1850–1935). Bulletin de l'Académie nationale de Médecine 1936;115:51–64.
2 Richet CH: Souvenirs d'un Physiologiste. Paris, J. Peyronnet, 1933.
3 Van Wijland J (ed): Charles Richet (1850–1935), l'exercice de la curiosité. Rennes, Presses Universitaires de Rennes, 2015.

Paul Sollier (1861–1933)

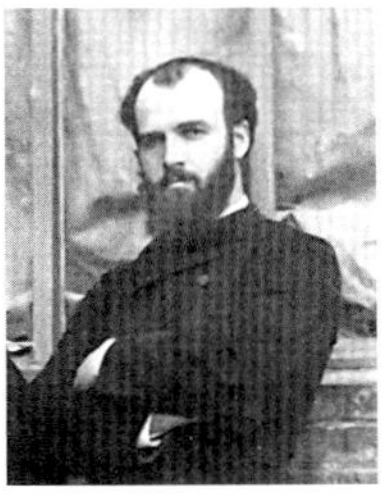

Paul Sollier, 1886
Olivier Walusinski, private collection.

Paul Sollier (1861–1933) was a student of Désiré-Magloire Bourneville (1840–1909), Jules Dejerine (1849–1917), and Auguste Voisin (1829–1898). He spent many years training as both a neurologist and a psychiatrist at Bicêtre Hospital and La Salpêtrière Hospital, where he worked alongside Joseph Babiński (1857–1932). In 1890, Sollier defended his thesis, inspired by Bourneville: Psychologie de l'idiot et de l'imbécile, which is one of the first theses on child psychiatry. In 1897, Sollier founded with his wife Alice Mathieu-Dubois (1861–?), who was also a physician, the Boulogne-Billancourt hydrotherapy center, near Paris. There, he developed new therapeutic methods, precursors to current cognitive-behavioral methods. His most famous patient was Marcel Proust, who consulted him at the end of 1905. Sollier was a prolific author, widely read and translated until World War II. He covered a variety of subjects, including doubt, psychic energy, conscience, morality, addiction to gambling, anorexia nervosa, and morphine withdrawal. He became professor of psychology at Université Nouvelle de Bruxelles in 1898 but never held this position in France. He was elected president of the Société Médico-Psychologique in 1926. As director of the neurological center of the 14th military region during the war, Sollier coordinated the preparation of a wartime clinical neurology treatise, published in 1918. His psychotherapeutic treatment of "war psycho-neuroses" was distinctly different from the more violent method using "persuasion by faradic currents," which soldiers referred to as "le torpillage" (torpedoing) and which was advocated by Clovis Vincent (1879–1947) and Gustave Roussy (1874–1947). At the end of his career, he devoted himself to mental health in the workplace and occupational therapy, which he named "la psychotechnique" [1].

In 3 domains, emotion, memory, and hysteria, his thinking is considered modern even by today's standards. Sollier developed a theory of memory based on neurological and psychological ideas. His main work on this subject was published in 1900. Sollier defined the conditions for memory stabilization (e.g., stimulus intensity, duration, repetition, attention, coexisting emotion, and will), cellular changes and plasticity during learning, and memory as a basic property of nerve cells. Memory organization centers are different than perception centers; the former are under the control of the frontal lobes. According to Sollier, neurophysiological mechanisms explained why a recalled memory is identified as memory rather than actual perception. Sollier was the first to analyze an involuntary surge of detailed memories and to use it during specific therapies for his patients. He linked memory with affective and emotional factors [2].

Marcel Proust (1871–1922), one of the greatest novelists of all times, is known for his extraordinary skills in analyzing the forms and psychological mechanisms of memory. With Proust as well as his other patients, Sollier used involuntary memories to trigger a kind of re-experiencing, so that the patient could reach a new mental and affective balance, which would then improve symptoms. Undoubtedly, several of Proust's ideas on involuntary memory appear to have developed from what he learned from Sollier, both from his books and from his personal experience as a patient [3].

Olivier Walusinski

References

1 Walusinski O, Bogousslavsky J: A la recherche du neuropsychiatre perdu: Paul Sollier (1861–1933). Rev Neurol 2008;164:F239–F247.

2 Bogousslavsky J: Memory after Charcot: Paul Sollier's visionary work. J Neurol Neurosurg Psychiatr 2007;78: 1373–1374.

3 Bogousslavsky J, Walusinski O: Marcel Proust and Paul Sollier: the involuntary memory connection. Schweizer Archive für Neurologie und Psychiatrie 2009;160:130–136.

Carl Wernicke (1848–1905)

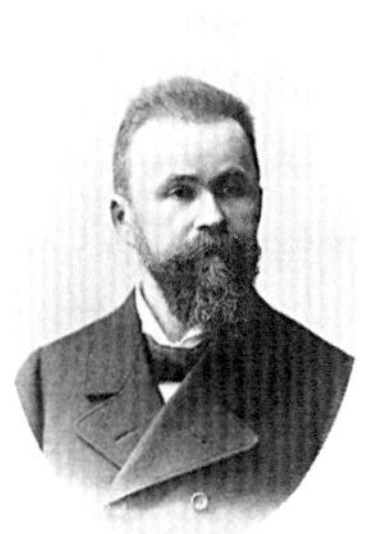

Carl Wernicke
By J.F. Lehmann, München – IHM, public domain.

Carl Wernicke (1848–1905), born in Silesia, studied medicine at Breslau University. After graduation, he served as an army surgeon during the Franco-Prussian war. He served in the Franco-Prussian war of 1870 as an army surgeon. He then became assistant to Heinrich Neumann (1814–1884) in the psychiatric department of the Allerheiligen Hospital in Breslau. Neumann advised him to study neuroanatomy under Theodor Meynert (1833–1892) in Vienna. From 1875 to 1878, Wernicke was assistant to Karl Westphal (1833–1890) in the Berlin Charité clinic. After working as a neurologist in private practice, he took over Neumann's position as head of the psychiatric department. In 1890, he became director of the neurology and psychiatry department at the university hospital, a position he held for 20 years, bringing together an outstanding team of scientists that researched apraxia, agnosia, and asymbolia [1, 2]. Wernicke died in 1905 from injuries sustained during a bicycle accident in the Thuringian forest.

Wernicke published, at the age of 26, the article that made him famous, which dealt with sensory aphasia localized in the temporal lobes (1874) [3]: "*Aphasische Symptomencomplex. Eine psychologische Studie auf anatomischer Basis.*" This disorder impairs comprehension of spoken language, the ability to read (silently) and write, and articulate speech. Hearing is intact. Patients may speak fluently with a natural language rhythm, but the result has neither understandable syntax nor meaning [1].

In 1877, Wernicke observed that lesions relatively limited to the 6th nucleus resulted in the paralysis of conjugate gaze on the side of the lesion. He was the first to postulate a center for conjugate gaze in the pontal tegmentum.

In 1881, Wernicke completed the initial description published by Charles-Alphonse Gayet (1833–1904) in 1875 [4] of an encephalopathy syndrome (Gayet-Wernicke encephalopathy) characterized by behavioral symptoms (listlessness, disorientation, confusion, hallucinations, Korsakoff psychosis), oculomotor paralysis (chiefly of the external recti, conjugate paralysis, and horizontal and vertical nystagmus), and ataxia. During the autopsies, Wernicke observed punctate hemorrhages of the grey matter around the third and fourth ventricles and aqueduct, which he called "polioencephalitis haemorrhagica superioris" [5]. The disturbance was primarily due to thiamine deficiency secondary to alcoholism and/or starvation.

Wernicke wrote a 3-volume textbook of nervous disease (*Atlas des Gehirns; Schnitte durch das menschliche Gehirn in photographischen Originalen*, 1881–1883) and a treatise on neuroanatomy (*Lehrbuch der Gehirnkrankheiten: für Aerzte und Studirende*, 1897–1900). In volume one, Wernicke described the vascular supply of the brainstem. With Georg Theodor Ziehen (1862–1950), he founded the journal *Monatsschrift für Psychiatrie und Neurologie* in 1897.

Olivier Walusinski

References

1 Keyser A, Carl Wernicke: Reader in the History of Aphasia; in Eling P: From Franz Gall to Norman Geschwind. Amsterdam, Philadelphia, J. Benjamins Pub, 1995.

2 Pillmann F: Carl Wernicke (1848–1905). J Neurol 2003;250:1390–1391.

3 Wernicke C: Der aphasiche Symptomencomplex. Eine Psychologische Studie auf Anatomischer Basis. Breslau, Cohn & Weigert, 1874.

4 Gayet CA: Affection encéphalique (encéphalite diffuse probable). Localisée aux étages supérieurs des pédoncules cérébraux et aux couches optiques, ainsi qu'au plancher du quatrième ventricule et aux parois latérales du troisième. Archives de physiologie normale et pathologique 1875;7:341 351.

5 Wernicke K: Die Acute, Hämorrhagische Polioencephalitis Superior. In Lehrbuch der Gehirnkrankheiten, Kassel, Fischer, and Berlin, 1881, pp 229–242.

Author Index

Subject Index